Safeguarding Children in Primary Health Care

Best Practice in Working with Children Series
Edited by Brigid Daniel, Professor of Social Work,
Department of Applied Social Science, University of Stirling

The titles in the Best Practice in Working with Children series are written for the multi-agency professionals working to promote children's welfare and protect them from harm. Each book in the series draws on current research into what works best for children, providing practical, realistic suggestions as to how practitioners in social work, health and education can work together to promote the resilience and safety of the children in their care. Brigid Daniel is Professor of Social Work in the Department of Applied Social Science at the University of Stirling. She is co-author of several textbooks and practice resources on child care and protection. She was a member of the multi-disciplinary team that carried out a national ministerial review of child protection practice in Scotland.

other books in the series

Safeguarding Children and Schools
Edited by Mary Baginsky
Foreword by Brigid Daniel
ISBN 978 1 84310 514 5

Child Neglect
Practice Issues for Health and Social Care
Edited by Julie Taylor and Brigid Daniel
Foreword by Olive Stevenson
ISBN 978 1 84310 160 4

Safeguarding Children Living with Trauma and Family Violence
Evidence-Based Assessment and Planning Interventions
Arnon Bentovim, Antony Cox, Liza Bingley Miller and Stephen Pizzey
Foreword by Brigid Daniel
ISBN 978 1 84310 938 9

Safeguarding Children in Primary Health Care

*Edited by Julie Taylor
and Markus Themessl-Huber*

Foreword by Brigid Daniel

Jessica Kingsley Publishers
London and Philadelphia

MT

First published in 2009
by Jessica Kingsley Publishers
116 Pentonville Road
London N1 9JB, UK
and
400 Market Street, Suite 400
Philadelphia, PA 19106, USA

www.jkp.com

Library of Congress Cataloging in Publication Data
Safeguarding children in primary health care / edited by Julie Taylor and Markus
Themessl-Huber ; foreword by Brigid Daniel.
     p. cm.
Includes bibliographical references and index.
ISBN 978-1-84310-652-4 (pb : alk. paper) 1. Child health services. 2. Child
abuse--Prevention. 3. Primary health care. I. Taylor, Julie, 1961- II. Themessl-Huber,
Markus.
RJ101.S25 2009
362.76'63--dc22

                          2008051577

British Library Cataloguing in Publication Data
A CIP catalogue record for this book is available from the British Library

ISBN 978 1 84310 652 4

Printed and bound in Great Britain by
Athenaeum Press, Gateshead, Tyne and Wear

5/4/10

Contents

Part 3 Strategic Interventions in and Beyond Primary Health Care

Part 4 Safeguarding Challenges in the Primary Health Care Context

List of Tables

List of Figures

Foreword

In the inter-disciplinary and inter-sectoral context the term 'health professional' is often used rather loosely to cover a vast range of specialisms and allied professions. Those within health care settings know that intra-disciplinary communcation may be as complex as inter-disciplinary communication. This book focuses specifically on the role of primay health care providers because of the key role they can play in safeguarding children, and it aims to support them in this vital role.

The UK and many jurisdictions with similar child protection and safeguarding systems are in the process of unprecedented reform and development. At the heart of the policy developments is an explicit articulation of the role of the universal services of education and health in the promotion of children's welfare and protection from harm.

Primary health care providers have always been concerned for the welfare of their child patients, and many children's lives have been significantly improved as a result of the actions of alert health professionals. However, there has been considerable variation in interpretation of roles and responsibilities. Quite understandably, many professionals have been concerned about the often uncomfortable collision of patient confidentiality and child welfare and protection. Over recent years extensive attention has been paid to this issue and health professionals have now been provided with much clearer support and guidance about the limits and extents of confidentiality.

The initial wave of reform focused on improving the recognition of abuse and neglect. There has been widespread 'awareness-raising' training across all universal services. This training, and associated guidance on 'referral' processes has been driven by the evidence of a disparity between prevalence rates of child maltreatment and official statistics. In other words, there are many children whose distress is not being identified. Of course, health professionals are in a prime position to recognize signs and symptoms of child maltreatment; they are also in a key position to identify aspects of parental health, behaviour and disposition that are likely to impact upon their children. There is no doubt that the level of awareness of child abuse and neglect has rocketed and that primary health care providers see the safeguarding of children as squarely part of their core activity. This awareness has gone hand in hand with, and been reinforced by, the increasing consensus that child abuse and neglect is best conceptualized as a public health issue.

The current wave of reform is building upon this to focus more on the ways in which primary health care providers play a role in being part of the response for children. The emphasis has shifted away from 'referral' on to social services towards an increasing expectation that primary health care professionals provide assistance and support to children.

This book provides invaluable insights for both aspects of the role. It offers detailed and practical guidance that will assist primary health care providers to be aware of the many factors that can seriously damage children's emotional and physical health and development. But, crucially, the book also sets out the many ways in which primary health care providers can actively contribute to the improvement of children's lives in the short and longer term.

Brigid Daniel, University of Stirling

Chapter One

Safeguarding Children in Primary Health Care: An Introduction

Markus Themessl-Huber and Julie Taylor

Introduction

More than 90 per cent of contact the public has with health services takes place in primary care. Accordingly, primary health care and child health are currently at the centre of WHO vision and policies (Horton 2008a; World Health Organization 2007a). Primary health care in general, but also particularly when aimed at children, is seen widely as being the most promising vehicle to address today's most pressing health concerns, such as health inequalities, cost-explosions or access to high quality care (Horton 2008b). Children in countries with a less developed primary health care system had poorer health and survival outcomes than countries with better developed systems (UNICEF 2007). Primary care professionals are very well-placed to monitor children's wellbeing and safety and to liaise with relevant agencies within and beyond primary care (Carter and Bannon 2002; HM Government 2006).

Despite its importance to health and health care, no universally accepted definition of primary health care exists. Lay people's as well as many health care professionals' understanding of primary health care is low. Interpretations of the concept of primary health care range from constituting the first level of care to representing a system-wide strategy (Muldoon, Hogg and Levitt 2008). Additionally, there is a growing tendency to distinguish between primary care and primary health care. The first is used to refer to general practitioner-type care provision and the latter to refer to individual as well as public health focused interventions (Muldoon *et al.* 2008). To avoid confusion as much as possible primary health care in this book will be defined in accordance with the World Health Organization's Alma Ata declaration of 1978. In this ground-breaking declaration primary health care was defined as:

> the first level of contact of individuals, the family and community with the national health system bringing health care as close as possible to where people live and work and constitutes the first element of a continuing health care process. (World Health Organization 1978)

In this declaration, primary health care was freed from a narrow understanding of medical care provision and conceptualized as an integrated bio-psychosocial system of care reflecting local socio-cultural, political and economic characteristics (see Box 1.1). It represented a radical shift from focusing almost exclusively on biomedical interventions to acknowledging the effects of social determinants on health (Lawn *et al.* 2008).

Box 1.1 Primary Health Care

1. reflects and evolves from the economic conditions and sociocultural and political characteristics of the country and its communities and is based on the application of the relevant results of social, biomedical and health services research and public health experience

2. addresses the main health problems in the community, providing promotive, preventive, curative and rehabilitative services accordingly

3. includes at least: education concerning prevailing health problems and the methods of preventing and controlling them; promotion of food supply and proper nutrition; an adequate supply of safe water and basic sanitation; maternal and child health care, including family planning; immunization against the major infectious diseases; prevention and control of locally endemic diseases; appropriate treatment of common diseases and injuries; and provision of essential drugs

4. involves, in addition to the health sector, all related sectors and aspects of national and community development, in particular agriculture, animal husbandry, food, industry, education, housing, public works, communications and

---

other sectors; and demands the coordinated efforts of all those sectors

5. requires and promotes maximum community and individual self-reliance and participation in the planning, organization, operation and control of primary health care, making fullest use of local, national and other available resources; and to this end develops through appropriate education the ability of communities to participate

6. should be sustained by integrated, functional and mutually supportive referral systems, leading to the progressive improvement of comprehensive health care for all and giving priority to those most in need

7. relies, at local and referral levels, on health workers, including physicians, nurses, midwives, auxiliaries and community workers as applicable, as well as traditional practitioners as needed, suitably trained socially and technically to work as a health team and to respond to the expressed health needs of the community.

Source: www.who.int/hpr/NPH/docs/declaration_almaata.pdf

In other words, this definition promotes an understanding of primary care which provides integrated, accessible health care services by clinicians who are accountable for addressing a large majority of personal health care needs, developing a sustained partnership with patients and practising in the context of family and community (Donaldson, Yordy and Vanselow 1994).

The declaration also emphasizes that in order to address constructively today's major health concerns, primary health care must be professionally, technologically, philosophically and politically equipped. Among other consequences this requires increased attention to the social determinants of health as well as intra- and intersectoral collaborations.

Social determinants of health have since been demonstrated emphatically to be of pivotal importance, albeit still not given the attention they warrant (Marmot 2008). The salience of social determinants of health, but also the call for more emphasis on prevention, demands that public policies across all sectors need to consider their effect on individual and public health (Marmot 2008).

While technological developments are not a primary concern of this book, the professional, philosophical and political equipment of primary health care very much is. Primary care consists of a broad range of services and professions working in a multitude of different settings. As a result, services and service providers within primary care are constantly evolving in order to improve the quality, scope and availability of care provided (Saltman, Rico and Boerma 2005). Points one, four, six and seven under Article VII of the declaration (primary health care), in particular, emphasize the reliance of primary health care on intersectoral collaboration, socio-cultural sensitivity and the expertise of a wide range of community-based professions (Walley *et al.* 2008). Primary health care is working best if it is provided for an identifiable population. For example, infant mortality rates of children born to parents in the routine and manual socio-economic group is still 17 per cent higher than in the population as a whole (Department of Health 2007c). This means both that the health characteristics of a population need to be monitored continually and that public (and, if possible, private) sectors need to contribute their expertise and information (van Weel, De Maeseneer and Roberts 2008). In fact, community partnerships aimed at protecting children from injuries, accidents, abuse and neglect is considered a basic practice of primary health care interventions (UNICEF 2007). Yet, despite being considered an essential element of effective primary health care provision, intersectoral collaboration is considered one of the major weaknesses of primary health care (Lawn *et al.* 2008).

Safeguarding children poses a significant professional, managerial and emotional challenge to primary health care providers. This challenge indicates the need to evaluate the status and priority primary care professionals allocate to safeguarding children vis-à-vis their other work commitments. The demand that 'a case of suspected child abuse and neglect should be treated with the same level of urgency as any other potentially fatal childhood disorder' (Bannon and Carter 2003, p.560) has been made. The questions remain whether this call has been heard; whether it is constructive; and whether professionals are equipped with the political, organizational and personal means to act accordingly.

Despite the many difficulties and challenges professionals and lay people face in this arena, good safeguarding practices in primary health care exist (see for example Bremberg 2006; Luig-Arlt 2004; Mckeown, Haase and Pratschke 2001). This book takes a closer look at the challenges of safeguarding children from abuse and neglect in primary health care. Practitioners, policy-advisors and academics present an overview of practical as well as strategic approaches deployed in primary health care to recognize and respond to concerns about child care and protection. The recognition and responses of primary health care professionals will be discussed in the context of competing professional priorities, the existing evidence base, the media coverage of child abuse and neglect, inter-professional collaboration, practical work-load decisions, as well as personal experiences, anxieties and available resources. The arguments and ideas presented in the different chapters are the authors' and may not always reflect the editors' opinions and perspectives.

Part 1: Roles and remits of primary health care professionals

Knowledge of signs and symptoms of potential sexual abuse is necessary for staff working in primary health care. However, such technical knowledge is only one factor in primary health care practitioners' decisions to enquire about, or protect, the welfare of vulnerable children. Whatever the level of knowledge of individual practitioners, potential or actual abuse in child patients usually evokes anxiety, stress and uncertainty in primary health care professionals. These personal reactions and the public backlash from highly publicized cases is thought to make many professionals reluctant to risk suggesting, or even contemplating, that they are facing an abused child, especially if the abuse is thought to be sexual. Thus, there is likely to be considerable under-reporting of the problem. In Chapter 2, Nelson discusses barriers to raising concerns about children in primary care and the kinds of training and support which may be helpful in overcoming them.

Nelson emphasizes that self-confidence, good support and supervision and an informed understanding of the topic are more important to primary health care professionals than learning lists of textbook signs and symptoms. She argues that in addition to the expected identifiable signs and symptoms of sexual abuse it is equally important for practitioners to recognize that a range of more amorphous health problems in children and adults, such as persistent medically-unexplained symptoms and behavioural problems, may be clues to a history of sexual abuse.

In many countries, general practitioners (GPs or family physicians) are at the centre of primary health care provision. They tend to be the gate keeper to other health services and carry the ultimate responsibility for the health of patients within the primary health care context. Due to their role, their knowledge of and confidence in dealing with potential and actual abuse and neglect is of consequence. Van de Laar and Lagro-Janssen in Chapter 3 discuss the roles and remits of family physicians in relation to safeguarding children from abuse and neglect within the Dutch health care context. GPs are described to be at the heart of a network of professionals and organizations intent on protecting and supporting children. They are often well acquainted with many of their patients and their families. This enables them to have information beyond the individual child or the presenting health issue. This level of familiarity, however, can impede as well as facilitate GPs' identification and management of potential and actual child abuse cases. Chapter 3 discusses these issues and describes promising ways forward.

Paediatricians, in some ways, have the opposite problem to GPs. Many primary health care professionals are not sufficiently familiar with the work and role remit of the paediatrician. Yet, their understanding of the paediatrician's role and relevant referral pathways is necessary for the effective preparation and management of child protection and safeguarding in the community. Skelton in Chapter 4 outlines the role of the paediatrician as well as the benefits and limitations of medical assessments following suspected child abuse, including the making of controversial decisions such as when to conduct an anogenital examination. Chapter 4 also focuses on the safeguarding-related responsibilities of primary health care professionals, barriers to referrals within and beyond the health care sector, the involvement of social care and confidentiality issues pertinent and specific to primary health care. Skelton further explores the effects of publicity and media coverage of high profile child abuse cases on the recruiting and retaining specialist health care professionals.

While the general remit of dentists is rarely questioned, relatively little is known about their role in safeguarding children. Freeman in Chapter 5 examines the role of primary health care dental practitioners in the safeguarding of children. Dentists have a key role in identifying abused or neglected children as such children may present first at the dentist and may be unknown to social or other health care services. Particular dental health problems in children may alert dentists that they are possibly working with a child and parent who are in trouble and in need of help. Children presenting with facial injuries, including fractured teeth, for example, may be abused and in need of protection. In addition to physical markers, Chapter 5 will explore the relationship between dental caries and the mother–child dyad as well as the correlation between dental fear and overall mental health.

The mother–child dyad is also of particular concern to maternity services. Domestic violence and the safeguarding of children are of particular concern over the course of a pregnancy. Community-based midwives along with other members of the primary health care team are well placed to identify pregnant women, young mothers and their children who have been abused or are at risk of abuse or neglect. The provision of care to families associated with possible or actual child maltreatment is one of the most difficult and challenging areas of practice that midwives and other primary health care professionals encounter. In Chapter 6, Lazenbatt examines the role maternity services can and need to play to safeguard women and their born and unborn children throughout and following a pregnancy. She explores professional and contextual barriers and facilitators of adequate midwifery responses to domestic and child abuse, as well as the challenges of effective inter-professional collaborations.

Part 2: Practical interventions suitable for primary health care

The prevalence of autistic spectrum disorder (ASD) in children is increasing. At the same time, so does the need for effective intervention and care. O'Neill, Zeedyk and Jones report on successes in working with children diagnosed with ASD who also experience significant difficulties caused by hyper-sensitivities. In Chapter 7, they propose that hypersensitivities are implicated in the behaviours and difficulties observed in ASD. They argue that in order to safeguard and promote the wellbeing of children with ASD, hypersensitivities must be taken into account when interpreting behaviour and designing and selecting interventions. Interventions are explored, which focus on children's hypersensitivities, reduce stress and subsequently decrease distressed behaviour. Additional benefits of these interventions include increasing positive social behaviours and promoting a child's autonomy and wellbeing in the course of simple interactions. Furthermore, primary health care practice is explored as a suitable context for offering such child-centred interventions.

In addition to ASD, primary health care professionals encounter children with a range of communication difficulties. Taking note of children's communication skills is important as a child's language and behaviour are usually early indicators of distress and abuse. However, Law and Mackie in Chapter 8 argue that it is often easier to engage parents in a discussion of their child's communication skills than it is to elicit their thoughts on their child's behaviour. Yet, addressing confidently a child's language and behaviour patterns requires primary care professionals to have some understanding of communication processes and difficulties. Chapter 8 presents definitions and illustrations of children's communication and behaviour difficulties and links them to potential abuse and neglect. Information about how these issues can be addressed in primary health care settings is provided as well as an overview of contributions speech and language therapists have to offer.

As illustrated in Chapter 8, emotionally available and sensitive caregivers are a fundamental basis of a child's safe development. Juen and Juen in Chapter 9 contend that providing preventive assistance for struggling parents constitutes one of the most important measures to protect a child's development. Emotionally responsive carers offer children a secure base for their emotional, social and moral development. In Chapter 9 the influence of emotional availability of at least one caregiver on reducing the risk of developmental and mental disorders to prevent disorders is explored. Emotional responsiveness is identified as a key factor in safeguarding children by way of providing them with a good base for a healthy development in often difficult social and economic contexts.

Irrespective of the presence of an emotionally responsive parent, abused children often have a history of trauma, which needs consideration in its own right. Feather and Ronan in Chapter 10 start by discussing the presentation and practical assessment of trauma in children. They highlight once more the importance of inter-professional collaboration in establishing a comprehensive understanding of individual children's experiences as well as in avoiding the drawing of inaccurate conclusions. This is followed by a focus on evidence-based interventions relevant to children who suffered from violence, abuse or neglect. In Chapter 10 they also describe and promote a manualized trauma-focused cognitive behavioural therapy approach to be used in primary health care.

Part 3: Strategic interventions in and beyond primary health care

Generally, in terms of child protection processes health care services tend to be reactive rather than being proactive. Health care services usually respond following the identification of a child who is thought to be suffering or at risk of suffering harm. However, messages from policies and research evidence are clear in calling for more emphasis on primary prevention and early intervention to ensure more positive upstream outcomes for children. In this spirit, Ferguson in Chapter 11 describes a conceptual framework that promotes a proactive public health approach to protecting children and builds on the capacity and capability of all health care practitioners to act in the best interests of children. Yet, to date health care practitioners are often not involved adequately or in a timely fashion. In this chapter, she illustrates a safeguarding model proposed in Scotland that supports the workforce in relation to training, education and supervision as well as robust management structures and clear lines of accountability. Moreover, the model aims to enable children and families to use local resources and to access services as necessary.

Mainstreaming child care commissioning is another way to address strategically the safeguarding of children. Effective safeguarding of children in and beyond the boundaries of primary health care requires coherent and comprehensive strategic plans and policies across public sectors. Selkirk in Chapter 12 promotes the role of the Child Health Commissioner in championing the strategic provision of child care in general and the safeguarding of children in particular. She demonstrates the processes and outcomes of applying a collaborative commissioning model to the safeguarding practices in primary health care.

Lessons to improve the safeguarding practice in primary health care can and should also be learned from child casualties. In the United Kingdom (UK), as in many other parts of the world, the death of a child or young person is a rare but highly significant event that will have a major impact on families, professionals and communities. These tragic events inevitably raise questions about the presence of avoidable or preventable factors. In acknowledgement of the sentinel importance of the death of a child or young person and the potential to learn lessons, the practice of systematically reviewing all childhood deaths is being introduced within the UK. Powell in Chapter 13 introduces new multi-agency child death review processes aimed to seek an understanding of why a child or young person has died, to use this information to gain insight into the individual death and to ensure that any messages for prevention and the future safety and protection of children are fed into policy, legislation and practice. This chapter informs and supports primary health care practitioners in how to make a full and meaningful contribution to the review process.

Part 4: Safeguarding challenges in the primary health care context

Many professionals and agencies are now involved in the care of children and families affected by parental problem drug use. The role of primary health care in this work is an important one and deserves special attention. Whittaker in Chapter 14 aims to provide primary care teams with a framework for care so that drug-using parents and their children can be offered appropriate and integrated help and support. Although the focus of her chapter is on safeguarding the welfare of children affected by parental problem drug use, a much broader approach is adopted. The wider role of primary health care is considered in promoting the health and wellbeing of the family as a whole and in delivering a range of harm reduction services to problem drug users. In this chapter an overview of the policy framework which underpins this approach is provided, along with guidelines of good practice for assessment and care as well as practical strategies and tools to assist primary health care teams in delivering high quality services.

Inter- and intra-professional collaboration is also the key to safeguarding the sexual health of older children and adolescents. Themessl-Huber and colleagues in Chapter 15 present the outcomes of the evaluation of a national demonstration project aimed at improving the sexual health of young people.

They demonstrate the need for partnership working in this area, describe a demonstration initiative and present the various effects of working in partnership on professionals and organizations involved in promoting young people's sexual health.

Ritualistic forms of child abuse cause sensational headlines, but are quite rare. Yet, in Chapter 16, Taylor and Cantrell elaborate that practices involving witchcraft and beliefs in spirit possession targeted at children constitute a worrying trend in some cultures and spiritual communes. Most cases of ritualistic abuse occur in the children's own homes and communities. Primary health care professionals, therefore, play a vital role in raising awareness of and identifying indicators of such forms of abuse.

As these chapters show, primary care plays an important and multi-faceted role in safeguarding children. Two themes, however, run through all chapters, regardless of how different some of them may otherwise be. First, primary health care includes a broad variety of health and social care professionals and second, the collaboration among these professionals is the key to guarding the safety, health and wellbeing of children.

Part 1
Roles and Remits of Primary Health Care Professionals

Chapter Two

Preparing for the Special Challenge of Sexual Abuse

Sarah Nelson

Introduction

What do most staff who work in primary health care now associate with the phrase 'child protection'? They think of written documents and training materials: for instance a list of signs, symptoms and behaviours which may be indicators of child abuse or neglect.

There is also extensive guidance, regulation and/or accounts of statutory responsibilities. These detail what health staff should do in the event of disclosures or their own suspicions and to whom they should report, within their own workplace and across inter-agency boundaries, since working together and sharing concerns are now key values in child protection.

Their own professional bodies (e.g. the Royal Colleges) will also have ethical requirements about confidentiality and guidance, informed by research, about child protection including controversial topics such as interpretation of reflex anal dilatation, or subdural haemorrhage in infants (for example RCGP 2005, 2008; RCN 2005; RCPCH 2008b). Because staff are expected to learn these documents (or to have them close by) for when the need arises, many unsurprisingly equate them with what 'child protection' is about. Modern emphasis on bureaucratic regulation can also imply that somehow if guidelines are followed closely, child protection failures and damaging criticism can be avoided.

These materials are all valuable, but in themselves neither protect nor identify children at risk. It is like giving people the furniture and fittings before the floors and walls of the house are built. They are particularly inadequate in preparing staff to deal with child sexual assault, because this form of abuse tends to raise the greatest anxieties in staff.

Research with health professionals has revealed more than 15 reasons for avoiding such inquiry. These include perceived lack of training, skills or time; fears about antagonizing, or wrongly accusing, families; and a widespread belief that it would be more distressing for patients to talk about abuse than to forget it (Nelson 2001; Nelson and Baldwin 2004; Nelson and Hampson 2008); with domestic violence, another major health issue, 'opening the can of worms' in local communities can be particularly daunting because the abuser might prove to be a patient, friend, neighbour, colleague, or relative. More widely, there has also tended to be a low rate of GP involvement in child protection case conferences and a low rate of abused children being identified by them (Bisset and Hunter 1992; Lea-Cox and Hall 1991; RCGP 2005).

Before health staff can pick up worrying signs they first need to see child sexual abuse (CSA) as a serious health and protection issue and to believe it is possible in that particular family. Otherwise they will reinterpret what they see (Festinger 1962). Before they can be alert, from often amorphous symptoms, that something might be seriously wrong, they need informed awareness on behalf of distressed children, which cannot come only from rote-learning. Before agencies can share concerns and information productively, someone needs to notice there is something to be concerned *about* and alert the others.

Before they can act to help protect abused children and make active use of their child protection procedures, staff need to reduce their own fears. They need confidence in their skills and access to supervision or at least to support and advice. They need to sense that their integrity in acting is likely to be supported by their managers and/or professional body – particularly given well-publicized criticisms, a media 'backlash' and disciplinary action against health care professionals such as senior paediatricians, in disputed cases of child abuse (Gornall 2008; Turton and Haines 2007).

Finally, simply waiting for victims to reveal sexual abuse, as a child protection strategy, will not adequately protect them. Most children and adults do not volunteer information about their own maltreatment, especially about the shameful, humiliating experience of sexual abuse. In research, young people have given numerous reasons for self-silencing, including deep shame, self-blame, fear of other children's rejection, fear of retaliation and the expectation (often realistic) of being disbelieved. Before a young person or worried non-abusing parent/carer can begin to confide within a health setting, they need to sense an atmosphere of respect, sensitivity and open minded, non-judgemental listening. That will help them take this huge leap of trust.

Therefore this chapter will concentrate not on esoteric symptoms of CSA, nor on the detail of written guidance and regulation, which you can all consult within your own localities and professions. Rather it will emphasize how to create the foundations for confident, informed and committed primary health care staff teams, working in a positive environment, to help protect young people from sexual abuse. These foundations enable people to work together knowledgeably and effectively, to interpret what they see more accurately and to use constructively their child protection guidelines.

This chapter will first explore why child sexual abuse (CSA) should be of concern in primary health care, as a major physical and mental health issue throughout life. It will summarize what CSA can involve and how common it is. It will consider key elements in confidence-building training; ways of creating a receptive respectful atmosphere for distressed children and their carers; and the importance of linking with local services, who can become informed support networks for both staff and service users.

Finally some general signs, symptoms, behaviours, comments and attempted communications which children and young people might display will be discussed. That also assists different professionals in primary health care to perceive more clearly the relevance of their own work and their own role in helping young people.

This chapter is informed throughout by the perspectives of adult survivors of CSA about their own experiences of primary health care as children and how they feel these relationships could be improved. These are drawn from my own experience of many years' research with adult survivors and from research and practice by others.

Health issues and the nature of sexual abuse

Why is child sexual abuse an important issue for primary health care?

Childhood sexual abuse is a major issue for primary health care because it brings severe trauma and distress to many children. It seriously affects many people's physical and mental health throughout their lives and currently these effects result in heavy, often unproductive use of health service resources. So it is important that recognition, intervention and protection comes for abused children as early in their lives as possible and that health services contribute their skills to playing an important role in this.

Primary health care staff are particularly important in the effort to keep children safe from sexual and other abuses and to notice changes, because like teachers, they are unusually well placed to observe children as they develop over time, seeing them and their families regularly over the years. GPs remain the first point of contact for most child health problems and most children are registered with one. *Simply noticing and being curious on children's behalf* are the most important things that we can do for children who have problems or who are distressed.

Primary health care professionals are also able to consult records over time. GPs with a particular awareness of CSA described how they felt frustrated when looking back into the records of adult patients with intractable depression and unexplained somatic symptoms, to find a 'trail' of indicators or even explicit reference to sexual abuse in childhood, which no-one appeared to have picked up at the time (Nelson 2001).

Wide-ranging effects on health

Mental health problems for people who experience childhood sexual abuse trauma have been very extensively researched over the years. For instance a CSA history is a significant risk factor for post-traumatic stress symptoms, depression and anxiety, severe loss of self-esteem (Beitchman et al. 1992; Briere and Elliott 1994), dissociation, suicide and attempted suicide (Bayatpour, Wells and Holford 1992; Oates 2004; Rew, Taylor-Seehafer and Fitzgerald 2001), self-harm (cutting, burning or otherwise physically injuring yourself) and prolonged or intractable substance misuse (Dube et al. 2003; Wilsnack et al. 1997). Sometimes the associations are very strong. For instance, a majority of people with histories of CSA trauma have consistently been found in those diagnosed with 'borderline personality disorder' (Herman, Perry and van der Kolk 1989; Kuritane 2005; Vincent et al. 1997).

Reasons for developing these symptoms can be complex. To take one example, many abused children and teenagers have problems with eating and develop anorexia, bulimia or compulsive eating – although of course there are many other reasons for these disorders too. Causes can include determination to exercise control over one's powerless life; self-hatred and self-disgust; self-comfort; but also attempts to be repugnant to abusers; reactions to oral sexual assault; efforts to avoid sexual relationships; the wish (with anorexia) to prevent pregnancy by abusers; sometimes a wish to die.

Direct physical effects of CSA can include genital and anal damage, sexually transmitted diseases (which can also reduce fertility), pelvic inflammatory disease and many gynaecological problems (Arias 2004; Kendall-Tackett 2002; Nelson 2002). Indirectly, poor health can be caused if a young person tries to escape abuse by a life of homelessness on the streets (Herman et al. 1997; Tyler and Cauce 2002). Young people and adults also suffer physical health impacts from psychological effects of abuse such as self-mutilation, depression, eating disorders, or high-risk sexual behaviour (Dube et al. 2002; Edwards 2007). Clinical depression, for instance, reduces mobility and exercise, proper diet or self-care. Other health effects can occur through the side-effects of prolonged psychiatric medication.

Self-medicating mechanisms for coping with or blotting out the trauma, such as alcohol, drug or solvent misuse and heavy smoking bring serious health risks as well as, often, the risk of caring inadequately for one's own children. Sexually abused people often fearfully avoid intrusive medical and dental examinations in sensitive areas of their bodies, which might detect disease at an early stage or safeguard a mother's and baby's health during pregnancy.

Finally, CSA survivors are also at higher risk than others for medically-unexplained conditions such as irritable bowel syndrome, chronic pelvic pain and other chronic pain, unexplained respiratory problems and non-epileptic seizures (Bhatia and Sapra 2005; Drossman *et al.* 1995; Kendall-Tackett 2001; Leserman *et al.* 1997; Nelson 2002; Spinhoven *et al.* 2004). These unexplained symptoms, some of which can appear in childhood or adolescence, often result in friction between doctors and patients and unproductive use of health resources.

All these long-term ill-health effects, then, provide many ethical and practical reasons why it is important for health professionals to contribute to identifying children at risk as early as possible.

What does sexual abuse involve?

Many people imagine sexual abuse is just 'a bit of fondling that shouldn't happen' or 'inappropriate touching'. This can be so, but CSA often involves more serious and degrading assault. Although it is unpleasant for any of us to think about, it is important to consider briefly what it can involve, in order to understand why some survivors experience serious long-term health effects for many years and why we should be open to considering risk in children of all ages. CSA may include:

- 'Non-contact abuse'. This can involve being watched (often daily) in private situations, like going to the toilet or having a bath; being forced to watch the abuser masturbating; being made to watch group sex, pornography and a range of perverse acts, including sex with animals or young children.

- 'Contact abuse' can include repeated vaginal, oral and anal assault by one abuser, a small or large group; penetration with objects or weapons; forced participation in group sexual activities; forced acts with animals; involvement in child prostitution and making of pornography; forced abuse of other children and other criminal acts.

- Additional physical violence during abuse which survivors have reported includes burning, scalding, electrocution, pulling of hair, beatings with weapons, tying of wrists and ankles, isolation, drugging and deprivation of sleep, food or drink.

The abusive acts or perverse scenarios might be filmed for the purpose of selling child pornography – whether to a local 'cottage industry' or via networks which through the internet now extend internationally.

How common is sexual abuse?

Perpetrators and victims of childhood sexual abuse are drawn from all social and geographic backgrounds and all ethnic groups. For instance, though CSA has often been seen as a working-class problem, the great majority of offenders found to be downloading, exchanging or making child pornography via the internet have been professional middle-class men with no criminal records. While most – though not all – offenders are male, victims may be both boys and girls, of all ages, including toddlers and even babies.

Studies of 'prevalence' (the proportion of any defined population who have been sexually abused in childhood) have produced varied results. Baker and Duncan's pioneering British study of 1985 suggested that 12 per cent of females and 8 per cent of males suffered CSA. Cawson's UK study (2000) found 16 per cent of females and 7 per cent of males had suffered contact sexual abuse (Cawson et al. 2000), while Irish figures were 20 per cent and 16 per cent respectively (McGee 2003).

Much higher than average high rates of CSA are found among certain groups such as among children in care, people with psychiatric problems or people with severe drink/drug problems. Wider considerations about prevalence can be found in, for instance Pilkington and Kremer (1995) and Tonmyr (1998).

Varied statistics result from differing definitions of CSA, different methodologies and the secretive nature of CSA. The questions asked, language used, privacy of setting, gender and skills of the interviewer affect people's willingness to disclose past abuse. Little sexual crime against children is detected and recorded. Thus we shall never know the *exact* extent of CSA and current knowledge is always likely to be an under-estimate. *The key point is that there will always be children and adults in your own practice who are experiencing, or have experienced, CSA.*

Staff issues

Elements of confidence-building training

I have found, over many years of work with sexual abuse survivors and with staff in contact with them, that by far the biggest obstacle across many caring professions to working with, or helping to protect, children and adults is staff reluctance to raise or address the subject. Awkwardness, fear of the consequences or a sense of inadequate training and skills can prevent action being taken or questions being asked which might protect young people, or bring adults therapeutic benefit (Bisset and Hunter 1992; Butler 1996; Lazenbatt and Freeman 2006; RCGP 2005; Tsang and Sweet 1999). Thus silencing is perpetuated and sometimes a professional paralysis which helps no-one. Thus anxieties, fears and myths need addressing before there is much point in discussing signs, symptoms, child protection guidance or ways to create a trusting atmosphere for survivors in health settings.

It is very important to give all staff in a primary health care setting time and opportunity for training in CSA issues and to ensure it is not narrowly confined to learning official guidance, but includes key elements (Nelson and Hampson 2008) such as:

- A basic knowledge and information about CSA and its health effects, such as that given in this chapter.

- The opportunity with a sympathetic skilled trainer to explore and talk through their own fears and their professional/personal anxieties about addressing CSA. A look at positive ways to overcome fears and to become self-aware about how the issue affects all of us individually. Many professionals for instance are themselves survivors of abuse and while this can give added empathy and understanding, it can also raise difficult memories for them.

- A challenge to implicit assumptions and prejudices which many people have, e.g. about who gets abused and who does not (such as prejudices about 'good' and 'bad' families in the area) and about who tells the truth and who does not (such as respectable professionals and delinquent teenagers!).

- An opportunity to test, against research and practice evidence, implicit assumptions which people may have about what abused children and adults 'want'. For instance this evidence does not support common beliefs that survivors would not wish to be asked about a CSA history, that all survivors need great amounts of time spent working with them after disclosure, or that high degrees of training and specialization are always needed for this work (Dale 1999; Nelson 2001; Nelson and Hampson 2008).

- Access to support and supervision. This is especially important for staff who work regularly and in more depth with children or adults on abuse issues, or whose job could involve hearing, at any time, painful and difficult revelations. They do need access to regular supervision either within your organization, or from an external supervisor. They need a safe place to discuss the work confidentially, offload feelings and receive consistent support. Managers should do their utmost to ensure this is available and health boards/authorities, who commission such services, need to build in funding for it.

- Access to the relevant local, national and professional child protection guidance and knowledge of one accessible person whom staff can consult for clarification on these.

Staff training and discussion can also raise awareness of successful ways of working. For instance some health professionals already explore, in a range of diplomatic ways, possible abuse issues when patients' symptoms or problems are worrying them.

One example was given by Dr Willie Angus, Scottish GP, recently retired (Angus 1996). More than 80 patients within the space of about two years revealed a sexual abuse history to him. He wrote about the issue for GPs in the *British Medical Journal* and about the symptom relief which occurred for many patients:

> I was never criticized by patients for asking them if they had suffered from abuse, or were sexually abused as children. I see no reason why, in suitable circumstances, the question cannot be sympathetically addressed to anyone...those to whom it did not apply seemed undisturbed and answered in the negative. Most survivors were considerably relieved when the question was asked as they had, in many cases, tried to bring up the subject but felt unable to do so in case they were disbelieved or rejected (Angus 1996, p.210).

Perhaps the single most important point which confidence-building training can impart is that while specialist skills are sometimes necessary the most important qualities in working with either abused adults or children are basic ones such as understanding, warmth, empathy and acceptance and the ability to listen. It is also about people having faith in their own strengths.

People throughout the caring professions often react fearfully to the prospect of someone revealing CSA, almost as if they or even the room might spontaneously combust! If someone chooses you to tell, it is a compliment. If you are used to encountering and comforting distressed people as a health professional, you would cope with a newly-bereaved person, with the parent of a very sick child, or someone crying with shock after a road accident. There's no reason to fear this particular disclosure or distress: use the skills, warmth and empathy which you would normally use.

A positive, encouraging environment for abused children and adults

Here are a few examples of how to enable staff to use their new awareness and confidence positively, to create a welcoming, respectful and sensitive atmosphere in settings such as health centres, dental practices, reproductive health clinics and so on. Often this first encourages women survivors to speak about their past in larger numbers, while men, teenagers and children and young people will usually confide more slowly.

This time, however, is not wasted, because helping adult survivors also helps vulnerable children. It enables adults better to protect and parent their own children, points the way to reducing substance abuse and persistent mental or physical symptoms and often enables adult survivors to tell police about abusers in the community who may still be a danger to children. The topic then becomes more 'speakable' for men, for teenagers and children.

Good practice in your own staff team

- A staff team should begin by expecting that childhood sexual abuse will already be affecting, either past or present, a significant percentage of patients/clients of all social, ethnic and family backgrounds. Expect it to happen – as you would other threats to health and wellbeing. You should especially expect it if dealing routinely with areas such as mental health problems and substance misuse.

- Managers should attempt to involve all staff of all levels in awareness raising and confidence-building training which gives enough time for consideration of all the issues. Likewise they should do their best to ensure support and supervision as described previously.

- Ensure that record-keeping in your own practice is as sound as possible and as able as possible to track records over time through childhood to adulthood. Have staff make a practice of reading a patient's past records carefully and thoughtfully, when they are worried or puzzled about the wellbeing of any patient.

- It increases confidence and diminishes fears if one staff member has a particular interest and knowledge regarding CSA, to whom people can go for advice, to discuss ideas and worries and, if they are particularly skilled at this, to inquire of a child or adult. He/she does not need to be the most senior person in the practice.

- That point links into the wider ethos of your practice and work setting. If the skills of different professionals of unequal status, such as practice nurses, occupational therapists, sexual health workers and many others are to be used to the greatest benefit of vulnerable children, they as staff need to work within an atmosphere of partnership and mutual respect.

- Staff should find a bit of time to read research about additional signs, symptoms and behaviours which should alert them in their own particular professions. To take one example, while dentists and health visitors should both be observant of 'frozen watchfulness' in young children, clearly there will also be different signs to note in the course of their services and different areas of the body will normally be the main focus of attention.

- Likewise different professions in a staff team can become alert to how the ways in which they meet patients/clients may make them more accessible. For instance health visitors, mental health nurses and other staff who visit mothers in their homes can find this is often a more private setting where they are better able to disclose problems such as domestic violence or child abuse inflicted by an intimidating partner.

Creating welcoming atmospheres for disclosure in health settings

CSA is surrounded by shame, silence and silencing and it is not often named in helpful leaflets about health. Simply seeing or hearing 'child sexual abuse' named can be crucial in encouraging people to get help. They think, 'Oh, it's OK to mention this?'

- Have posters and leaflets available in surgeries, clinics and dental practices for people to pick up and read, with contact details of organizations which support adults and children. This is much easier when good links have been made with other agencies (*see next*). You could include information leaflets about reporting sexual crime and about the local child protection committee. Some organizations such as NSPCC and 'Stop it Now' also provide very useful leaflets and pamphlets, with information for parents on how they can better protect their children from danger or abuse (NSPCC 2007; Stop it Now! UK 2008).

- Many health centres and clinics have space that can be used for lectures, talks or discussions, for workers only or more widely for the local public. This is an opportunity to invite speakers who work with child protection or domestic violence, support for adult survivors, etc. Health staff could also help initiate a public information event at a local community centre if their premises were unavailable.

- Be fully aware of particular fears survivors may have and build reassurance into your routine practice: for instance by inquiring before reproductive health checks if people have particular worries about the test, or by asking dental patients if they want a nurse present, or would prefer the chair not to be placed in a horizontal position.

- A counselling service in a health centre can be very helpful to people with a wide range of problems, including sexual abuse. It also helps other staff to use their own time to best effect, because they can offer to refer people when this is appropriate.

Making links with other relevant agencies

The guidance material on child protection liaison and contacts in your area can seem dry and unreal and usually sits around until there is some pressing need to use it. Personal contact turns names into real people, making processes more understandable.

- Ask the senior police officer, social worker or relevant paediatrician to meet all staff at some point. Ensure a senior member of staff also has a personal contact. This effort should not be arduous. After all, others such as pharmaceutical companies make numerous contacts with primary health care staff!

- Primary health care teams should, in particular, develop close links with local primary and secondary schools, especially with guidance teachers and others working with child welfare in schools.

- It is good practice to be aware of a few good national and local voluntary organizations who work with adult survivors, with victims of sexual crime (such as rape) generally and of domestic violence; and with vulnerable or abused children. This also gives staff far more confidence, when they can suggest names of other organizations to patients. Have someone make a printed list, for anyone who might find it helpful. Established adult survivor groups in your area might also be interested in doing a presentation for primary health care staff and users, or in helping to make a training video.

- Likewise awareness of statutory services which are knowledgeable and interested in sexual abuse work is valuable. For instance are there local mental health services or addiction services, or committed individuals within these, which routinely address sexual abuse issues? Unfortunately, these services do not necessarily do so.

- Are you aware if your local/regional hospital specialists who receive referrals for persistent urinary, bowel or unexplained respiratory problems in children routinely consider the possibility of child abuse among the causal factors they explore? Can a senior practitioner raise this with them if they do not?

Signs, symptoms and comments to notice in children and young people

Why it's hard to volunteer the secret

All the previous measures will encourage an atmosphere where children and young people and adults will feel safer to confide. However, since most children and teenagers do not volunteer, unprompted, that they have been sexually abused, staff also need to be more sensitive to other cues and to confused attempts to communicate. Children – especially boys – tend not to tell readily in any case, through shame, humiliation, fear, not knowing the words and many other reasons.

Adult survivors have talked about why they felt unable to speak to medical staff when they were children. Children are usually with a parent, carer or older sibling at a health centre or clinic so cannot speak freely. The carer may not be abusive themselves, but the child may not want them to have the information, or may want to protect them from it.

Adult survivors talk of how they were convinced that the doctor would tell their family, even if this was untrue. Sometimes a GP, dentist or nurse, especially in rural areas was friendly socially with the family or the abuser, so again they did not risk trust. In a few cases unfortunately they had been abused by a health professional and could not trust others. On the other hand adult survivors often say they much appreciated kind and helpful health professionals whom they met as children and wished that they could have confided in them. So it is important to be receptive and welcoming; to be informed and responsible about confidentiality issues and prepared to explain them.

If children and young teenagers do say something, it will often sound vague. Younger children may repeatedly complain, 'My tummy hurts', 'My bottom hurts', 'My throat hurts', while teenagers might ask, 'If I told you something would you have to tell someone else?', or 'My friend has got this problem and doesn't know what to do'. They might also keep coming in about apparently small things without being able to say what is actually bothering them, or be repeatedly about to reveal something.

These are situations where it's important to be observant, to be receptive and sensitive and to take a few minutes' extra time rather than hurrying the consultation along. With such young people it can also be important to give them a choice of staff to tell and some opportunity to speak without a carer present.

Sexual and reproductive health issues

A simple but often overlooked point is that sexual abuse leaves sexual evidence. Professionals have been so busy arguing over whether or not physical signs such as reflex anal dilatation, anal tissue scarring or certain changes to the hymen are reliable indicators of CSA that they often miss what is in front of them. They re-interpret it, accept other explanations, or do not consider that sexual assaults occur beyond genital and anal areas.

Most obviously, if there is unexplained injury or soreness or sexually transmitted infection present in genital, anal or throat areas, especially if this is repeated, sexual abuse should seriously be considered as a possible cause. There is now a considerable literature on physical signs in sexually abused children, although this also reveals how research conclusions still vary on the percentage of abused children who do show physical signs (Bruni 2003; Delago et al. 2008; Heger et al. 2002; Hobbs, Hanks and Wynne 1999; RCPCH 2008b). However, many suggestive signs can still be missed or dismissed in pre-teen children who have reached puberty and in young teenagers.

This comes from a mistaken assumption that they are all simply deciding to take part in consensual sex at an early age: even though adults would consider them incapable of taking other significant decisions about their lives (even about smoking!) until after 16 or 18. Amorphous responsibility for pregnancy by some unknown unspecified boyfriend is often accepted at face value. There has also been a libertarian ethos in much sexual health work, which genuinely seeks to be young person-centred but which has underplayed the role of coercion. Because, unfortunately, government-led emphasis in sexual health programmes has always been more about technical prevention of pregnancy and sexually transmitted infections (STIs) in young people than about protecting them from coercion, technical preventives or solutions to unwanted pregnancy and STIs have been more readily supplied than skilled advice about the quality and safety of sexual relationships.

Pregnancy, miscarriage, abortion requests, anal sexual damage in boys, or STIs in 11–13 year olds should always warn of likely present or past sexual abuse (since the impact of catastrophic loss of self-respect often leads to apparent 'promiscuity' in young people). These same signs in 13–15 year olds (older in the case of learning-disabled youngsters) should still raise concerned curiosity. The relationships may well be consensual or they may not. *Many adult survivors have described these (often repeated) events in their medical history as clues to their abuse which were not picked up, or where vague explanations were accepted.*

Because health professionals in sexual health matters usually have a wider degree of confidentiality (unless very directly told about abuse) than other agencies working with young people they have an advantage – less likely to 'scare off' abused children who are silenced through knowing that other agencies must report immediately.

They can for instance routinely tell under-16s gently that they are always concerned that young people are safe and have not been pressured into sex. They can tell younger teenagers why they are worried and ask if anything has been making them sad, hurt or frightened. They can routinely give out leaflets to both girls and boys whose sexual/reproductive health is affected, with the names of agencies and with 'sexual abuse' actually named. They can ask if there is someone within or beyond the practice they would like to speak to and they can continue to monitor these young people, which is particularly important. Often when young people are given a little time and space to think and to realize the professional is sincerely concerned, they do find the courage to reveal what is happening and let the case be taken forward.

Unexplained, or suspiciously explained, physical symptoms

Very many adult survivors describe having had medical histories, as children and teenagers, of frequent illnesses, injuries, hospitalizations, examinations, unexplained physical symptoms or mysterious pains and psychiatric referrals to psychiatrists or psychologists. This was especially so when they also experienced frequent physical violence, as many did (Arias 2004; Kendall-Tackett 2002; Leserman et al. 1997; Nelson 2002). In some cases people suffered severe injuries without questions apparently being asked about maltreatment. Many survivors feel insufficient questions were asked or notice taken when these incidents happened over years and that observant, concerned practitioners might have helped bring about protective intervention.

If children have frequent unexplained pain such as persistent stomach-aches or headaches, don't dismiss these too quickly as psychosomatic without full checks, or without getting them to show exactly where the pain is (younger children in particular may describe pain in their genital area as a 'tummyache'). Do not dismiss such symptoms as anxiety-driven without being curious about the *source* of their anxiety or of what may indeed be a psychosomatic process. One adult male survivor has described how he would pull his eyebrows and hair out in anguish and fear when he was eight. This was seen as anxiety at his school and in the surgery, yet the cause of such extreme emotion and such distressingly visible effects was never sought.

Of course, many children have perfectly innocent reasons for a history of poor health. It is not about suspecting everyone: it is about including possible abuse among background reasons where there are years of frequent visits and hospitalizations – most especially if infections, pains or injuries tend to be in areas vulnerable to sexual assault and if there are also behavioural and psychiatric symptoms present.

Mental health and behaviour

It would also, of course, be wrong to jump to conclusions that young people with various mental health symptoms or behaviours must have been sexually abused. Depression in particular is worryingly common among young people. There are many things which upset, anger or depress young people and underlying reasons including bullying, bereavement, parental divorce or separation and many others.

However, the possibility that a young person is being abused or has been should *always* be among your considerations if they have clusters of symptoms such as depression, an eating disorder, early drink and drug misuse, self-mutilation, persistent sadness and withdrawal, or alternatively persistent behavioural symptoms of anger and defiance. Suicide attempts and running away should always be taken very seriously, with careful, continuous monitoring of their wellbeing.

Many adult survivors have described fairly extreme behaviours in which they indulged as children or teenagers in the sometimes desperate hope that someone would ask what was wrong. These included throwing chairs and tables at school, repeatedly stealing in the hope of being taken into care, or even in one instance running along the roof of their school. In none of these cases was an accurate conclusion drawn (Nelson 2001).

Campaigning for the future

Health professionals genuinely committed to addressing CSA and other child abuse may feel frustrated at reading this chapter, because at present some of the suggestions will be difficult for them or their managers to implement: the resources and time given for training and supervision, employment of counsellors and other supports will be inadequate, local services for child and adult survivors will be scarce, other pressures will appear endless and child protection regulations too tight to allow sensitive, more gradual work with abused young people. These do not seem reasons to avoid stating what is important for abused children and what kinds of things need to happen in primary health care. Up to a point at least, partners in GP practices and dental practices will be able to decide that this should receive greater priority.

It will be hugely helpful to future health services, to other caring professions, to the voluntary sector and to abused children and adults, if health staff can join campaigns for improvement in these under-resourced areas. Unions and professional associations can pressurize for better support and supervision. There is much need for better trauma-based mental health and drug/alcohol services for children and adults; for more and better-funded voluntary sector survivor support agencies; and especially for children's agencies where young people can be referred or self-refer, where they are given some 'confidential space' to talk through their options and gain strength before cases are publicly pursued (Children 1st 2007).

Protecting children and reducing child abuse, as well as providing counselling facilities in primary health care, need to become recognized priorities nationally for primary health care, with their own set of targets, so that staff work in this area is rewarded and funded just as much as (for instance) GPs' success in persuading women to have regular smear tests. Who could doubt that it is equally valuable, as well as equally important to our public health?

Chapter Three

Child Protection: A Dutch GP's Perspective

Floris van de Laar and Toine Lagro-Janssen

Introduction

The difficulties of recognizing child abuse in general practice are demonstrated in the following anecdote about Frans Huygen, a well-known professor of family practice. In the late 1970s, a colleague and admirer congratulated Huygen on his book *Family Medicine: the Medical Life History of Families*. The colleague told Huygen that he was especially impressed by his case report of an incest victim who killed herself. Although Huygen was flattered, the compliment also shocked and surprised him because he was not aware of a case of incest in his book. Instead of arguing, Huygen carefully re-read his chapter about the dramatic case as soon as he arrived home. It was the story of a young girl ('a typical father's child') who had suffered severe depressions and pre-occupation with dieting and weight from an early age. He literally wrote that finally at the age of 24 years she hanged herself in the barn 'ten minutes after having been lying in bed with her father, something she often did' (Huygen 1978). Although he had accurately observed every fact, the possibility of sexual abuse had never crossed his mind.

Frans Huygen's book demonstrates how general practitioners have knowledge of, and involvement in, the families for whom they care. It also shows that this does not guarantee a crystal clear insight into the dark aspects of human behaviour. In this chapter we will give an overview of the occurrence and management of child abuse in general practice in the Netherlands. Further, we will discuss some opportunities and challenges in the methods of approaching child abuse.

Definition and scope

The Dutch Act on child care provides a definition of child abuse which is broadly adapted in research and care on this topic:

> for a child any form of threatening or violent interaction of physical, psychological or sexual nature, forced upon actively or passively by parents or other people to whom the minor has a dependent relationship, through which serious damage is being caused or runs the risk of being caused to the minor in the form of physical or psychological damage. (Act 28 168 2006)

In daily practice, the definitions are:

- sexual abuse
- physical abuse
- emotional/psychological abuse
- physical neglect
- emotional/psychological neglect
- being witness to domestic violence.

A recent Dutch study about the occurrence of child abuse in the Netherlands indicated a prevalence of 107,000 cases in 2005 (IJzendoorn *et al.* 2007). This boils down to 30/1000 children aged 0–17 years. The majority of the cases were physically and/or emotionally neglected and almost 25 per cent were victims of sexual and/or physical abuse. Compared with such numbers, death as a result of abuse is relatively rare. Data from a survey among general practitioners (GPs) and paediatricians showed an incidence of 1.14 deaths per 100,000 children 0–17 years, of which 4.13 deaths per 100,000 children were 0–2 years old (Kuyvenhoven, Hekkink and Voorn 1998). If we translate these data to an average practice with approximately 2350 patients listed, there will be about 16 children who have been abused the past year, four of them sexually and/or physically. One in five GPs will have a fatal case of child abuse in a career of 35 years.

Position, approach and tasks of the GP in Dutch health care

In the Netherlands the GP is the 'gatekeeper' of health care. With the exception of prisoners, people living in institutions and the military, every Dutch citizen (aged 0 upwards) is registered with a GP. Patients may consult their GP with every health problem they feel help is necessary. About 96 per cent of all contacts are settled by the GP and the remaining 4 per cent are referred to other workers in primary health care (e.g., physiotherapists, psychologists) or secondary care (Cardol *et al.* 2004). Although GPs are trained traditionally as doctors within a biomedical model, GPs use their knowledge of family history, psychosocial context, socio-economic status and environmental factors (e.g. pollution, neighbourhood trouble) in the assessment and treatment of the problems they encounter. This generalistic approach, the position in the centre of society and health care and the fact that in most cases the GP provides care for all members of a family, makes the GP especially equipped to recognize and manage child abuse.

Collaboration with other care providers

Most, if not all, Dutch GPs are attached to, or have working relations with, social workers. Sometimes, collaboration takes place in so-called 'home-teams', which are teams where GPs work together on complex cases with (for example) social workers, nurses or psychologists. In the Netherlands, social work is freely accessible for every citizen, is free of charge and aims to support people in coping with problems and disturbances in the interaction with their social environment (NVMW 1999). In daily practice social workers will see people and families with a wide variety of problems such as unemployment, marital problems, difficulties in raising children, or difficulties in coping with disease. Consequently, social workers will encounter many families at increased risk of child abuse. Therefore, social workers may play a role in the prevention, detection and management of child abuse.

In the Netherlands, paediatricians are part of secondary care and thus based in general or academic hospitals. Access takes place after referral by a GP or, in some cases, through an emergency department. Paediatricians and workers on emergency wards may play a role in the detection of child abuse, especially physical or sexual abuse. Hospital Child Abuse Teams, guidelines on how to deal with child abuse and standard registration forms for suspicion of child abuse have shown to increase the number of reported cases of child abuse in a Dutch academic hospital (Bleeker *et al.* 2005). Within such a structured approach, evidence for child abuse from physical examination, history taking and diagnostic tests are combined with information from other professionals such as the GP.

The Dutch Child Health Care (CHC; in Dutch: Jeugdgezondheidszorg) system covers care for all children and minors 0–19 years old. The main tasks of CHC are to gain insight into the health conditions of children, to prevent and detect diseases, to attune health care needs to health care supply, to promote healthy behaviour and to identify possible health threats in the physical or social environment. Their tasks are conducted through Children

Welfare Centres (CWC) for the age 0–4 years and mainly through schools in the age groups 5–19 years. All newborn babies with their parents or caregivers are invited to a nearby CWC. Doctors and nurses check and measure children, screen for a series of disorders, give vaccinations and supply advice and support in a wide range of issues referring to child health, safety and upbringing. For treatment of a possible disorder, children are referred to their GP. In some places the GP also acts as a CWC physician.

Bureau Youth Care (BYC; in Dutch: Bureau Jeugdzorg) is the main entrance for children and caregivers who need special care, for example when a child has abnormal behaviour or parents experience serious problems in upbringing. Access may be through own initiative or through referral by a professional (e.g., GP, CHC). BYC makes an inventory of the problem(s), assesses the urgency and gives advice on further treatment. Short-term treatments will be conducted by BYC itself, but in most cases the actual help is given by other specialized institutions who offer a wide range of extra- and intramural programmes. When a child is placed under custody BYC delivers (temporary) guardians to protect the child and to oversee the process.

A special role in the management and prevention of child abuse is provided by 'Advies and Meldpunt Kindermishandeling' (CPS). Translated this means 'Bureau for Reporting and Advice on Child Abuse' and it is comparable to the American Child Protection Services (CPS). The CPS offer access for everyone, professionals (e.g., GPs, teachers, social workers) and non-professionals (e.g., victims, family, neighbours), who knows or has a suspicion that a child is being abused. Cases may be reported anonymously, but this is not recommended for professionals. CPS investigates every report of suspected child abuse and will initiate proceedings of help if necessary. In severe cases the CPS will bring the police or the Child Protection Counsel into action.

Detecting child abuse in general practice

Detecting abnormalities is a matter of knowledge and common sense. Both consciousness and intuition supports the ability to signal when something is not in order. Signals that may raise the suspicion for child abuse may come from the family history, specific physical problems or injuries, medically unexplained complaints or behavioural problems.

Rarely, one sign will be enough to draw definitive conclusions. However, one sign should be enough reason to be on the alert. In this view it is an advantage that the GP is familiar with the family members and their (medical) histories. Therefore, the GP may have knowledge of risk factors for child abuse related to the whole family, such as domestic violence, unemployment or financial problems, or risk factors related to an individual family member such as alcohol abuse or violence or neglect in someone's own parental situation.

Among the physical problems that are encountered during surgery hours and that may point to abuse are physical injuries or stuntedness and venereal disease, the latter being a very specific sign. In case of injury the GP should always question whether the explanation about the cause makes sense. Poor personal hygiene, dishevelled appearance or inadequate dental care may be indicative of neglect. A home visit will bring information about a dirty or untidy living situation.

Next, medically unexplained complaints and a number of behavioural abnormalities may occur, pointing at possible child abuse. For example, headache, stomachache, or frequent fainting, may be a sign of the pressure under which the child lives. Examples of abnormal behaviour are noticeably aggressive or anxious behaviour during physical examination, or when the child behaves differently than may be expected from its age (e.g., enuresis or encopresis). Also, parents may indicate that there are problems, for example when a father or mother 'complains' about the upbringing methods of the other parent.

Historically, the Netherlands is a country of immigrants; this is reflected in the fact that about 20 per cent of the population is of non-Dutch origin, half of them being of non-western descent. Hence cultural aspects should be taken into consideration when dealing with (possible) child abuse. The different values in western and non-western countries will be reflected in the way people raise their children. Especially in non-western cultures the GP may have great authority and consequently play an important role in establishing a working relation with the parents. It is important to have knowledge of specific rules and habits when the GP wants to start a dialogue. For example, it may not be appropriate to speak with the mother alone, but always in presence of the father, being the head of the family. Sometimes an interpreter is needed to communicate, in which case it should be avoided that one of the children acts as a translator. Child abuse is always a topic that is surrounded by a sense of shame and may also be experienced as a loss of dignity in some cultures.

Signals of sexual abuse

Even more often than with other forms of abuse, a child only very rarely speaks out about sexual abuse. After all, the child will be pressurized by the perpetrator into remaining silent about what is or was going on between them. The perpetrator will know that his behaviour is unacceptable and will deny as long as possible.

Usually, sexual abuse will not leave lasting physical traces. Damage caused to the genitals or anus recovers fast. Vaginal infections, discharge or itch may be a sign of sexual abuse, but sexually transmitted diseases as a result of sexual abuse are rare. Sometimes the child is forced to undergo an abortion in case of pregnancy, but more likely the signals are much more diffuse and present as psychosomatic complaints such as stomachache or other medically unexplained symptoms. Repeated urinary tract infections or secondary enuresis should lead to vigilance. In adolescents, symptoms such as self-mutilation or bulimia could be suggestive of sexual abuse.

When the child raises the subject, the response of the GP is very important: believe the child. Children hardly ever lie about abuse. Moreover, battered children are more likely to trivialize what has happened rather than to exaggerate its occurrence.

Impact of witnessing domestic violence

Often victims can be unaware of the impact of the abuse on children. Witnessing violence may have damaging effects on children and young people (Victorian Government Department of Justice 2006). When either victim or perpetrator has disclosed partner violence in the home, it is important for a family physician to ask about the risk for and impact on children. Discussing the impact on children may encourage parents to seek additional help to make beneficial changes.

If there is an opportunity to speak to children or young people by themselves, the GP should consider asking if they feel safe at home. If they choose to disclose and discuss issues further, this may offer opportunities to discuss their personal safety. It is also important to explain to children and young people that the violence is not their fault and, if appropriate, that the GP is available to help and support them. In some cases, the GP may be the only person in whom children or young people will confide. When a child discloses, do not document this in any records to which the perpetrator has legal access. It is also important not to breach confidentiality (Lo Fo Wong and Lagro-Janssen 2005).

Statute for the reporting of child abuse

In 2004 the Royal Dutch Medical Society published a 'Reporting statute concerning child abuse'(KNMG 2008). The purpose of this statute is to ensure efficient diagnostic strategies in cases of suspected child abuse and to initiate immediate help in cases of a threatening situation. In this statute the CPS plays an important role in supporting physicians who encounter child abuse and the initiation and co-ordination of their subsequent care.

Based on this statute the Rotterdam region developed a protocol 'Statute for the reporting of child abuse' (GGD Rotterdam 2008). This protocol is an example of a stepwise approach for all professionals that encounter possible cases of child abuse. The protocol contains clear guidelines with respect to early signalling, management and reporting of child abuse. It offers clarity on what is expected from professionals in order to improve their help for victim and perpetrator.

The protocol consists of the following basic steps:

1. Discuss the (suspected) abuse with your patient(s). Candour is an important value in medical aid. Only if this step may lead to danger for victim(s) or professional, or if it may be expected that the patients will completely turn their back to the professional, this step may be skipped.

2. Discuss with an expert or with the CPS. If step 1 does not take away your concerns discuss the (anonymous) case with a colleague with special expertise or with the CPS.

3. Always report (suspected) severe abuse to the CPS. In order to reduce the risk that multiple professionals are working at cross-purposes, severe abuse always needs to be reported to the CPS in order to co-ordinate the various actions. The severity of the abuse may appear from the duration and intensity, repetition, the severity of the physical or mental damage.

4. If a professional chooses to manage the case of abuse alone, he or she should monitor the patient, arrange regular appointments and stay alert for signals pointing at new abuse. The case should be reported to the CPS after all if the abuse does not stop.

The statute is explicit about how to deal with professional secrecy. Information should remain confidential where possible, but this confidentiality should be broken if necessary. Answering five basic questions may guide the decision whether or not to break the professional secrecy. (1) What is the aim of talking to someone else about my patient? (2) Is there another way to reach this goal without having to break the confidentiality? (3) Why is it not possible to get permission from the patient to discuss his/her case with a third person? (4) Do the interests of the child weigh up to the interests of the person whose secret I am about to break? (5) If I decide to break the professional secrecy to whom should I give what information in order to help my patient?

Challenges and opportunities in the management of child abuse in general practice

The GP should be well-equipped to identify and manage child abuse: the GP delivers care for a limited number of listed patients nearby the practice; the GP has knowledge of families and the (social) environment; and he follows patients over a long time-span. Ideally, the GP has an open and non-judgemental attitude which facilitates easy and accessible opportunities for patients to discuss difficulties in raising children and possible child abuse. Still, there are some concerns. The incidence of child abuse in morbidity registration networks is significantly lower than expected from other data sources. And next, GPs have difficulties in recognizing signs of child abuse and subsequent reporting it.

Under-registration or blind spot?

Data from a Dutch continuous registration network, based on what GPs register in the medical files, indicated in 2001 a number of 52 cases of child abuse per 100,000 children. These data are in contrast with data from the CPS, who reported about 300 cases of abuse per 100,000 children in 2001 (Maat-Van Manen *et al.* 2005) and the previously mentioned Dutch study indicating 30/1000 children aged 0–17 years (IJzendoorn *et al.* 2007). Remarkably, in the continuous registration network one third of the victims are boys, whereas the CPS reports as many boys as girls. The reasons are unclear as to why there is a significant discrepancy between incidents of child abuse recorded with the registration network and the likely number of victims. It is possible that some cases remain completely out of the GP's sight. Another possibility is that the GP only reports the type of injury (e.g. bruise) and not the possible cause; after all parents always have the right to see the files of their children. Another possible explanation might be that (early) signs of child abuse are not recognized at all, due to lack of knowledge or failing continuity when patients are seen by other GPs in the evenings or at weekends.

Pitfalls in evaluating and reporting child abuse

Doctors are trained to help people and the basic attitude is to believe and trust people, rather than to be suspicious. Therefore, doctors do not easily question whether the information patients give them is true and may think of alternative explanations for complaints or injuries, such as child abuse. It is thus no surprise that in most medical curricula forensic aspects are absent or have only a very limited place. Consequently, it is also not very surprising that skills in interpreting injuries and diagnosing abuse show room for improvement. In a

Dutch survey among 250 practising GPs who received photographic material of three cases, only 15 per cent doubted the given cause in a child that had been abused (Reijnders, van Baasbank and van der Wal 2005). Nevertheless, (post-academic) education has shown to improve knowledge and performance with respect to child abuse. A 1997 American survey among 370 paediatricians, family physicians and emergency physicians showed that the knowledge level about socio-economic and behavioural aspects of sexual abuse increased in the past 10 years, probably as a result of increased education opportunities (Lentsch and Johnson 2000). Moreover, another American study among 98 primary care paediatricians showed that education about child abuse was the only physician-related variable that affected the likelihood that a practitioner would suspect abuse (Flaherty *et al.* 2002). This concords with a Dutch study about GPs signalling intimate partner abuse that improved significantly after training (Lo Fo Wong *et al.* 2006).

Even if child abuse is suspected, this does not always lead to subsequent action. In Australia, 25 per cent of medical practitioners reported that they failed at least once to report a suspected case of child abuse or neglect, although this was mandatory in their country. Non-reporting was predicted by the belief that the suspected abuse was a single incident (Schweitzer *et al.* 2006). Other possible reasons not to report to official institutions include the possibilities that physicians are reluctant to risk their relationship with parents; pessimism with regard to the effectiveness of CPS; and fear of legal claims if the suspicion turns out not to be true (Vulliamy and Sullivan 2000). Data from focus group research in a group of paediatric primary care physicians asked for their experiences in identifying and reporting child abuse. Two main themes emerged. First, past subjective experiences strongly influenced their personal practices. In particular, negative experiences with the CPS reduced the physicians' confidence in detecting abuse. Second, doctors felt an enormous responsibility to make a correct assessment within the limited time of an office visit. Moreover they reported that their relationships with the families involved both facilitated and hampered their assessment of possible child abuse. On the one hand a close relationship made it more difficult to think of abuse. On the other hand their knowledge of possible difficulties in families increased awareness of abuse. When they reported suspected abuse to the CPS this permanently affected their relationship with the families. It was found helpful to discuss decisions with colleagues or to consult child abuse experts (Flaherty, Jones and Sege 2004).

Final considerations

The GP may play an important role in (early) detection and management of child abuse because of their position at the centre of the health care system, knowledge and lengthy relationships with families and easy accessibility for all possible health problems. Nevertheless, detection and management of child abuse is capable of improvement as can be concluded from the under-registration in GP research networks. Awareness of the problem and better education seems paramount. On the one hand, awareness might be increased by ongoing attention for the problem on a societal and policy level. GPs and GP-registrars should be trained regularly in the recognition of risk factors and physical and psychological signs of child abuse. Moreover, exploration of own past experiences might be useful in order to identify potential obstacles in managing child abuse.

If a GP signals or suspects child abuse he or she is not alone. Consulting a colleague or an expert on child abuse helps in making the diagnosis and supporting the child and the child's family. The GP should not act as a soloist, but as a team player instead. Paediatricians, social workers, BYC or CPS are other important players and may take over the body of work once the diagnosis is made. Protocols such as a statute for the reporting of child abuse could be an important tool in bringing the final goal closer: a safe childhood for all.

Chapter Four

The Role of the Paediatrician in Safeguarding Children

Ruth Skelton

Introduction

All professionals are familiar with the heart sinking feeling as the possibility of child abuse or neglect comes to mind in the middle of a busy clinic. This may be a baby with a small unexplained bruise on the cheek; the thin grubby two-year-old brother with nits and an old burn on his hand; or the older girl who is 'sore down below' again. You may know the family and have been concerned about family dynamics for a while, you may have information on the partner that Mum does not know, or the family will be new to the area and there is no information. What do you do? Should you let the concerns go or is there enough to refer? What will be the reaction of the family? Do you contact social work or paediatrics? What training is available? To whom do you turn for advice and support?

Child protection work is often quoted as the most stressful part of any work (although it can be the most satisfying). The paediatrician is part of a multi-disciplinary team and has a number of roles in the safeguarding of children, many of which can help the child in the previous scenarios. Recognition and acceptance that abuse may have taken place is important. A strong back-up service, clear referral and advice pathways and availability of further training are essential for the confidence to carry through the required medical investigations and be involved in the team who will manage the care of such children. The paediatrician is pivotal in this service.

Understanding the role of the paediatrician and referral pathways can help primary health care professionals manage the medical needs and prepare the child and family for the ongoing assessment which will be required. Getting it right at the beginning is crucial to maintaining co-operation and understanding in the family. It is therefore of concern that the number of paediatricians willing to do this work is falling. This chapter will also consider availability of paediatricians for such work and the possible consequences for children and their families.

Referral pathways

In his enquiry into the death of Victoria Climbié, Lord Laming found a reluctance of all professionals, including medical staff, to consider and treat a child with suspected abuse with the same level of care as a child with a medical condition (Laming 2003). One of his 108 recommendations was that 'the investigation and management of a case of possible deliberate harm to a child must be approached in the same systematic and rigorous manner as would be appropriate to the investigation and management of any other potentially fatal disease' (p.53).

If a child has unusual bruising, most primary health care physicians will be comfortable taking a history and examining for leukaemia or clotting disorder and will know the referral pathways to specialist paediatric services. However, there appears to be a reticence to undertake a detailed history, examination, investigation and referral for possible abuse.

When starting in a new practice most professionals familiarize themselves with basic emergency policies such as fire, anaphylaxis protocols and contacts for admissions. Finding out the local safeguarding arrangements and in particular who to contact should be considered an equally important priority.[1]

Responsibility for child protection services is usually headed by a statutory governmental body, in liaison with the police. The medical service, including the paediatrician, is part of a wider multi-disciplinary team. In some countries, e.g. Australia and the USA, child protection medical services tend to be based in a large team in specific premises, rather than linked with a trust or hospital. In the UK current child protection guidance and services have been heavily shaped by enquiries into children's deaths. Most recently Lord Laming's first report led to more specific government guidance for both social care and medical services (Laming 2003), and his second report (2009) is likely to result in further changes. Similar provision of joint responsibilities of health, social work and police is in place in Scotland (Scottish Executive 2005a).

Local details of the service may vary, but the following basic structure is common. The pathway normally involves referral to social work and/or a paediatrician. If abuse is likely social work should be contacted first.

---

1   Richard Balmer, personal communication.

Paediatricians are usually happy to discuss cases and take referrals directly for an opinion, which can make referral easier for the GP. Paediatricians also take referrals from other areas including police, Accident and Emergency, colleagues in other specialties and sometimes the courts, who will order a paediatric assessment, particularly for children for whom neglect is a concern.

Child protection referral and advice during office hours is usually managed by a rota of local hospital or community paediatricians who vary from specialists to general paediatricians. While physical abuse and neglect are usually well-covered, services for sexual abuse, especially acute, may be less robust. General paediatricians are rarely trained in this area. Sexual abuse is usually dealt with by a combination of paediatricians and forensic medical examiners (FMEs): GPs or paediatricians who have had training in taking forensic specimens and who work for the police. They have experience in sexual assault work, but they may have limited paediatric training. In the UK joint examinations are common. There are recommendations which outline the balance of forensic and child-centred requirements (RCPCH and The Association of Forensic Physicians 2007). However, some areas have insufficient funding and staffing to offer such a joint service.

Designated and named professionals

While paediatricians of all grades and experience staff the rotas, designated and named doctors and nurses take on service, training and strategic responsibilities in the UK. Primary health care in England is managed within Primary Care Trusts (PCTs). PCTs have a responsibility for employing a designated doctor and nurse, usually experienced paediatricians and paediatric nurses 'to take a strategic professional lead on all aspects of safeguarding' (HM Government 2006). In addition each individual trust employs a named doctor and nurse; a paediatrician, GP or other appropriate professional. They are involved in the day-to-day operational management of cases.

Roles of named and designated doctors overlap considerably and include (HM Government 2006; RCPCH 2005a,b):

- Inter-agency responsibilities, representation on Local Safeguarding Children Boards (LSCB).
- Advisory responsibilities for planning services, training, procedures and policies.
- Clinical role and advice.
- Monitoring and supervision.
- Involvement in internal audits and case reviews.
- Informing Trust Boards on safeguarding issues and risks.

Medical assessment

Traditionally the medical assessment for abuse has involved giving a specific opinion as to whether or not abuse has occurred. However, this assessment now has to be part of a more thorough holistic assessment of the child (RCPCH 2006), allowing a more effective assessment of possible abuse or neglect and any other aspects of medical care required. For the child and family this can be difficult and stressful. Good preparation makes a huge difference. Understanding the process of the medical assessment can help prepare the family.

The following is a guide as to what an ideal child protection medical assessment should cover. However time, availability and training may in practice restrict this to a much briefer assessment, reducing the effectiveness of the holistic approach.

The aims of the child protection medical assessment include:

- Assessment for evidence of other abuse or neglect.

- Assessment of alternative medical condition.

- An holistic assessment of the child's needs, including growth and development, medical conditions, uptake of basic screening and immunizations and a basic assessment of psychological and emotional state.

- Reassurance of child and family.

- An opinion regarding abuse or neglect.

- Collection of forensic evidence.

Discussing referral with parents

Opening the subject of possible abuse is probably one of the hardest areas to broach. Timely advice can help. If referring a child where concerns have been raised, it is very helpful to be as clear and honest as possible as to the reasons for referral. A common complaint is not that abuse was considered, but that parents were not told what was happening. Most parents realize that abuse has to be considered; they just need to know what is happening and why. Explaining that routine further opinion is needed for an unusual injury is often enough.

Interpreters

If a carer, including either parent, has difficulties understanding English, an interpreter with experience and understanding of child protection work is essential. It is not appropriate to rely on family members. The interpreter must also be briefed and prepared.

Consent

If the parents are not present, consent should be sought from whoever has 'parental responsibility' for example natural parents or the local authority. This should include consent for a full medical including anogenital examination, photographs, blood tests and X-rays if required. If no consent is available and it is thought to be in the child's interest the medical may be done, but it is best practice to obtain consent and work with the parents if possible. It is usually possible to perform a full medical assessment with the alleged perpetrator present.

History

A full detailed history is taken regarding the injury, preferably from the carer at the time. This may help unravel the circumstances and may lead to an understanding of an accidental event. A full background history including previous medical and social history, a detailed systemic enquiry including a search for behavioural changes is taken (RCPCH 2006).

Measurement and observation

A reliable height and weight measurement is undertaken. Parent-held records can give useful previous measurements and a pattern of growth. An experienced nurse or play specialist can give vital observations, e.g. 'The mother kept leaving the baby where he could roll off'; 'She only paid attention to the child when in with the doctor and ignored her in the waiting area.'

Examination

A detailed assessment of the injury and full examination of the child will be requested. This requires the child to be fully undressed. It greatly benefits all if the parents are aware that this will happen before the medical assessment.

Investigations include clotting screen for children with bruising and skeletal survey for children under two years. Infants may be admitted for a more thorough assessment for non-accidental head injury. Skeletal surveys usually include repeat chest X-ray or full survey as particularly rib fractures may not show up immediately (RCPCH 2008b).

Anogenital examination

Anogenital examination, often referred to as 'intimate examination', is the most controversial part of the medical assessment. The main purpose is to detect and document evidence (clinical and forensic) of sexual abuse. It also offers other benefits for the child (Hobbs *et al.* 1999), including detection or exclusion of other medical problems (skin conditions, undescended testes) and sexually transmitted infections. It has been shown to be reassuring (Kellogg 2005b). However, it is extensively debated within the child protection field.

Guidance stresses that the assessment should not be traumatic for the child. The actual examination is an external inspection using a colposcope with video or still photograph recording and is generally well-tolerated (Hobbs *et al.* 1999). Only in sexually active teenagers is it sometimes necessary to examine internally and this would only be done with full consent.

Current UK guidance (RCPCH 2006, 2008a) recommends that an anogenital examination should be part of the assessment for children with suspected physical abuse and neglect as well as sexual abuse. Some paediatricians feel uncomfortable with this and reserve examination for those with identified problems. This is more in line with American guidance: anogenital examinations are performed only when concerns arise during the assessment of children with physical abuse or neglect (Kellogg 2005b).

Reporting

Feedback is usually given to parents at the time of examination, followed by a report which may be shared with the parents. Questions often arise about confidentiality and storage of these reports. While confidentiality is important, multi-agency sharing of information for the protection of the child must take precedence (HM Government 2006). Lack of communication is identified as a major problem in serious case reviews carried out on children who die following maltreatment (Dodsworth *et al.* 2008). Reports should be stored in the main file or a clear link made to them. Files for siblings should again be linked. Paediatricians should not keep separate child protection records.

Confidentiality and reporting

Current guidance is quite clear. The needs of the child are paramount and all information which may help to protect the child must be shared with relevant agencies (BMA 2004; Department of Health 2007a; RCPCH 2004b) The professional has a clear duty to protect the child and must act in the child's best interest (GMC 2007).

The line between under- and over-reporting is fine and the consequences of overstepping dire on either side. However, a balance can be found if it is remembered that in primary health care the responsibility is to raise concerns about *possible* abuse or neglect and refer for further assessment. The primary health care team will rarely be in a position to confirm a diagnosis of abuse. They should pass on concerns and assist enquiries by other agencies. 'You will be able to justify raising a concern even if it turns out to be groundless, if you have done so honestly, promptly, on the basis of reasonable belief and through the appropriate channels' (GMC 2007).

Barriers to child protection work and media attention

This section looks at why professionals sometimes fail to recognize and deal appropriately with possible signs of abuse and examines what can be done to try to stem the flow of paediatricians and other professionals away from child protection. The barriers are common to most professions.

Child abuse is complex, requiring a commensurate degree of multi-agency co-operation. Basic awareness and knowledge of abuse and neglect is necessary and acceptance that abuse does occur. Confidence in referral mechanisms is equally important. This is much more dependent on the professional's background and experiences. Fear of repercussions is also a very powerful barrier to safeguarding children. This has grown out of some high profile cases.

Even when professionals believe that abuse may have occurred, they may not always take action. Studies show that professionals in many countries fail to report children they suspect of being abused, even in those countries with mandatory reporting (Kilpatrick, Scott and Robinson 1999; Sege and Flaherty 2008). The proportion of children suspected to be abused but not reported, varies from only 5 per cent (Flaherty *et al.* 2000) to 71 per cent (Cairns, Mok and Welbury 2005). Lazenbatt and Freeman (2006) found 13 per cent non reporting and noted that community nurses were more likely than doctors to report and appeared to be more comfortable in this work. Reasons for non-reporting include uncertainty, lack of training and confidence, fear of repercussions and lack of confidence in statutory referral organizations.

Insufficient training and knowledge

Studies report consistently that professionals feel their training in abuse is inadequate (Cairns *et al.* 2005). Further training has been shown to improve recognition and reporting (Flaherty *et al.* 2000; Lazenbatt and Freeman 2006).

Currently in the UK there are no specific requirements or qualifications for paediatricians in child protection, as for example the American System of Board recognition. A more formal process is being developed in the UK. A training day recently developed by the Royal College of Paediatrics and Child Health (RCPCH) and the NSPCC emphasizes the barriers to recognizing and managing Child Protection (RCPCH, NSPCC and ALSG 2007). Safeguarding boards offer multi-agency training. Resources and training courses for other professionals are emerging (Department of Health 2007a; RCGP 2007).

All professionals working with children now have a responsibility to acquire appropriate training and knowledge of child protection and are increasingly required to show evidence of it (HM Government 2006; RCPCH 2005b).

Evidence base and guidance

Like many other paediatric sub-specialities, the medical evidence base for child protection has been relatively poor. Attempts are being made to address this. In the UK current literature is currently being collated (Welsh Child Protection Systematic Review Group 2008).

There is a danger, however, of over-reliance on literature. The injury should not be looked at in isolation. Context, age of the child, history given and background are all important in assessing the likelihood of abuse. A torn frenulum in a baby is of more concern than in a toddler with a clear history of running into a table, whatever the predictive value of the injury claimed in the literature (Maguire *et al.* 2007).

Firm guidance also helps to increase the confidence of professionals in managing child abuse. Child protection guidance is increasingly being published in the UK (BMA 2004; Department of Health 2007a; RCGP 2007; RCPCH 2006). The BMA and GMC have recently published further child protection guidance (BMA 2004; GMC 2007). In the USA the move has been more towards consensus statements (American Academy of Pediatrics and American Academy of Pediatric Dentistry 1999; Kellogg 2005b).

Complaints

Complaints are stressful and unpleasant. Numbers, although still small, are increasing. In most specialities complaints usually arise from missed diagnoses and lead to an increase in investigation. In child protection the risks appear to be greater for correct diagnosis leading to a reduction in investigation. When abuse is missed few parents complain and the voice of the child is rarely heard. Clearly there are, at times, valid grounds for complaints and a system is necessary to protect the public from poor practice. However, aggrieved parents or relatives may complain after child care proceedings due to a lack of understanding and acceptance of child abuse and neglect rather than due to poor practice. Within the court system a 'diagnosis' of abuse will be questioned. Parents may understand this to be casting doubt on the diagnosis and perceive it to be grounds for a complaint against the doctor. However, 'diagnosing abuse' is not the same as diagnosing measles (for example). Paediatricians may have to live with uncertainty and state only that the forensic evidence points to the possibility or likelihood of abuse, rather than a certainty.

A study in 2003 showed that both the threat and reality of complaints may deter paediatricians from child protection work (RCPCH 2004a). The number of complaints increased five fold over eight years. Fourteen per cent had received a complaint against them, 11 per cent of these were referred to the General Medical Council (GMC) and 16 per cent received adverse publicity. The GMC figures show that that disciplinary proceedings for child protection are rare (Catto 2008). In the RCPCH study only 3 per cent of complaints overall were upheld and, at the time, none by the GMC.

A further qualitative analysis of 72 of the above paediatricians who received complaints showed that while most paediatricians understand and accept the risk of complaints, for some the repercussions made it unacceptable. Almost a third had been put off such work (Haines and Turton 2008).

In a small study, Lalanda and Haslam (2008) showed that the numbers of complaints dealt with by the Medical Protection Society (a defence organization) for child protection are still reassuringly small. In a sample of 526 complaints notified to the Medical Protection Society, 13 per cent involved children. Two were for child protection, one for delay in referral and one for inappropriate referral (Lalanda and Haslam 2008).

The highest level of complaint for a doctor is referral to their regulatory body (in the UK the GMC). Referral may result in being seen before a fitness to practice (FTP) panel. If found guilty of gross professional misconduct (GPM), disciplinary measures include limitation of practice or withdrawal of licence to practice. Recent high profile cases of prominent paediatricians referred and severely disciplined for their child protection work have concerned many professionals.

The GMC rulings in such cases have been controversial. The appropriateness of investigations, correctness of procedure and findings have been questioned (Chadwick, Krous and Runyan 2006; Williams 2007). The GMC, however, is clear that its fitness to practice panels are conducted according to strict guidelines and that numbers of complaints that reach this level are extremely small, most being filtered appropriately long before (Catto 2008). The GMC have issued further advice concerning acting as an expert witness recently (GMC 2008). However, in his last report in 2009 Laming noted that paediatricians are still reluctant to engage in this work.

Media reporting

Balanced reporting of such an emotive subject is difficult. When children are seen to have suffered and died from abuse or neglect professionals may take the blame. However, the same professionals are held to account when abuse is thought to have been wrongly diagnosed. Publicity has been commonplace for social workers and other professionals in the many cases where abuse has been missed leading to children dying. The Cleveland case is a prime example.

In 1987, paediatricians were forced into the media spotlight when sexual abuse came to society's attention. A total of 121 cases of suspected child sexual abuse were diagnosed in Cleveland over five months by two paediatricians. Most children attended for other reasons and had not made disclosures. This was a difficult area for agencies to investigate, particularly for those who were inexperienced. The children were often removed from their parents suddenly. This increase in new referrals overwhelmed the services. The subsequent court cases were controversial with paediatric and police doctors' opinions opposite and polarized. Multi-agency working broke down. Many, but not all of the children were returned home, some on court orders. Widespread reporting of the crisis lead to a major enquiry chaired by Dame Elizabeth Butler-Sloss.

All doctors involved in the Cleveland case were plagued by media attention. Liam Donaldson, in a thorough analysis, demonstrated the bias in the reporting showing greatest coverage of evidence for the parents and least for the professionals. Use of 'emotive headlines to imply blame or support for the main protagonists' was common (Donaldson and O'Brien 1995).

Butler-Sloss (1987) noted that, 'Social workers need the support of the public. It is time the public and the press gave it to them.' She saw the dangers and urged professionals not 'to stand back and hesitate to act to protect children'. This applies equally to paediatricians.

Media confusion is compounded by theories about child abuse which emerge in court. In 2001 Geddes suggested that minor trauma may result in injuries characteristic of shaking injury and doubted the validity of shaking injury (Geddes and Plunkett 2004; Geddes et al. 2001). Patterson, a biochemist, gave expert evidence on his theory of temporary brittle bone disease, casting doubt on many cases of abusive fractures (Dyer 2004). Both theories were used in court, often successfully, to disprove allegations of abuse.

However, both theories were later discredited, but this has received little publicity (Lord Goldsmith 2006).

Solutions

Where does this leave the paediatrician involved in child protection work? Many designated doctor posts are unfilled (RCPCH 2004a). Few paediatricians are entering child protection and there is a severe national shortage of expert opinions (Bosely 2008). How can children still be protected?

Child protection does not appear to result in the same level of difficulty in America as in the UK to date. An American doctor writing in support of British paediatricians picks up on this stating that the public and press need to be 'educated responsibly about the realities of the diagnosis of child maltreatment' (Jenny 2007, p.799). Jenny suggests that their mandatory reporting system, more formalized training and subspecialty recognition of child protection give American paediatricians more protection, although not immunity.

The UK government has recognized and tried to respond to some issues. A recent statement noted that the concerns of professionals about legal action are 'understandable' but should not deter reporting provided they have 'acted in good faith and within their own sphere of competence' (Brennan and Keen 2007).

Child protection workers need good robust support, emotionally and clinically. This must include the support of their employer, multi-agency support such as the LSCB, clear guidance and confidence in the employer's handling of complaints and support from professional colleges. It also involves regaining confidence in the GMC, wider society and the media. The RCPCH and GMC are currently working together on this. Until this happens, primary health care may be left with inadequate support and many more children may be left without a robust service to safeguard them.

In 2008 Lord Laming spoke about his distress about the lack of progress since his report into Victoria Climbié's death (Laming 2003). The opportunity to report on progress came all too soon with the death of another child in the same borough. Laming's second report noted that paeodiatrician's needed to be 'confident in carrying out their role' and this required work with the Department of Health (Laming 2009). While training is important, until society and the media fully accept child abuse and neglect, and understand and suppoort professionals in their difficult role, further tragedies are likely to happen. It is important to end on a positive note. Craft states, 'Child protection should not be a burden... There can be few greater achievements than to see a child restored to an environment where they can grow and develop safely' (Craft 2007, p.573).

Chapter Five

The Role of Primary Care Dentist in Safeguarding Children

Ruth Freeman

Introduction

One of the first papers to comment upon the role of the dentist in the identification of the abused child was written in 1968 (Wald 1968). This case report suggested that dentists might be the first health professional to see a child and parent in trouble and in need of help (Wald 1968). In 1960s America there were 662 reported cases of child abuse; by the 1990s that number had increased to be in excess of 3 million (Kenney and Laming 2006). With the increasing prevalence of child abuse it was proposed that dental health professionals should be able to identify the abused child and be knowledgeable about legislation and referral procedures (Kenney and Laming 2006). Consequently, a series of policy documents and guidelines were issued in America. The first of these was a joint statement between the American Academy of Pediatrics and the American Academy of Pediatric Dentistry (American Academy of Pediatrics and American Academy of Pediatric Dentistry 1999). It stated that in all states of America dentists must recognize their responsibility to report cases of childhood abuse and/or neglect (CAN). In order to achieve this aim the statement reviewed the physical and psychological signs of child abuse and set out a series of recommendations to enable the referral of such cases for specialist care. The recommendations included that general dental practitioners must refer suspected cases of CAN to specialist paediatricians, paediatric dentists and maxillo-facial surgeons whose training included 'a mandated child abuse curriculum' (American Academy of Pediatrics and American Academy of Pediatric Dentistry 1999). The call for dentists to undergo training programmes in child abuse and neglect was made.

In 2005, Kellogg (2005a) revisited the 1999 statement and evaluated the importance of oral physical signs (e.g. lacerations of the tongue) in the recognition of child abuse. Kellogg concluded with the need for education for dental health professionals and collaboration between all those providing health care for children.

In the UK, two cases highlighted the need for dental health professionals working in the primary health care sector to be aware of child abuse and neglect in their paediatric cases. The first of these cases, in Scotland, was the death of a three-year-old boy (Cairns, Murphy and Welbury 2004), the second was the 'torture, starvation and eventual murder' of Victoria Climbié (Hall 2003, p.293). Both cases resulted in Scottish (Laming 2003; Murphy and Welbury 1998; Scottish Executive 2002, 2004c) and UK-wide (Department of Health 2003a; Laming 2003; Murphy and Welbury 1998; NICE 2006) recommendations to improve the protection of children from physical, sexual and emotional abuse. In Scotland, the Scottish Executive (Scottish Executive 2002; 2004b) called for co-ordination between groups caring for children; similar recommendations were made following the death of Victoria Climbié (Laming 2003). There has been a plethora of recommendations and mandatory requirements[2] for dental health professionals to be educated, not only on how to recognize and identify the abused and/or neglected child, but also how to refer a suspected case of child abuse (Department of Health 2005; General Dental Council 2005; Murphy and Welbury 1998; University of Glasgow and NHS Greater Glasgow 2005; Wood 2006). Calls were made for this educative process to begin at the undergraduate level, from which it is currently absent (Cairns et al. 2004).

While dental health professionals became ever more aware that head and neck injuries were suggestive and in some cases pathognomonic of child abuse, they were still anxious about referring parent and child to the appropriate authorities. In response to Hall's editorial on the lessons from Climbié (Hall 2003), Freeman and colleagues stated their concerns:

> Knowledge of the roles key professionals can play in child protection, are now clearly defined, however as health professionals do we recognize the new and serious challenges we are facing? What is our understanding of the complexities surrounding identifying and reporting child abuse cases and preventing further abuse? (Freeman et al. 2003)

In order to answer these questions, Lazenbatt and Freeman (2006) surveyed primary health care professionals including general medical and dental practitioners and community nurses working in the primary health care sector. This

---

2   It is considered to be professional misconduct in Scotland, for dentists not to report cases of child abuse and neglect (Cairns et al. 2004)

work concluded that while doctors and community nurses felt more confident in the recognition and the procedures to report suspected cases, dentists were anxious not only in their recognition of child abuse but also in the consequences upon parent, child and family. These findings reflected those found elsewhere (Cairns *et al.* 2004; Ramos-Gomez, Rothman and Blain 1998).

Therefore while it was recognized that dental health professionals might be the first to encounter the maltreated child, their attitudes and fears had the potential to result in the child and parent in trouble being overlooked. The following quote, from a general dental practitioner, is illustrative:

> As a dentist, I don't think I come in contact with children who have been abused. Going to the dentist is generally initiated by parents as a caring aspect of parenting, so I think it is unlikely that a child who is being physically abused will be taken to the dentist. (Lazenbatt and Freeman 2006 p.232)

It seemed that those working in primary health care dentistry did not appreciate that an abusive parent may bring their child for dental treatment (Mezzich *et al.* 2007; Moran and O'Hara 2006). The dentists' misapprehension together with fears of misdiagnosis acted as barriers with regard to referring the abused child presenting with decayed and painful teeth to social services (Lazenbatt and Freeman 2006).

The aim of this chapter is to present three different groups of children who present for dental treatment whose physical and emotional state betrays the difficulties they are experiencing in their interactions with their parents. It is proposed that dentists and their teams may be the first to see the physically and/or sexually abused child, the neglected child and the child presenting with overwhelming anxiety indicative of emotional difficulties. All of which suggest that they are seeing children and parents in trouble and in need of help. This chapter is in three sections. The first will describe the types of injury associated with physical abuse as well as describing procedures for identification and referring suspect cases of abuse; the second section, explores the role of the parent–child dyad as a factor and comments on the possible causes for delaying accessing treatment for dental decay; the third section sets out the argument for the need for separation of dental anxiety from dental phobia and proposes the need to acknowledge that the dentally phobic child represents a child and parent with emotional and family difficulties.

The physically abused child

Examining the relationship between 'traumatic dental injuries' and life experiences, Nicolau, Marcenes and Sheiham (2003) suggested that the child presenting with dental injuries could be a child experiencing physical abuse.

The home circumstances of children, presenting with dental injuries, tended to be different to the home circumstances of children presenting without dental injuries. The parents, of children with dental injuries, were more likely to have emotional difficulties and to have experienced physical abuse (Dixon, Browne and Hamilton-Giachritsis 2005). This section will examine (i) the home circumstances of the abusive parent-abused child dyad; (ii) provide a description of the types of dental injury associated with child abuse; and (iii) describe the steps that should be taken by primary health care professionals when they suspect child abuse.

The physically abused child: the child and family characteristics

The abused child tends to be younger and may suffer from a physical and/or learning disability. Although over 75 per cent of children who are at risk from physical abuse are above age two (Naidoo 2000), the majority of actual physical abuse occurs within the period from birth to the second birthday (Naidoo 2000). Infant boys experience more physical abuse than infant girls, with equivalent proportions of boys and girls experiencing physical abuse following infancy and until puberty; after puberty girls are more likely to be subjected to sexual abuse and boys to physical abuse (Kenney and Laming 2006; Naidoo 2000; Nicolau *et al.* 2003). It is of interest, therefore that in an investigation by Nicolau *et al.* (2003), adolescent boys, rather than adolescent girls, experienced 'parental punishments' and presented with traumatic dental injuries. Nicolau *et al.* suggest that traumatic dental injuries, such as fractured incisors, could thus, be a consequence of physical punishments – a manifestation of physical abuse.

The family environment, for the abused child, is one which is often characterized by conflict and poverty. According to Kenney and Laming (2006) and Nicolau *et al.* (2003) many children, at risk of abuse, live in one-parent households or in households with step-parents and step-siblings. Often their parents are young, have experienced early separation from their own families; have experienced physical abuse in childhood and are in abusive and violent relationships (Kenney and Laming 2006; Nicolau *et al.* 2003). In addition, these parents may have a history of mental ill-health, substance abuse and low self-esteem (Dixon *et al.* 2005; Fonaghy 2001; Mezzich *et al.* 2007). In all aspects of their lives these parents may re-enact their own unhappy childhood experiences with their partners and children (Kenney and Laming 2006; Nicolau *et al.* 2003). This is reflected in their current life circumstances – and the belief that physical abuse ('punishment') is of 'value' to the child (Kenney and Laming 2006; Nicolau *et al.* 2003). Therefore the evidence concerning the characteristics of the abused child suggests that they exist within an

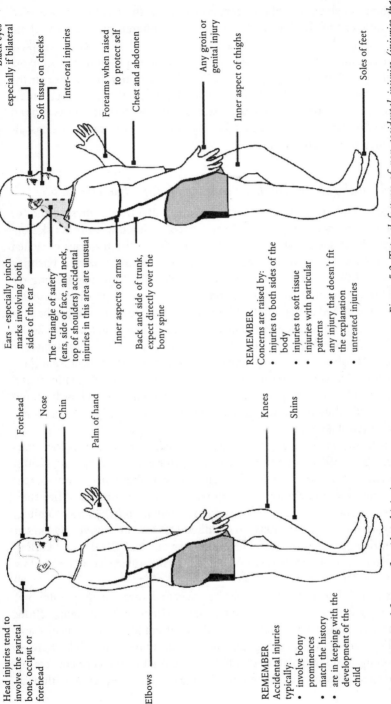

Black eyes especially if bilateral

Soft tissue on cheeks

Inter-oral injuries

Forearms when raised to protect self

Chest and abdomen

Any groin or genital injury

Inner aspect of thighs

Soles of feet

Ears - especially pinch marks involving both sides of the ear

The "triangle of safety" (ears, side of face, and neck, top of shoulders) accidental injuries in this area are unusual

Inner aspects of arms

Back and side of trunk, expect directly over the bony spine

REMEMBER
Concerns are raised by:
- injuries to both sides of the body
- injuries to soft tissue
- injuries with particular patterns
- any injury that doesn't fit the explanation
- untreated injuries

Figure 5.2 Typical features of non-accidental injuries (injuries that should raise concerns

Forehead

Nose

Chin

Palm of hand

Knees

Shins

Head injuries tend to involve the parietal bone, occiput or forehead

Elbows

REMEMBER
Accidental injuries typically:
- involve bony prominences
- match the history
- are in keeping with the development of the child

Figure 5.1 Typical features of accidental injuries

Figures reproduced with the permission from Harris, J. Sidebotham, P. Welbury, R. et al. (2006) Child Protection and the Dental Team: An Introduction to Safeguarding in Dental Practice. *Sheffield: COPEND.*

abusive and emotionally distressed parent–child dyad (Fonaghy 2001; Kenney and Laming 2006; Nicolau *et al.* 2003).

The physically abused child: the physical and emotional signs of abuse

Over 50 per cent of child physical abuse is around the face, outside and inside the oral cavity (Cairns *et al.* 2004, 2005; Maguire *et al.* 2007). Figures 5.1 and 5.2 show the differences between accidental and non-accidental injuries.

The importance of the torn frenum[3] as pathognomonic of child abuse has been questioned by Maquire and colleagues (Maguire *et al.* 2007). Reviewing the literature these authors have concluded that: 'a torn frenum in isolation cannot be described as pathognomonic of [child] physical abuse. Clearly the finding of an unexplained torn frenum in a young child warrants full investigation' (Maguire *et al.* 2007, p.1115).

Therefore the types of non-accidental orofacial injuries, associated with child physical abuse include (Cairns *et al.* 2005; Maguire *et al.* 2007; Naidoo 2000):

- bruising to the head, face and neck
- abrasions to the head, face and neck
- laceration to head and face
- eye injuries
- bites, slap marks
- facial fractures
- intra-oral injuries: torn frenum injuries to lips, gums, tongue, palate, intrusions, extractions of teeth.

While the physical signs of abuse can be readily identified, the emotional aspects of the abused child are harder to discern. While some abused children are overtly anxious others hide their distress. The PANDA or Prevent Abuse and Neglect through Dental Awareness programme developed in America provided a series of behaviours which were indicative of child abuse. For details about these behaviours see the PANDA programme website (Delta Dental 2008).

Examining the ability of physically abused children to recognize facial emotions Masten *et al.* (2008) noted that physically abused children tended to

---

3   A frenum is a small fold of tissue inside the mouth that ties the upper lip to the upper gum above the upper front teeth.

be hypervigilant, identifying menacing situations more quickly than non-physically abused children. Moreover since physically abused children were also 'quicker to infer a threatening intention in an ambiguous situation' (Masten *et al*. 2008) it was proposed that they would react with aggression and anxiety when presented with the prospect of dental treatment. Thus, on a visit to the dental surgery, unguarded comments from dental health professionals could be construed as intimidating, menacing and threatening by both parent and child.

The physically abused child: the role of the primary health care professional

Government (Laming 2003; Scottish Executive 2002; 2004b) and professional (Murphy and Welbury 1998; Wood 2006) recommendations and the recognition that dentists were in an ideal position to identify children experiencing abuse have been voiced by many (Cairns *et al*. 2004; Kenney and Laming 2006; Naidoo 2000). Consequently child protection has become part of undergraduate curricula (McCartan and McCreary 2006) and dental health care professionals have been encouraged to undertake postgraduate training in child protection. As part of this continuing education the 'British Society of Paediatric Dentistry and the Royal College of Paediatrics and Child Health' have provided a check-list for when a dentist suspects a case of child abuse (British Society of Paediatric Dentistry and Royal College of Physicians 2005).

The Department of Health has also provided the dental team with practical guidance, a child protection strategy and policy for the dental practice, all of which can be found on their website (www.cpdt.org.uk/indexhtm). Using a flowchart (Figure 5.3) the dental health professional is taken on a journey which starts by asking the question 'You have concerns about a child's welfare?'

Following a detailed examination and assessment of the child the dentist is invited to discuss her findings with experienced colleagues including child protection nurses, social services and the child's general medical practitioner. From this juncture the primary care clinician will be able to decide upon what action to take. From the examination of the child and parent and discussions with experienced colleagues, the dentist may decide that the initial concerns were unsubstantiated. Nevertheless detailed notes of the child and parent must be made with a dental follow-up appointment being mandatory. When the dentist's concerns have been substantiated then urgent action is necessary for the dentist to:

- Provide urgent *dental* care.

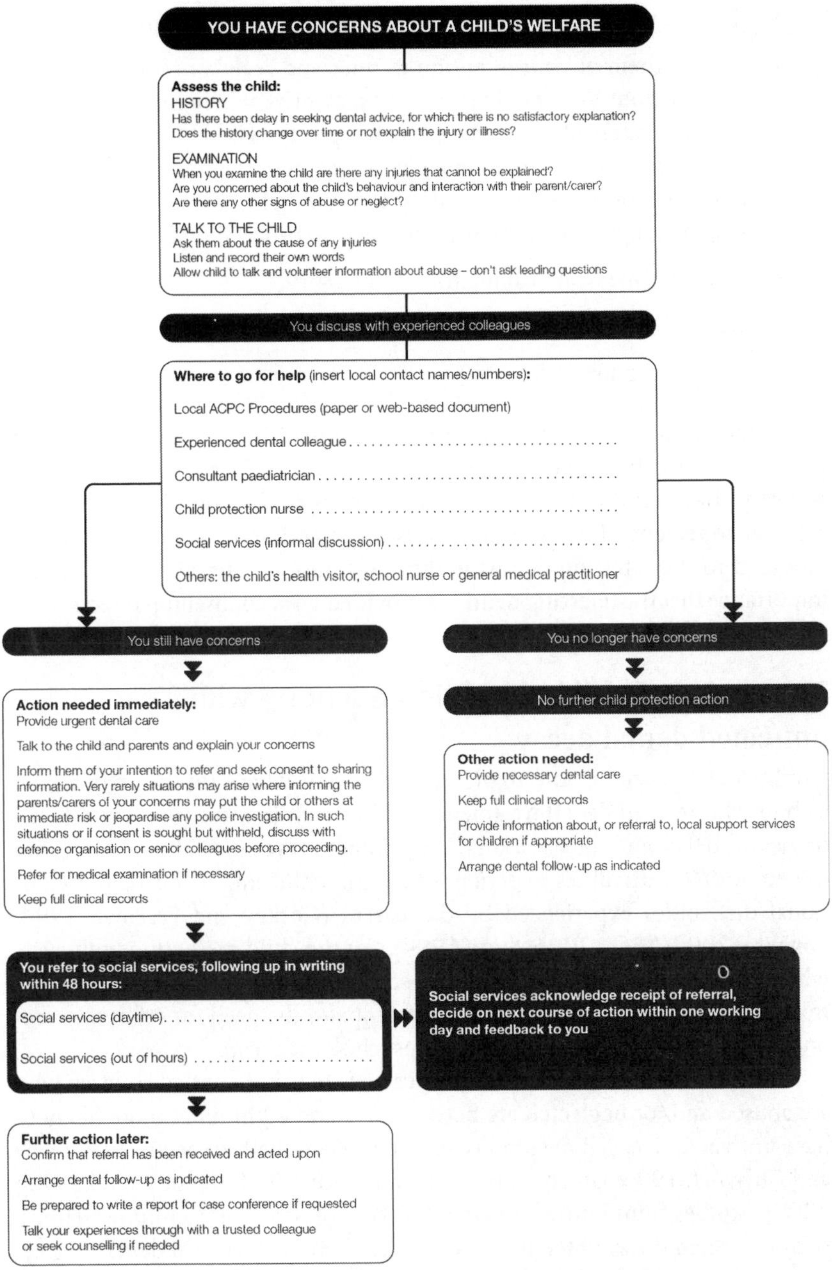

YOU HAVE CONCERNS ABOUT A CHILD'S WELFARE

Assess the child:
HISTORY
Has there been delay in seeking dental advice, for which there is no satisfactory explanation?
Does the history change over time or not explain the injury or illness?

EXAMINATION
When you examine the child are there any injuries that cannot be explained?
Are you concerned about the child's behaviour and interaction with their parent/carer?
Are there any other signs of abuse or neglect?

TALK TO THE CHILD
Ask them about the cause of any injuries
Listen and record their own words
Allow child to talk and volunteer information about abuse – don't ask leading questions

You discuss with experienced colleagues

Where to go for help (insert local contact names/numbers):

Local ACPC Procedures (paper or web-based document)

Experienced dental colleague . . . .

Consultant paediatrician . . . .

Child protection nurse . . . .

Social services (informal discussion) . . . .

Others: the child's health visitor, school nurse or general medical practitioner

You still have concerns

Action needed immediately:
Provide urgent dental care

Talk to the child and parents and explain your concerns

Inform them of your intention to refer and seek consent to sharing information. Very rarely situations may arise where informing the parents/carers of your concerns may put the child or others at immediate risk or jeopardise any police investigation. In such situations or if consent is sought but withheld, discuss with defence organisation or senior colleagues before proceeding.

Refer for medical examination if necessary

Keep full clinical records

You no longer have concerns

No further child protection action

Other action needed:
Provide necessary dental care

Keep full clinical records

Provide information about, or referral to, local support services for children if appropriate

Arrange dental follow-up as indicated

You refer to social services, following up in writing within 48 hours:

Social services (daytime) . . . .

Social services (out of hours) . . . .

Social services acknowledge receipt of referral, decide on next course of action within one working day and feedback to you

Further action later:
Confirm that referral has been received and acted upon

Arrange dental follow-up as indicated

Be prepared to write a report for case conference if requested

Talk your experiences through with a trusted colleague or seek counselling if needed

Figure 5.3 Child protection and the dental team: flowchart for action
http://www.cpdt.org.uk/f_info/dload/CPDT_Doc4.pdf

Figures reproduced with the permission from Harris, J. Sidebotham, P. Welbury, R. et al. (2006)
Child Protection and the Dental Team: An Introduction to Safeguarding in Dental Practice. *Sheffield: COPEND.*

- Talk to the child and parents and explain your concerns.

- Inform them of your intention to refer and seek consent to sharing information. Very rarely situations may arise where informing the parents/carers of your concerns may put the child or others at immediate risk or jeopardize any police investigation. In such situations or if consent is sought but withheld, discuss with defence organization or senior colleagues before proceeding.

- Refer for medical examination if necessary.

- Keep full clinical records.

(www.cpdt.org.uk/index.htm)

The referring dentist must confirm that the referral has been received and further action is being taken by social services. The Department of Health advice is for referral in writing within 48 hours of the original referral with acknowledgement of referral and decision regarding the next steps to be provided to the referring dentist within 24 hours of referral. It is of central importance that the referring dentist is provided with counselling if required.

The neglected child: the child presenting with untreated dental decay

Psychoanalytic formulations to provide a theoretical basis for the premise that a child who refused dental treatment could be a child presenting with developmental delay and/or emotional disturbances (Freeman 2007). Moreover the emotional difficulties experienced by the child might mirror the emotional difficulties experienced by the parent (Corkey and Freeman 1994; Fonaghy 2001; NICE 2006; Stern 1994). For the child presenting with overwhelming dental anxiety, there is the need to recognize their emotionally distressed state, together with that of the parent and the need for referral to secondary specialist paedodontic and/or psychological care.

Case controlled studies from America have highlighted that children who are abused and/or neglected are between five and eight times more likely to have untreated decayed deciduous and permanent teeth respectively (Greene and Chiswick 1995; Greene, Chiswick and Aaron 1994; Kenney and Laming 2006). Studies from Europe (Olivan 2003) suggested that a child presenting with untreated decayed teeth was a neglected child. The term dental neglect was coined and defined by the American Academy of Pediatric Dentistry as: 'the wilful failure of parent or guardian to seek and follow through with treatment necessary to ensure a level of oral health essential for adequate function and freedom from pain and infection' (Kellogg 2005a, p.1566).

Although Kellogg acknowledges that the role of parental oral health knowledge is central to this definition, the definition, nevertheless, suggests that the neglect of a child's dentition is a conscious decision ('wilful failure') made by a knowledgeable parent. However parents may neglect their children not through acts of commission (wilfulness) but as an act of omission having experienced neglect in their own childhood.

The parent who has been neglected, in her own childhood, will not wilfully neglect her child but might, without knowing, relive her own childhood experiences of neglect by neglecting her own children (Freud 1914; Shengold 2006). This potential perpetuation of neglect between the generations (Hendricks, Freeman and Sheiham 1990) may be a consequence of misunderstanding the influence of past experiences upon the parent–child interaction of the present. There is a need to examine the various types of parent–child interaction as this might provide a clue as to why dental neglect continues throughout the generations.

Ways of interacting: the parent–child dyad

Meta-analyses to examine the ways parents and children interact were conducted by Coren and Barlow (2001) and later Barlow and Parsons (2002). Both analyses suggested that parents and children interact in different ways. These patterns included warm and nurturing interactions; permissive interactions and authoritarian interactions which were associated with three types of parent–child dyad – (1) the competent parent–child dyad; (2) the aggressive parent–child dyad; and (3) the anxious parent–child dyad (Black and Logan 1995; Bloomfield et al. 2005; Hummel and Gross 2001).

1. The competent parent–child dyad is characterized as a parent who is consistent in her manner towards her child, who can contain her child's fears and who provides positive and emotional support. The competent parent nurtures and encourages independence and promotes social skills.

2. The parent of the aggressive parent–child dyad is inconsistent, unable to set clear boundaries and remains emotionally distant and uncontactable to her child (Black and Logan 1995; Bloomfield et al. 2005; Hummel and Gross 2001). Consequently much of a child's negative and controlling behaviours are thought to be a consequence of the parent's non-responsiveness to the child's demands (Fonaghy 2001; Stern 1994).

3. The parent of the anxious parent–child dyad is ambivalent towards her child and within a matter of seconds may shift from being

intrusive and authoritarian, to being punitive and distant (Barlow and Parsons 2002; Black and Logan 1995; Bloomfield et al. 2005; Coren and Barlow 2001).

Children caught up in the aggressive and/or anxious parent–child dyad become increasingly mistrustful as a consequence of the parent's ambivalence which results in an emotional disconnection between parent and child (Chorpita, Albano and Barlow 1996; Fonaghy 2001; Hummel and Gross 2001). In order to 'recapture and reanimate' the parent, children bombard their parents with demands for attention which instead of gaining their parents' attention and love result in parental retaliation and anger (Fonaghy 2001; Stern 1994). Thus the parent inadvertently reinforces their children's anxious and aggressive behaviours by being both overprotective and being aggressive at the same time (Chorpita et al. 1996; Hummel and Gross 2001).

Nursing caries, neglect and parenting

Tooth decay or dental caries is caused by an increased frequency of the consumption of non-milk extrinsic sugars (NMES). The sugar is converted to acid by *Streptococcus mutans* and it is the acid that burns a hole in the tooth which allows the bacteria to cause tooth decay. Examples of NMES include sucrose, fructose, glucose and lactose which are contained in confectionery, cakes, biscuits and soft drinks. Sucrose is the most cariogenic of all NMES and lactose the least cariogenic, however, even lactose (milk sugar) can cause tooth decay. For lactose to cause tooth decay special circumstances must be fulfilled which are (1) for the milk to be in close proximity to the teeth for a prolonged period of time and (2) for the saliva flow to be reduced. In children who have prolonged use of the feeding bottle into their toddlerhood all the conditions for lactose (in the milk) to cause tooth decay are fulfilled. The result is a particular form of tooth decay, known as early childhood caries or nursing caries. We conducted an investigation to understand why mothers and children persisted in the prolonged use of the feeding bottle. It became apparent that although the mothers were quite knowledgeable about the causes of their young children's tooth decay they still continued to give their children milk in feeding bottles. Was this the neglect of their children's dentition another expression of a conscious decision ('wilful failure') made by a knowledgeable parent?

The findings from our qualitative exploration are supported by Wilkins (2006) who found that concerns associated with parenting interfered in the parents' ability to use their health knowledge in the service of their children's health. The main concerns of the mothers whose child has nursing caries were about having time. The feeding bottle enabled them to buy quiet time away from their children while, at the same time, buying extra time with their 'baby-toddler': 'The bottle is really a comfort. At night, he just holds onto the bottle and I have him in my arms. I keep him there until he goes to sleep and I look at him and I think he's still my wee baby.'

Despite the mothers believing that closeness and prolonging their child's time in 'babyhood' would ultimately benefit their children they also found their child's slow progression to greater independence as onerous. These observations suggested that the mothers' behaviours reflected many of the characteristics of the ambivalent mother. Almost simultaneously the mother would cling onto her child, fearful of separation while in the next second wish for her child to have greater independence from her. The mothers' anxieties about the effect they had upon their children – physically and emotionally – gave way to feelings of self-reproach and questioning of their parenting role.

What relevance can this have for the neglected child? Children who experience parental ambivalence, tend to perceive new situations as threatening and punishing (Barrett et al. 1996). The child presenting with decayed and painful teeth and whose parents screen their own anxiety with hostility, may perceive dental treatment as punishing and threatening (Freeman 2007). Such fears of reprimand and discipline may result in the avoidance of routine dental treatment and the propensity for emergency, pain-only attendance. Hence the child with a neglected dentition with the tendency to present in pain may be indicative of a child and parent ensnared in an ambivalent and neglectful interaction.

The emotionally disturbed child: the child presenting with intense dental anxiety

The need to make a differentiation between dental anxiety and dental phobia was highlighted in earlier work (Freeman 2000). Burke and Freeman (2004) proposed that a differentiation existed between patients who were dentally anxious and those who were dentally phobic. Although both sets of patients presented with the affect of dental anxiety it was the intensity of the anxiety experienced and the underlying history which differentiated dentally anxious patients from dentally phobic patients. For those who are dentally anxious a history of a previous frightening dental experience is easily elicited. For those with dental phobia it was not necessarily true that they had had a frightening dental experience. In some instances these patients had made a 'false connection' (Freeman 1999) between experiences outside the dental surgery with those experienced inside the dental surgery. Therefore a false connection was made because something that they have seen, heard or experienced outside the dental surgery had something in common with what they have seen, heard or experienced inside the dental surgery. The combined intensity of the anxiety was so great that the dentally phobic patient was unable to accept treatment (Kavle et al. 1997).

What relevance can a child's intense dental anxiety have with regard to identifying the child and parent dyad in trouble and in need of help? It is postulated (Freeman 1999) that dental phobia is a not a disease entity in its own right but a symptom of an affective disorder in childhood and adolescence which results in lower psychosocial functioning. Intensive work with child patients supports this view (Freeman 2007). Moreover, the intensity of the dental fear does not lie with the reality of the treatment but with the imaginings or fantasies stirred up by it. Therefore, it is the real event of dental treatment which provides the nexus for fearful fantasies which are a combination of real and imagined events:

> The role of the actual experience of dental treatment will lend 'a feeling of reality' to the child's fantasies resulting in increased anxiety as a consequence of environmental experiences (such as discomfort during treatment) and internal and emotional dangers (such as bodily harm) to the self. The more painful and the more frightening and traumatic the dental experience is, the greater will be the weight of reality that reinforces the child's fantasies of harm, maltreatment and attack. (Freeman 2007, p.416)

The child presenting with intense dental anxiety may be a child who has emotional difficulties which may be due (1) to an affective disorder; (2) to problems within the parent–child dyad; and (3) to sexual abuse.

The child presenting with intense dental anxiety: a symptom of an affective disorder

In her seminal paper 'The role of bodily illness in the mental life of children' Anna Freud (1952) suggested that children react in different ways to surgical intervention. There are those children who seem to be able to toughen it out, those who become angry and those who become overwhelmed with anxiety. She suggested that childhood fears of school, of the doctor and the dentist may be part of a wider emotional disorder (Freud 1952). Using this theoretical framework it is suggested that the child who presents with dental phobia is a child whose imaginings of harm, maltreatment and punishment are so great as to represent an internal danger to the self. These children fear that they will be so harmed and so maltreated as to result in their disintegration. However, what becomes apparent when working with these children is that they do not only fear dental treatment, but experience food fads, separation anxiety, in short all their anxieties and behaviours are suggestive of a falling back or 'regression' to early and more infantile forms of functioning. A child who presents with intense fear of dental treatment, who has fears of separation from mother, who experiences food fads and does not provide a positive history of a fearful dental treatment experience, should be referred to their general medical practitioners for referral to psychological services.

Another group of children may present with intense dental fears. These patients are usually in their late adolescence. They present to the dentist with dental fears associated with the appearance of their teeth and the intensity of their fear (that others are looking at them), is so great that they become secondarily agoraphobic. Descriptively, these patients are dysmorphophobic (i.e. a delusion that some part of the body is ugly and/or deformed when in reality it is normal). The importance of dysmorphophobia presenting in late adolescence (or early adulthood) is that it may be prodromal of schizophrenia (Freeman and Kells 1996; Gipson and Connolly 1975). An adolescent presenting with this combination of symptoms is clearly in need of help and should be referred to their general medical practitioner for secondary referral to psychiatric services.

The child presenting with intense dental anxiety: difficulties in the parent–child dyad

The interaction of parent with child can result in a number of recognized behavioural patterns which are the competent, anxious and aggressive parent–child dyads. It was suggested that the parent's anxiety and ambivalence towards the child, could affect the child's ability to react appropriately to the potentially frightening or threatening situations such as dental treatment. It also seemed, however, that real events out-with the child's influence could also act to influence or exacerbate difficulties in their interactions with their parents. The NICE guidelines (2006) support this hypothesis. *Depression in Children and Young People* suggested that family factors such as parental depression/mental ill-health, the impact of divorce, separation and bereavement as well as feelings of hopelessness and family dysfunction could affect the child and that children whose parents were depressed or anxious were 2.6 times more likely to experience a major depressive disorder than children whose parents had no affective disorder. It seemed to indicate that the emotional state of the parent affected the emotional state of the child. Thus, it may be proposed that the child who attends for dental treatment whose parents experience depression, whose parents may have recently become divorced or separated or where there has been a family bereavement may react with increased anxiety due the accompanying parent being unable to react in a positive and supportive manner to their child's emotional needs.

Although the evidence remains ambiguous there are research findings (Carson 1998; Corkey and Freeman 1994; Freeman 2007) which support the view that the emotional difficulties experienced by the parent affect the child's ability to respond appropriately to the dental treatment intervention. Observations of children's reactions to dental treatment suggest that they are connected with the parent's ability to respond in a supportive and positive way to her child's fears. In essence the reassurance provided by the parent reduces the intensity of the anxiety experienced by the child and reduces the potency of the child's fantasies of harm, maltreatment and punishment. However, when the parent is too anxious or too ambivalent or has emotional difficulties she may be unable to provide her child with reassurance and emotional support. Faced with dental treatment, a child in this family situation is bombarded by internal fears (fears of abandonment by the parent) and the external fear of dental treatment (Freeman 2007). This child will present for dental treatment with an intensity of anxiety to suggest that she is in trouble and in need of help.

The view that the child's ability to cope with dental treatment is a consequence of difficulties in the parent–child dyad was supported by a study of 60 mother–child dyads which examined dental anxiety in six-year-old children (Corkey and Freeman 1994). Fifteen per cent of the children were dentally phobic, also had separation anxieties, poor bowel/bladder control, depressive moods and aggressive behaviours. Their behavioural problems were indicative of developmental delays. With their mothers scoring high for psychiatric morbidity this suggested that the mothers' psychiatric morbidity was mirrored in the child's dental anxieties and developmental delays (NICE 2006).

Therefore the dentally anxious child and parent may be in need of psychological help. Moreover this may be a population of mothers and children who may be unknown to service providers.

The child presenting with intense dental anxiety: the sexually abused child

Willumsen (2001, 2004), among others, has shown that adult dental phobia may be a symptom of child sexual abuse. In her studies of sexually abused women, Willumsen showed that 75 per cent of the women had experienced forced oral penetration as part of their abuse. Her results suggest that this abuse was relived and re-experienced as if happening in the here and now when the women attended for dental treatment, since they mistrusted the information provided by the dental team and were intensely anxious of the local anaesthetic injection and drill.

Kenney and Laming (2006) writing on domestic violence highlighted the relationship between dental anxiety and the sexually abused child. He stated that sexual abuse was 'a progressive action over a long period of time' with the abuser being someone well known to the child. As with other investigators he noted that the oral cavity was a frequent site for child sexual abuse (American Academy of Pediatrics and American Academy of Pediatric Dentistry 1999; Kellogg 2005b; Kenney and Laming 2006) and the requirement for the dental health professional to be aware of the physical signs of forced fellatio (petechial palate: particularly at the junction between the hard and soft palate) and the oral manifestations of sexually transmitted diseases. Kenney and Laming (2006) also commented upon the behaviour of the sexually abused child in the dental surgery. He emphasized that where there was a sudden change in the child's acceptance of a dental examination accompanied by intense dental anxiety, refusal to be reclined in the dental chair, refusal to be alone with the accompanying adult and 'subtle signs such as difficulty in sitting or walking' (Kenney and Laming 2006, p.124), then the dental health professional may be seeing a child who has suffered sexual abuse. It may be suggested, therefore that when a child presents with this change in her behaviour with or without oral signs of sexual abuse then the dental practitioner should be alerted to the possibility of child abuse.

Conclusions

This chapter has provided information regarding the role of the dental health professional with respect to child protection. It has proposed that when an abused/neglected child is identified, the referring practitioner has to consider not only the child, but also the abusing and neglectful parent. It has been suggested that the abused child lives in an abusive and neglectful home environment in which parent(s) unable to cope relive their own difficult life experiences. Thus both child and parent are in trouble and in need of help.

The idea that the knowledgeable parent who brings her child with untreated decayed teeth will have made a conscious decision to neglect their child's dentition must be treated with caution. It has been hypothesized that the parent whose child presents with untreated decay represents a parent and child experiencing difficulties and problems arising from their interaction. Communication difficulties exist and for those caught up in the anxious and/or aggressive parental–child dyads the result may be observed as regressive and disruptive parent–child behaviours. Consequently, these parents and children delay in seeking dental care and the child thus presents with dental neglect. A cogent example is the mother whose child has nursing caries due to prolonged feeding bottle use.

Similarly the child who presents with intense dental anxiety may be a child who is experiencing both internal (emotional) and external (emotionally disturbed parents, divorce parents etc.) difficulties. The ability of the child to withstand the onslaught of threats from her internal world (her fears of harm, maltreatment and punishment) will be influenced by her personality development and parental support to reduce the potency of these childhood fears. The child whose parents are emotionally disturbed and/or who have experienced bereavement, may be unable to recognize their child's emotional needs. Consequently they react inappropriately increasing rather than decreasing their child's fears and anxiety. The child presenting with intense dental anxiety may represent a parent–child dyad in need of help.

For the sexually abused child the actual experience of abuse will lend a reality to the child's fantasies of hurt and maltreatment. The degree of trauma experienced by the sexual abuse will reinforce the child's fears of attack and disintegration. Thus when sexual abuse is suspected or diagnosed a multi-disciplinary child abuse evaluation should be carried out (American Academy of Pediatrics and American Academy of Pediatric Dentistry 1999; Kellogg 2005a).

Dental health professionals are in a unique position and may treat children presenting with orofacial injuries, disturbed behaviours or with an intensity of anxiety which together may be suggestive of child abuse. The child and parent may be unknown to social services and the dentist may be the first one to see a child and parent in difficulty and in need of help. Therefore it is necessary for dental health professionals and those who come in contact with children including, specialist paediatric dentists, doctors and community nurses to appreciate that the abused, neglected and anxious child together with her parent represents a child and parent in need of help. It is of central importance that both child and parent are provided with care and assistance in order that current and future generations of children will be safeguarded from harm.

Chapter Six

Violence in the Community

Anne Lazenbatt

Introduction

Violence is a major public health issue internationally, and domestic violence or abuse in particular, represents a serious public health issue for women and their children all over the world (Tjaden and Tjaden 2000; WHO 2000, 2002). In the United Kingdom (UK) one in four women experience domestic abuse, at some point in their lives (Bacchus, Mezey and Bewley 2002; BMA 1998) and this violence accounts for almost a quarter of all crime (Department for Education and Skills 2006; Home Office 2003). The term *domestic abuse* is used to describe violence perpetrated by an adult against another with whom they have or have had a sexual relationship. This abuse can take many forms including physical (hitting, kicking, restraining), sexual (including assault, coercion, female genital mutilation), psychological (verbal bullying, undermining, social isolation) and financial (withholding money, unrealistic expectations with the household budget). The Department of Health's definition is, 'Any incident of threatening behaviour, violence or abuse (psychological, physical, sexual, financial or emotional) between adults who are or have been intimate partners or family members, regardless of gender or sexuality' (Home Office Circular 2000, p.14). Its prevalence in society is shocking and unacceptable, and disturbingly, in many instances the violence is hidden (Gazmararian *et al.* 1996; Jewkes, Levin and Loveday 2002). Women remain silent and excluded however, what is clear from the literature is that it is likely to escalate in frequency and intensity over time and may increase at specific critical points, especially during pregnancy and the postpartum period.

Midwives, health visitors, obstetricians, general practitioners (GPs) and other staff who work as members of the primary health care or hospital maternity team have a safeguarding role to play in the identification of babies and children who have been abused, those who are at risk of abuse and in subsequent intervention and protection services. In the UK we expect that every pregnant woman will have access to, and engage with, high quality maternity services. It is also increasingly acknowledged that for the majority of women, pregnancy and childbirth are normal life events and that care of these women and their babies may be exclusively midwifery-led. Community midwives in particular take a key role in caring for mother and child from diagnosis of pregnancy to the immediate period after birth, and many visit families at home and in doing so gain a unique level of access to the mother and her family. These midwife-led services are provided primarily outside hospitals in community-based primary health care settings.

The Royal Colleges and Professional Bodies including the Royal College of Midwives (RCM) were part of an advisory group to take forward the *National Service Framework for Children, Young People and Maternity Services* (DfES 2004b) with a commitment to provide a supportive and enabling environment within antenatal care for women and their children experiencing violence. Child protection is also fundamental to the role of the midwife, as they have a duty of care to the child as well as to the mother. Recent UK guidance (HM Government 2006) acknowledges this and the importance of midwives in contributing to the identification of care of vulnerable women, especially those suffering from domestic abuse, in itself an important risk factor for child maltreatment. Community midwives are seen as the primary health professional working with and supporting and safeguarding women and their families throughout pregnancy. However, the provision of care to families where issues of possible or actual child maltreatment have been raised is now seen as one of the most difficult and challenging areas of contemporary midwifery practice (Protheroe, Green and Spiby 2001; Smith 2003).

Domestic violence as a child protection issue

Violence during pregnancy should be seen as a complex problem because of its dual risks to both a mother and her unborn child (Coker, Sanderson and Dong 2004; McFarlane, Parker and Soeken 1996a; McFarlane 1996b). However, assessing domestic abuse as a child protection issue has been relatively slow in gaining health professional acceptance, even though the international evidence suggests that there is a clear and irrefutable link between domestic violence (DV) and the co-occurrence of child abuse (Edelson 2001; Hall and Elliman 2003; Jones, Gross and Becker 2002; Lundy and Grossman 2005; McGuigan and Pratt 2001; Ramsay *et al.* 2002). If a woman is being abused by a current or former partner and she has other children living with her, the likelihood is that they are being abused too. Although pregnant women may experience domestic abuse in the same ways as women who are not pregnant, it has only been recently that attention has been paid to the intricacies of the relationship between pregnancy and child protection (Jasinski 2004). Evidence suggests that domestic abuse during pregnancy and the first six months of child rearing, is significantly related to all three types of child maltreatment: child physical abuse, neglect and emotional abuse, up to the child's fifth year, with children under one year being at the highest risk of injury, or death (Butchart and Villaveces 2003; Goodall and Lumley 2007; Kotch 1999; McGuigan and Pratt 2001). In addition, where it is believed that a child is being abused; those involved with the child and the family should be alerted to the possibility of domestic abuse. An association of between 45–70 per cent has been found between a father's violence to the mother and his violence to the children (Goodall and Lumley 2007). The evidence shows that domestic violence is a child protection issue:

- Almost a third of domestic violence starts during pregnancy and existing violence often escalates during it (Freel and Robinson 2005; Women Equality Unit 2004).

- There is a co-occurrence of domestic violence and child abuse in 40 per cent of cases (Appel and Holden 1998; Walby and Allen 2004).

- Domestic abuse during pregnancy and the first six months of child rearing, is significantly related to all three types of child maltreatment: child physical abuse, neglect and emotional abuse up to the child's fifth year (Butchart and Villaveces 2003; Goodall and Lumley 2007).

- Children under one year are at the highest risk of injury, or death (Bradley *et al.* 2002; Goodall and Lumley 2007; McVeigh *et al.* 2005).

- Domestic abuse can have direct and indirect impacts upon children (including the foetus) and is likely to have a damaging effect on the health and development of children (Goodall and Lumley 2007).

- The situation where a woman and her children are both abused by the same male perpetrator is common (Lucas *et al.* 2002). The more severely a woman is harmed, the more severely her child is likely to be harmed (Goodall and Lumley 2007; Hartley 2002).

- Domestic violence is a contributory factor in half of all serious case reviews (Hartley 2004; Hester, Pearson and Harwin 1998; Mullender 2004).

- Domestic violence is a factor in 75 per cent of cases on the child protection register (Fleck-Henderson 2002; Hester et al. 1998; Mullender 2005).

- In 90 per cent of incidents, children are in the same, or next room (Kolbo, Blakely and Engleman 1996; McGee 2000; Mullender et al. 2003c).

- It has been suggested that foetal morbidity from violence is more prevalent than that from gestational diabetes or pre-eclampsia (Casanueva and Martin 2007).

- Foetal abuse can have effects on the developing infant's brain leading to anxiety and hyperactivity (Osofsky 2003).

- Women who have suffered domestic abuse are: 15 times more likely to abuse alcohol; 9 times more likely to abuse drugs; 3 times more likely to be diagnosed as depressed or psychotic; and 5 times more likely to attempt suicide (Stark and Flitcraft 1995).

Co-occurrence of domestic and child abuse

Children in violent homes face three risks: the risk of observing traumatic events, the risk of being abused themselves and the risk of being neglected (Mullender et al. 2003a). According to published studies, there is a 30 per cent to 60 per cent overlap between violence against children and violence against women in the same families (Edelson 2001). Although the studies on which these ranges are based employ different methodologies (e.g., definitions of child and domestic abuse, case record reviews, case studies and national surveys), use different sample sizes and examine different populations, they consistently report a significant level of co-occurrence (Lundy and Grossman 2005; Ramsay et al. 2002). These results point to the importance of protecting the abused parent to ensure the safety of the child. Co-occurrence of domestic and child abuse occurs in 40 per cent of cases (Walby and Allen 2004) and many child deaths occur in situations where domestic violence is also occurring. Indeed, children under one year are at the highest risk of injury, or death (Goodall and Lumley 2007; McVeigh et al. 2005).

Although system responses are primarily targeted towards adult victims of abuse, recently, increasing attention has been focused on children who witness DV, as studies estimate that between 10 and 20 per cent of children are at risk for exposure to domestic abuse (Carlson 2000; Carter and Schechter 1997; Cawson 2003; Creighton 2004). A growing body of research suggests that children who live in a household where mothers are being abused by a partner are significantly affected and experience considerable emotional and psychological distress (Hester, Pearson and Harwin 2000; McGee 2003; Mullender *et al.* 2003b). Living with or witnessing domestic abuse is identified as a source of 'significant harm' for children by the Adoption and Children Act (2002). In the USA child abuse and maltreatment have been reported to be a risk marker of DV with each year seeing an estimated 3.3 million children exposed to family violence and abuse (Filipas and Ullman 2006). There is also evidence to suggest that in 75–90 per cent of cases, children are in the same or next room when their mother is being abused (BMA 1998).

Understanding the impact of domestic abuse in pregnancy

Pregnancy is identified as a 'high-risk' period for domestic abuse, prompting the initial episode, or an escalation of a pre-existing abusive relationship (Scobie and McGuire 1999; Shadigian and Bauer 2004; Sidebotham 2001; Silverman *et al.* 2006; Stewart and Cecutti 1993). Almost a third of all domestic violence (37%) starts in pregnancy (Bacchus, Mezey and Bewley 2005; Women Equality Unit 2004); and the findings of a review by Jasinski (2004) highlight the factors associated with pregnancy-related abuse such as: poverty, low socio-economic status; low levels of social support; first-time parenting; unexpected or unwanted pregnancy; ethnicity; drug and alcohol abuse. Prevalence rates for domestic violence during pregnancy range from 1 per cent to 20 per cent depending on the definition of violence in the study, although most studies report prevalence rates between 3 per cent and 14 per cent (Gazmararian *et al.* 1996; Jasinski 2004). The Confidential Enquiry into Maternal and Child Health (CEMACH 2008) estimates that 30 per cent of domestic abuse commences during pregnancy.

Although a causal relationship between exposure to violence during pregnancy and adverse perinatal outcomes has not been clearly demonstrated, pregnant women who experience abuse are more likely than are non-abused women to have conditions that place their unborn child at serious risk (Jasinski 2004). Studies have shown that women attending accident and emergency departments with physical injuries owing to domestic violence are more likely to be pregnant than women attending with accidental injuries (McWilliams and McKiernan 1993). Physical violence and trauma during pregnancy increases the risk of foetal abuse and the risk of adverse pregnancy outcomes such as antepartum haemorrhage, urinary tract infections, premature birth, low birth weight, placental damage, a prime cause of miscarriage or stillbirth, chorioamnionitis, foetal injury and foetal death (Bacchus *et al.* 2002; Craig 2003; Mezey *et al.* 2005; Mezey *et al.* 2003; Mezey and Bewley 1997).

Domestic abuse also produces a range of psychosocial effects upon the mother such as alcohol and drug dependence, unemployment, homelessness, suicide attempts, depression, anxiety and post-traumatic stress disorder and heightened maternal and foetal stress (Amaro et al. 1990; Lemon, Verhoek-Oftedahl and Donnelly 2002; Richardson et al. 2002). In addition, pregnant women experiencing violence are at a higher risk of becoming victims of homicide than are pregnant women not experiencing violence (Campbell, García-Moreno and Sharps 2003; Lewis and Drife 2001; McFarlane et al. 2002) and domestic abuse has been cited as a prime cause of maternal deaths during childbirth (Lewis and Drife 2001). Evidence shows that within the six weeks following birth, 11 new mothers were known to have been murdered by their male partners during 2000–2002, and 14 per cent of all the women who died during or immediately after pregnancy (43 women) had reported domestic violence to a health professional during the pregnancy (Lewis and Drife 2005). Furthermore 12 per cent of the 378 women whose deaths were reported to the Confidential Enquiry on Maternal Deaths had voluntarily reported domestic violence to a healthcare professional during their pregnancy (Lewis and Drife 2001). None had routinely been asked about domestic violence so this is almost certainly an under-estimate.

Impact of foetal abuse

Domestic abuse is clearly a child safety issue, and the unborn child is at significant risk from harm. Violence against pregnant women has been referred to as 'child abuse in the womb' (Hunt and Martin 2001). There has been concern for some time, particularly in the USA about the issue of 'foetal abuse', where a foetus may be damaged in-utero by acts of omission or commission (Mezey et al. 2005; Mezey and Bewley 1997; Mirrlees-Black 1999). Men can physically harm a foetus by physically assaulting a mother and evidence suggests that controlling men may be particularly violent to women when they are pregnant (Hobbs et al. 1999). Also abdominal trauma resulting in placental damage, uterine contractions, or premature rupture of membranes can directly lead to low infant birth weight (Campbell and Lewandowski 1997).

Women who experience abuse are more likely than non-abused women to have conditions that place their foetuses at risk (McFarlane et al. 1996a,b; Murphy et al. 2001; Tuten et al. 2004). Domestic abuse in particular causes heightened maternal stress (Lemon et al. 2002; Richardson et al. 2002), which is of critical importance during pregnancy because the consequences extend to her foetus and, later, her newborn. Chronic maternal stress increases cortisol levels (Sandman et al. 2007), and during pregnancy, elevated cortisol levels lead to decreased uterine perfusion and a decreased transfer of essential nutrients for foetal growth, a contributory factor to intrauterine growth retardation. Cortisol also increases uterine irritability, contributing to the increased number of preterm births (Hoffman and Hatch 2000; Orr, James and Blackmore Prince et al. 2002).

However, a causal link between domestic abuse during pregnancy and adverse perinatal outcomes has not been clearly demonstrated. These risks can be considerable as violence may increase rates of miscarriage, antepartum haemorrhage, premature birth, low birth weight, chorioamnionitis, placental damage, sexually transmitted infections, effects on the developing infant's brain, foetal injury and even foetal death (Bacchus et al. 2002; Connolly, Katz and Bash 1997; Hosking and Walsh 2005; Mezey and Bewley 1997; Shumway, O'Campo and Gielen 1999).

The Domestic Violence, Crime and Victims Act (2004) was introduced to increase the protection, support and rights of victims and witnesses. It was the biggest overhaul of domestic violence legislation for 30 years. The Act aims to ensure better protection for victims and bring more perpetrators to justice through civil and criminal law. Legally, according to this Act if a miscarriage is caused by abuse, the assailant can be charged under S.58 of the Offences against the Person Act, 'using an instrument with intent to cause a miscarriage' and if a baby is born prematurely as a result of an assault and then dies, the assailant may be charged with manslaughter (Crime and Victims Act 2004). One of the most consistent empirical findings, however, is the delay of antenatal care among victims of violence (Dietz et al. 1997; Goodwin et al. 2000), which often results in inadequate care during pregnancy. Research indicates that many abused women only begin antenatal care in the third trimester (McFarlane et al. 1992) and this may be a serious risk factor for the foetus with the risk of pregnancy complications such as low birth weight and premature birth (Norton et al. 1995).

The role of primary health care professionals

Primary health care professionals for some time have been acknowledged as having a key role in child protection and family violence (Birchall and Hallett 1995; Cawson 2003; Lupton, North and Khan 2001). They may be the first to detect that a child is at risk, and the consequences of their failing in this recognition can be dire. However, until recently the NHS has largely ignored the problem of identifying women who access health services for injuries caused by domestic abuse, while historically primary health care professionals have experienced difficulties when attempting to identify an abused child (Goodall and Lumley 2007; Lazenbatt and Freeman 2006; Leventhal 1999). There are now many clear messages from government, professional organizations and research to indicate that health professionals, such as midwives, should be actively involved in tackling these significant public health and primary health care issues (BMA 1998; Community Practitioners' and Health Visitors' Association 1998; 2004b; Department for Education and Skills 2006; Department of Health 2004a, b; Home Office 2006; Home Office and Cabinet Office 1999; RCM 1997; RCN 2000).

However, in a review of fatal child abuse cases by the Department of Health (Sinclair and Bullock 2002), it was found that health professionals were more likely than any other group to have knowledge of the child and over a quarter of children who died at the hands of their parents were unknown to social services. Also a NSPCC publication, *What Really Happened?* (Dale, Green and Fellows 2002) highlights how many infant deaths and serious injuries could be prevented if all professionals within primary health care were better informed and equipped to identify family abuse. Although research in this area is increasing, it is often difficult to determine the exact nature of the pregnancy-related violence, and this is posing difficulties for both practitioners and researchers, who need a clear understanding of the relationship between domestic and child abuse and pregnancy in order to develop risk assessment and screening tools and effective prevention and intervention programmes. Worryingly, although abuse may begin or accelerate during pregnancy, few women report the problem to their primary health care providers (Gazmararian *et al.* 1996; Gielen *et al.* 1994; Lazenbatt, Taylor and Cree 2008).

Midwives' response to domestic and child abuse in pregnancy

Community midwives have always had a role in primary health care; however, there is now an explicit need for the profession to direct its attention to issues such as domestic abuse. Even though evidence suggests that 35 per cent of women already suffering domestic abuse experience an increase during pregnancy and the postpartum, they are rarely identified by midwives (Bacchus *et al.* 2002, 2005; Espinosa and Osborne 2002; King and Ryan 1996; Lazenbatt, Cree and McMurray 2005; Lazenbatt *et al.* 2008; Nasir and Hyder 2003; Thompson *et al.* 2000).

Historically, midwives have experienced certain difficulties when attempting to identify, either, or both, domestic and child abuse (Bewley 1997; Bewley, Friend and Mezey 1997; Lazenbatt *et al.* 2008; Leventhal 1999). This finding may represent a reluctance by midwives to discuss the topic of domestic violence with their clients, arising in many cases, from fears and anxieties about causing offence; revealing something which may escalate out of control; of not knowing what to do if abuse is disclosed; of embarrassment; or at a personal level identification with abuse either as a victim or perpetrator (Bacchus *et al.* 2002; Department of Health 2000).

However, this reluctance may also correspond in general to: midwives' attitudes towards victims of abuse (Lazenbatt *et al.* 2005); their general lack of knowledge, education and training and available information about questioning and screening protocols (Lazenbatt *et al.* 2008; Taket *et al.* 2003); and a lack of understanding of their perceived professional role in addressing both forms of abuse (Lazenbatt *et al.* 2008; Parsons *et al.* 1995; Peckover 2003). Importantly, at a more basic level the opportunity to 'ask the question' may not always be available, i.e. a partner or other family member may be present (Price, Baird and Salmon 2005; Ramsay *et al.* 2002; Shadigian and Bauer 2004; Taket *et al.* 2003).

To assess and intervene appropriately to situations where domestic or child abuse are known or suspected, midwives, managers and supervisors must have a willingness to identify and report the abuse. They need to have had opportunities to undertake up-to-date education and training and skills necessary to ask questions, and to offer the appropriate multi-professional help and inter-agency support required (Paluzzi and Houde-Quimbly 1996) as well as an understanding of domestic violence risk assessment and safety planning in child protection (Radford, Blacklock and Iwi 2006). In addition, regular continual professional development updates should be available for all. The Department of Health publication *Domestic Violence: A Resource Manual for Health Care Professionals* (Department of Health 2000, 2006) supports the need for education and training of health professionals, as the majority of women will use the health care system at some stage in their lives.

The most important factor in identifying domestic and child abuse is the awareness that it often commences or escalates during pregnancy. There are a number of physiological, psychological/emotional and behavioural indicators which can alert a midwife to the possibility of potential or actual abuse. Where abuse is suspected, the midwife has a duty of care to routinely ask the woman about problems with relationships, but only when it is safe to do so, i.e. not when a partner or other person is present. The midwife must not put the woman or her/himself at any further risk.

The questioning must be undertaken very sensitively and very carefully. The midwife's role and responsibility is then to provide the appropriate response, believing the woman, showing her that someone cares, not judging her, respecting her reasons and decisions to stay or leave the relationship, offering her support, providing her with helpful information, referring her to appropriate agencies, or any other action that may be required (Taket *et al.*

2003). All midwives should be aware of the services and resources (statutory, community and voluntary) available both locally and nationally to a woman and children suffering domestic abuse. Maternity services should be active in developing a multi-agency, inter-disciplinary approach in local procedures and services, to ensure a seamless and effective response to a woman seeking help (Protheroe *et al.* 2001).

It must also be remembered that victims of domestic abuse may also be reluctant to disclose abuse for a variety of reasons which include: reprisals from their partner; an outsider becoming involved; embarrassment; and importantly fear of losing their children if social services become involved. Research, however, has shown that often these women hope that someone will realize that something is wrong and ask them about it (Bacchus *et al.* 2002; Department of Health 2000; Mezey *et al.* 2003; Taket *et al.* 2003). Many women may not spontaneously disclose the issues of child or domestic abuse in their lives, but often respond honestly to a sensitively asked question (Bacchus *et al.* 2002). For midwives routinely to ask women about domestic abuse and to offer support and information is therefore an extremely important issue in both community and primary health care settings.

However, although midwives approve in theory of routine questioning about domestic violence and also broadly agree that it is their responsibility; in practice, only about two-thirds are happy to do it (Price 2004). It appears that routine enquiry about domestic violence during antenatal booking is infrequent despite such enquiry being included in clinical practice recommendations and is made less frequently than any other aspect of social history taking (Buck 2007). Practical and personal difficulties, including lack of time, staff shortages and difficulty in obtaining sufficient privacy are frequently cited.

Midwifery settings – differences in community and hospital-based midwifery

Findings from research show that significantly fewer midwives in hospital settings are addressing the issue of domestic abuse with their clients, as they appear to be driven by more medically dominant organizational structures and targets, which result in their using a more standardized form of care that stresses measures of efficiency, effectiveness and risk management (Lazenbatt *et al.* 2008). According to this study, hospital midwives work in a setting that has an ideology which places less emphasis on the psychosocial needs of the individual woman and her child and more on providing care for women experiencing complications, and thus public health issues are seen as low priorities. These findings are consistent with work by Hunter (2004), whose results suggest that the occupational ideology of the hospital midwife is 'with the institution' rather than with a more 'woman-centred' approach (Hunter 2004). On the other hand, more midwives from community-based settings appear to follow more women-centred and child-focused care.

First, community midwives are able to create a healthy living environment for women experiencing domestic violence, by asking about 'abuse' with their clients (Poland, Green and Rootman 2000). Second, they integrate health promotion and health empowerment into the primary health care setting by working in partnership with the woman in their own homes, frequently talking to them about issues such as domestic and child abuse, and are more aware of providing private facilities in which woman can discuss violent relationships. Third, they develop links with other settings and with the wider community (Whitelaw, Baxendale and Bryce 2001). Community midwives are more empowered to use a joined-up approach that includes an understanding of evidence-based research in the area, a clear knowledge of local and national multi-professional support agencies and inter-agency networks and refuges that allows them to give ongoing and appropriate information that in itself can empower women to make their own informed choices about how to deal with abuse (Lazenbatt *et al.* 2008). The Code of Professional Conduct exhorts midwives to work collaboratively, to enable them to strengthen areas of practice by liaising with other professionals and learning from them (Nursing and Midwifery Council 2004).

However, the biggest hindrance recorded for both hospital and community midwives is the reluctance of a partner to leave the consultation. Recent changes in midwifery practice designed to 'empower women' and demedicalize childbirth may in reality be reducing the possibility of effective intervention, i.e. the traditional concept of women-only space is rapidly disappearing as more and more men are now accompanying their partners to their antenatal and postnatal visits. Women now hold their own notes, eliminating confidential documentation of suspicions of/or identified cases of domestic violence. This can lead women themselves to feel emotionally unable to, or physically prevented from, accessing support, either from their family and friends, or from statutory and voluntary agencies. International research evidence illustrates that maternity services are no longer woman-only spaces because women are now accompanied by their partners when attending antenatal clinics and partners are often present in primary health care appointments (Hester and Radford 1996; Hunt and Martin 2001; Protheroe *et al.* 2001; Taket *et al.* 2003).

Multi-agency pre-birth child protection procedures

Research and experience indicate that very young babies are extremely vulnerable to abuse and that work carried out in the antenatal period to assess risk and plan intervention will help to minimise harm. Any concerns about the welfare of an unborn baby, or about the future care of the baby when born should be shared with the appropriate agency at the earliest opportunity, as plans for safeguarding may need to be put in place before the baby is born. Antenatal risk assessment is a valuable opportunity to develop a proactive multi-agency approach to families where there is an identified risk of harm (Table 6.1). The aim is to provide support for families, to identify and protect vulnerable children and to plan effective care programmes; recognizing the long-term benefits of early intervention for the welfare of the child. The UK Local Safeguarding Children Board (LSCB) have produced a set of procedures that explain the action any person should take when they think a child needs protecting because they may have been abused, or are at risk of abuse or significant harm (Radford *et al.* 2006). They also take into account any risk to the unborn child. They clarify the responsibility of the various agencies involved, for reporting and investigating allegations of abuse. However, the process of assessment is consistently criticized in inquiries particularly in relation to professionals' understanding of risk factors (Brandon *et al.* 1999). In assessing risk there is sometimes a tendency to overlook the mother's male partner.

Table 6.1 Antenatal risk factors to be considered when undertaking a pre-birth assessment of risk

Unborn baby	
Premature birth	Poor antenatal care
Unwanted/concealed pregnancy	No plans
Lack of awareness of baby needs	Special needs
Unattached to unborn baby	Inability to prioritize baby needs
Unreal expectations	
Stressful gender issue	

Parental capacity

Negative childhood experiences	Postnatal depression
Abuse in childhood	Previous care proceedings
Drug/alcohol abuse	Very young parent
Violence/abuse of others	Mental disorder/illness
Abuse neglect of previous child/ren	Learning disability
Physical disability/illness	Past antenatal/postnatal neglect

Family/household/environmental

Family violence	Relationship instability
Unsupportive family network	Multiple relationships
Frequent house moves	Lack of community support
No commitment to parenting	Poor engagement with professional services

Conclusion

Domestic abuse is a damaging social problem affecting the health of many women and children within the maternity setting. It cannot be solved by midwifery alone; however, the midwife's role in identification and referral plays a critical part in primary health care co-ordinated response. In order for such a response to be effective, midwives need greater exposure to and familiarity with recommended good practice; and must be able to identify and support women and children who are experiencing abuse with a joined-up approach that has adequate resources and support of health service managers. Close inter-agency liaison is required with midwives who are accountable and not afraid to challenge historical working practices, and who are willing to work across traditional boundaries.

Concerns over inadequate record keeping, poor information sharing and communication have been raised by the Commission for Health Improvement (CHI 2004) between NHS organizations and other agencies with respect to violence and abuse (Truman 2004).

Developing a system that allows the sharing of information and statistics on abuse would immensely benefit midwives and the families with which they work, as it could provide interpretation of the multiple contributing factors associated with domestic and child abuse. This information would provide baselines to establish education, prevention and treatment programmes

(Creighton 2004), to formulate benchmarks for performance evaluation, as well as allow professionals to collaborate and provide assistance and protection to victimized children in a more efficient and effective way. As Lord Laming states in his report:

> Improvements to the way information is exchanged within and between agencies are imperative if children are to be adequately safeguarded... Effective action designed to safeguard the wellbeing of children and families depends upon the sharing of information on a multi-professional, inter-agency basis. (Department of Health 2003b)

Finally the co-occurrence of risk factors for violence in pregnancy, where the health and safety of two potential victims are placed in jeopardy (Mezey *et al.* 2003, 2005; Mezey and Bewley 1997) stresses the importance for midwives to be able to recognize and report domestic and/or child abuse at this time. Identifying domestic abuse, however, may be a useful risk factor for recognizing child abuse, which is clearly within the appropriate domain of midwives (see Table 6.1). Although tensions between the 'best interests of the mother' and the 'best interests of the child' are not always easily responded to, Fleck-Henderson (2002) suggests that best practices for families, where both children and women are at risk of violence, requires professionals to 'see double'; drawing from the knowledge and values of both perspectives to best meet the needs of these families. 'Seeing double' should therefore apply to all midwives in every child abuse case involving domestic violence.

Part 2

Practical Interventions Suitable for Primary Health Care

Chapter Seven

Safeguarding and Promoting the Wellbeing of Children with Autistic Spectrum Disorder

Michelle B. O'Neill, M. Suzanne Zeedyk
and Martyn C. Jones

Introduction

As the prevalence of autistic spectrum disorder (ASD) is now estimated to be as high as around 1 in 100 children, there is growing demand for care and provision on education, social work, health and voluntary services. For high quality care to be provided, clear information is needed about the ways in which ASD affects children and about effective approaches for safeguarding and promoting their wellbeing. A particular area of importance is the deleterious effect that ASD has on social interactions. Engaging with other people is often ambiguous, challenging and distressing for children with ASD. The aim of this chapter is to provide workers in primary health care with information which (i) increases their understanding of how ASD affects children in communicative, psychological and sensory terms; and (ii) heightens awareness of effective approaches to enhancing communication and interaction for children with ASD. Increasing such understanding of ASD allows professionals, as well as family members, to better interpret the behaviours they display and to respond to these children in ways that are more sensitive and conducive to promoting a sense of safety and wellbeing.

This chapter starts with a description of ASD, including a discussion of the information-processing styles associated with it. The use of imitation as an approach to communicating with children with ASD is then explored, both in terms of the current evidence base and in terms of its potential for workers in primary health care settings.

What is autistic spectrum disorder?

In the UK, ASD is diagnosed using the International Classification of Diseases 10 (World Health Organization 2007b). As detailed by the Public Health Institute of Scotland (2001) and the ICD-10, there are three categories of ASD: childhood autism, atypical autism and Asperger's syndrome. The type of ASD is diagnosed according to the age of onset and behaviours. Childhood autism (also known as classical autism) occurs before a child is three years old and consists of abnormalities in the development of reciprocal social interaction, communication and restricted, stereotyped, repetitive behaviour (also referred to as the 'triad of impairments'). There may also be problems relating to phobias, sleeping, eating and distress (which can sometimes be interpreted by others as misbehaviour or even aggression) for children who have this form of ASD. Atypical autism is characterized by significant difficulties in only one or two of the three areas of the Triad of Impairments, with the onset of the difficulties occuring after three years of age. Finally, Asperger's syndrome results in some impairment in the triad of impairments, but there is no delay in the development of spoken or reciprocal language and there is no apparent delay in cognitive abilities. The main features of Asperger's include social impairment, all-absorbing restricted interests and a lack of appreciation for humour (Trevarthen et al. 1999).

The severity of the problems experienced by individuals with ASD in relation to the triad of impairments vary from person to person and have been described extensively by a range of authors (e.g. Frith 2003; Public Health Institute of Scotland 2001; Trevarthen et al. 1999; Wing 1996). Problems in relation to reciprocal social interaction include difficulties and anxieties in relating to others and difficulties in recognizing social cues and signals. In terms of communication and language, there may be difficulties in using semantic and pragmatic language structures. Analogy and sarcasm can prove challenging, with many people with ASD interpreting such statements in a literal fashion. Difficulties in relation to thought and behaviour include problems with pretend and imaginative play, ritualized and obsessive behaviours and distress in adapting to change.

Although the precise prevalence of ASD is uncertain, it would appear that there has been a dramatic increase over the last 25 years (Public Health Institute of Scotland 2001). The prevalence of ASD reported above (Baird et al. 2006) could now be as high as 1 in 100 children, contrasting with figures in 2001 which estimated the rate to be 0.6 in 100 (Chakrabati and Fombonne 2001). The causes of these apparent increases are not fully understood, although key factors are likely to include changes in diagnostic criteria and also recording systems (Volkmar et al. 2004; Wing 1993; Wing and Potter 2002).

The economic cost of ASD in the UK is very high. The socio-economic cost of ASD in the UK is now estimated to exceed £1 billion each year (based on a rate of 5 people per 10,000, Järbrink and Knapp 2001). The lifetime cost for an individual with ASD, who also has developmental delay, is thought to reach almost £3 million, the majority of the cost resulting from living support expenses (Järbrink and Knapp 2001). The cost to parents ranges from £689 to £855 per week (Järbrink, Fombonne and Knapp 2003). Such financial figures highlight the need for society and the health care sector to increase the attention given to this condition.

The care of children with ASD can incorporate a multitude of professionals, including GPs, community paediatricians, health visitors, community nurses, school nurses, speech and language therapists, occupational therapists, physiotherapists, psychiatrists, clinical psychologists, educational psychologists, early years practitioners, teachers, social workers and social care officers. The Public Health Institute of Scotland (2001, p.31) states that, 'it is important that parents who have concerns over the development of a child have access to appropriately trained health visitors, community nurses and GPs. These concerns should be listened to, taken seriously and addressed in all cases.' The report then argues that it is vital that, 'all key front-line professional groups (health visitors, nursery/pre-5 education staff, general practitioners, teachers and others) receive training to increase their awareness of the presentation of ASDs at various ages and their confidence in referring on for further investigations' (ibid) Thus, professionals require information on how ASD is likely to present in children and how and why it affects their behaviour.

Processing of psychological and sensory information in ASD

A central component of ASD is the way in which incoming information is processed in cognitive and sensory terms. The most popular theories currently explain ASD as some type of cognitive dysfunction, with the three predominant theories being the Theory of Mind Deficit (Baron-Cohen, Leslie and Frith 1985), Executive Dysfunction (Hill 2004a) and Weak Central Coherence (Frith 1989, 2003; Happé 1999a). Notably, though, as will be highlighted, all of these cognitive accounts give rather cursory attention to the considerable sensory problems associated with ASD.

The Theory of Mind Deficit account (Baron-Cohen *et al.* 1985) proposes that at the core of ASD lies an impairment in the ability to understand that a person's behaviour is related to their own thoughts, desires and beliefs. That is, individuals with ASD are not regarded as having what has come to be known as 'a theory of mind'. Their (perceived) difficulties in understanding the link between a person's behaviour and their mental states is seen as the cause of their avoidance of social interaction. In effect, if they cannot see the 'sense' of such interactions, they would be unlikely to participate in it (Messer 1994).

The Executive Dysfunction account claims that the difficulties observed in ASD are a result of more general impairments in executive functions – the cognitive processes that underlie behaviours such as planning, shifting and directing attention and execution of actions. In short, this view sees ASD as explained by wider cognitive dysfunction (see Hill 2004a,b for a fuller discussion).

Finally, the Weak Central Coherence account (Frith 1989, 2003) emphasizes the tendency of people with ASD to pay attention to details, as opposed to the overall meaning of information. People without ASD tend to process information according to the Gestalt principle of 'the whole being greater than the sum of the parts', while people with ASD tend to process information in terms of 'the individual parts being greater than the whole' (Frith 1989, 2003; Happé 1999a,b).

Francesca Happé (1999a,b) has used the Weak Central Coherence account to argue that ASD should be conceptualized as a cognitive *style*, rather than a cognitive *impairment*. She draws attention to the superior abilities that present with ASD and argues that these should not be overlooked in our attempts to explain the impairments associated with the condition. Many commentators see this approach as less restrictive, even less judgemental, than the alternative cognitive accounts. The evidence certainly shows that individuals with ASD have a tendency to perceive local information rather than the global context and that they have a detail-driven automatic processing preference (Happé 1999a). Happé has grouped the existing research findings into three main categories, which she terms perceptual coherence, visuo-spatial-constructional coherence and verbal-semantic coherence. Her review leads her to conclude that 'because weak central coherence provides both advantages and disadvantages, it is possible to think of this balance (between preference for parts versus wholes) as akin to a cognitive style' (Happé 1999a, p.220). The possible interpretations offered by the wider landscape of cognitive theories highlight the important implications that any particular theoretical stance holds for professionals' understanding of the behaviours observed in ASD.

When we engage in social communication, we observe, interpret and respond to numerous behaviours such as facial expression, eye contact, body language and tone of voice. Our interpretation of another person's engagement with us is driven by context. For example, a raised voice is understood in relation to what is being communicated; it might mean excitement or it might mean anger, depending on the context. Grasping the context and interpreting the meaning of such social actions can be confusing and upsetting for people with ASD. This may be due to the piecemeal processing of information in ASD – pulling numerous behaviours together to form one overall meaning (e.g. the gist) is hugely problematic when information is processed in detail (e.g. the expressiveness of a person's face separately from their tone of voice, their posture, or the event in the wider environment that prompted the raising of the voice). It is these challenges that cause people with ASD to experience such difficulty when engaging in social interaction. Happé (1999a, p.220) summarizes this view by stating that 'failure to integrate information in context might contribute to everyday social difficulties'. It helps one to begin to realize how complex the social functions that we take for granted actually are. Interpreting another person's emotional state is not straightforward, even though people without ASD achieve it effortlessly.

It is at this point in a theoretical discussion that the importance of accounting for sensory processing emerges. Lawson (2001) has become well known in the field of autism, as a consequence of her ability to articulately describe her own ASD. That is, her accounts are drawn somewhat from her personal experience of the condition, rather than on the results of empirical studies that have given rise to cognitive accounts of ASD. She argues that ASD causes the processing of social stimuli to be channelled through only one sensory modality at one time, a process known as 'monotropism'. Knowledge of this phenomenon can help to explain why the integration of diverse elements such as eye contact, touching and changes in tone of voice becomes so problematic. Lawson points out that for information to be perceived and processed, people with ASD may need to focus on only one element at a time, for example by looking away from the person who is talking, in order to avoid being distracted by eye contact and facial expression.

Indeed, the extreme distress often displayed by individuals with ASD may be a consequence of sensory overload. (Caldwell 2004, 2006) is among those theorists who now argue that ASD results in hypersensitivities – to taste, sound, touch, vision and proprioception – which often leave individuals in a state of sensory confusion. She suggests that those individuals with the most profound levels of ASD are at constant risk of sensory confusion and that the 'challenging behaviour' exhibited by them is actually an indication of their stress and pain. Being unable to make sense of one's relation to the world around one's self is a frightening, indeed terrorizing, experience. Caldwell maintains that sensory confusion and hypersensitivities are at the root of many of the social problems observed in people with ASD. When one is 'rooted in sensory confusion', it undermines the brain's ability to function (Caldwell 2006, p.280). Once one is overwhelmed with sensory input, the systems become overloaded and the person goes into 'fragmentation', where the images, sounds and other sensory feedbacks, both from inner and outer worlds, 'break up' (Caldwell 2004, p.20). An impending state of overload is exacerbated when carers who do not understand what is happening to the individual push their sensory systems even further (for example, by trying to encourage face-to-face gaze or by insisting that they get up and walk into a noisy room). Interestingly, Happé (1999a, p.218) seems to be approaching some synthesis with Caldwell's analysis when she discusses autobiographical accounts of what she terms 'fragmented perception'.

It is clear from this brief review that there is continuing debate about the nature of ASD. This is an important discussion, for theoretical frameworks guide future investigations of the condition, both in terms of discovering its causes and in developing effective interventions. In the next section, we will discuss an intervention approach in which there is growing interest as a result of its rapid effectiveness and its ease of implementation: imitation.

Imitation as an approach to creating shared communication

Being able to promote the ease and confidence with which children with ASD engage in social interaction and communication would be a significant step in fostering their wellbeing. It is therefore encouraging that the technique of imitation seems to offer such a possibility.

Interest in imitation has been growing within both research and practitioners' literatures. For practitioners, the draw is that it seems to generate rapid increases in children's social abilities and costs little to implement. Research interest comes from the fact that the abilities demonstrated by children, under imitative conditions, cannot be accounted for within particular theoretical frameworks and this process helps to drive theoretical debates forward.

Early studies exploring the effectiveness of imitation for children with ASD were able to demonstrate that imitation of the child's behaviour results in positive shifts in social behaviours such as eye gaze and social responsiveness (e.g. Dawson and Adams 1984; Dawson and Galpert 1990; Harris, Handleman and Fong 1987; Lewy and Dawson 1992; Tiegerman and Primavera 1984). Such work began to be incorporated into therapeutic programmes, such as those devised by Ingersoll (Ingersoll and Schreibman 2006; [The] Sonrise Program® 2001; Sussman 1999) and others (e.g. Hwang and Hughes 2000; Salt et al. 2001; Seung et al. 2006).

The work of Jacqueline Nadel and colleagues, based in France, offers a novel example of the way in which this work has been conducted (Nadel, Croué et al. 2000). Her team used what is known as the 'still face paradigm', in which experimenters become non-responsive in social interactions, holding their face rigid and statue-like. The experiment was comprised of three sessions, each of which lasted three minutes. In the first, the experimenter adopted a still-face pose, followed by a play session in which the experimenter imitated the behaviours of the child and finally returning to the still-face pose. Nadel was interested in the amount of social interest that the children displayed in the two still-face sessions. This is an interesting question because, if children with ASD do have some cognitive dysfunction that makes it fundamentally impossible for them to be interested in or engage with others socially, then a brief, three-minute session of imitative play should not be expected to produce any change in their behaviour. Surprisingly, Nadel's findings showed just the opposite. In the first still-face session, the children showed virtually no interest in the experimenter. In the second still-face session, a monumental shift was observed; they spent most of the session looking at the experimenter, moving closer to them, touching them and generally trying to interact with them.

The findings show how quickly and dramatically imitation can foster not only children's own social behaviours, but also their expectancies about the behaviours of others. That is, having experienced responsive imitation from the adult, the child now expected the adult to interact. They therefore reacted strongly and insistently when the adult failed to meet with their new expectation. In short, within only a few minutes, they had developed a social interest (and perhaps even a theory of mind) about their partner. This work has since been replicated by others with similar results (Escalona *et al.* 2002; Field, Sanders and Nadel 2001; Heimann, Laberg and Nordren 2006). It is a line of enquiry that suggests that the social capacities of children with ASD may not be as 'limited' as they are frequently portrayed.

The types of insights that are coming out of this empirical work can also be seen in the intervention field. A good example here is the approach known as 'intensive interaction'. Intensive interaction uses elements of an individual's own behaviours in a responsive, imitative way, with the aim of initiating and maintaining communicative contact with them. Initiated by Ephraim (1986) and Nind and Hewitt (2001) for working with children and adults with profound learning disabilities, the approach is increasingly being used with individuals with ASD. This focus has been led by the efforts of Phoebe Caldwell, who has now written several books on the use of intensive interaction with this population (e.g. Caldwell 2004, 2006, 2007, 2008; but see also Nind (1999, 2000). Evaluations have shown the approach to be effective in establishing social interaction (e.g. Zeedyk, Caldwell and Davies, in press) and in reducing distressed behaviours such as rocking, self-harm and screaming (e.g., Nind and Kellett 2002). These are encouraging results, for these are arguably the two most challenging aspects of working with and caring for individuals with ASD.

Our research team has been drawing on this literature to develop a programme that teaches parents to use the technique of imitation (O'Neill 2007). We will describe these efforts by reporting on a case study of a pre-school child with ASD and his mother. We filmed a series of play sessions that took place at the child's preschool centre. The research design involved three different conditions: standard free play which involved singular toys, free play with a duplicate set of toys and play with a duplicate set of toys following imitation training. In each session, a set of toys were provided (e.g. balloons, children's umbrellas, cymbals, hats, sunglasses) and the mother was invited to play as she wished with her child. In the standard free play condition, only one of each toy was provided (as would be usual in most children's playrooms). In the duplicate toys condition, we provided two sets of these toys, the purpose of which was to allow us to see the extent to which the parent's imitative acts spontaneously increased. In the final condition, the parent was given a brief training session in the use of imitation and demonstrations were provided as to how the parent could make use of imitation while playing with her child. The video-taped play sessions were analysed using microanalytic coding techniques, which allowed a detailed analysis of specific social behaviours.

The first comparison involved the standard free play and duplicate toy free play sessions. The findings showed shifts in three key behaviours: the number of imitations produced, the physical proximity of the child in relation to his mother and the amount of turn taking. As shown in Figure 7.1, the child's and mother's imitations of each other increased from 0 to 11 and from 1 to 12 respectively, suggesting that simply providing a duplicate a set of toys to parents and children spontaneously encourages imitative exchanges. There was also a noticeable increase in the physical proximity of the mother and child (Figure 7.2), with a clear increase in their physical closeness from 40 per cent in the standard play condition to 85 per cent in the duplicate toys condition. Finally, there was a slight increase in the amount of turn taking that occurred, from only one instance to a total of four instances (Figure 7.3). Overall, these data suggest that the use of a duplicate set of toys increased the parent's imitation of the child which, in turn, increased the physical closeness and turn taking behaviours of the pair.

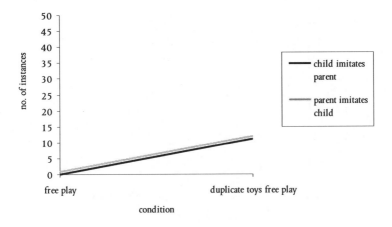

Figure 7.1: Frequency of parent and child imitations of each other in the free play and duplicate toys free play conditions

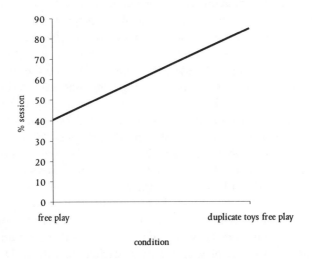

Figure 7.2: Proportion of session the parent and child spent in close physical contact in the free play and duplicate toys free play conditions

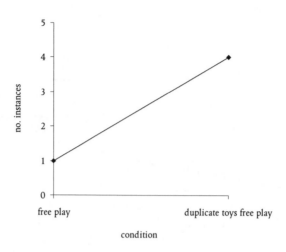

Figure 7.3: Frequency of turn taking between parent and child in the free play and duplicate toys free play conditions

Once the mother had been trained in imitation, the findings showed even further increases in the communicative interaction of the pair. The number of imitative acts produced by the parent increased under these conditions from 12 to 53 (Figure 7.4), confirming that the imitation training had been successful. The proximity of the pair also increased – to 93 per cent, as compared to 85 per cent during the duplicate toys play (Figure 7.5) – and the amount of turn-taking rose noticeably to 24 instances (up from four instances) (Figure 7.6). These findings indicate that the imitation training encouraged the parent to imitate her child, which nurtured increases in physical closeness and turn taking between the pair. Interestingly, such positive changes did not necessitate an increase in the number of imitative acts produced by the child himself, which actually reduced in the final imitation training condition to four instances, as compared to 11 instances in the earlier duplicate toys condition (Figure 7.4). This decrease was not to the original levels, however, given that there had been no imitative acts at all during the standard play session.

This set of findings is most encouraging. It suggests that promoting the use of imitation within the play of parents and children with ASD brings positive benefits. Proximity and turn taking both increase. Such shifts can be generated simply through the provision of duplicate sets of toys, although providing training to parents in the technique of imitation produces further positive change. This outcome should be of significant interest to professionals who work with ASD, for it suggests that the communicative experiences of children with ASD can easily and inexpensively be improved.

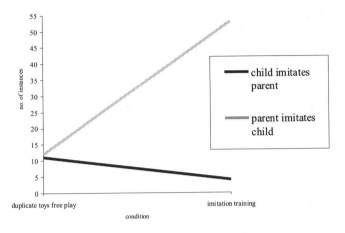

Figure 7.4: Frequency of parent and child imitations of each other in the duplicate toys free play and imitation training conditions

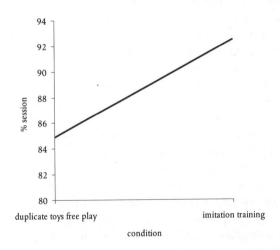

Figure 7.5: Proportion of session the parent and child spent in close physical contact in the duplicate toys free play and imitation training conditions

Why should an act as simple as imitation prove to be so effective in promoting communication? First, the use of imitation can be seen as reducing the amount of sensory chaos experienced by the child. Caldwell (2007) argues that this is

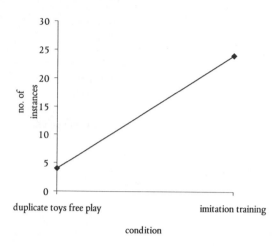

Figure 7.6: Frequency of turn taking between parent and child in the duplicate toys free play and imitation training conditions

key to facilitating social engagement. Such shifts occur because the body language that the adult is using is now recognizable to the child. The highly predictable nature of the adult's behaviour, and thus the flow of the interaction, enables them to experience it as a safe and non-threatening context. The content of an imitative interaction is now interpretable to the child; their attention is drawn to features that are salient and intriguing – experiencing the familiarity of their own body movements, but now being produced by another person. The child's sense of distress at being presented with unfamiliar or ambiguous actions by another person is diminished. In essence, the adult and the child are 'talking the same language', a language which is intelligible and reassuring to the child because it is his own. The child-led nature of imitation does more than promote the child's ability to predict the flow of the interaction, though, it also enables the child to identify more readily the impact that they are having on another person. That is, their awareness of the link between self and other is strengthened, and new pathways for the development of social abilities are opened up.

The second reason that imitation is likely to be so effective is that it involves the 'conversation' being focused on the detailed aspects of the child's behaviours. This explanation accords well with the detail-driven and monotropic processing styles of ASD. The focus of the interaction is on specific components of the child's behaviour (i.e. a noise they produce, twirling string, hand flapping, facial movements) and does not depend on taking account of the wider social context of the interaction. The topic of conversation can range from a single behaviour, such as string or finger twirling, to a combination of behaviours, such as vocalizations, facial expressions and physical gestures and actions. As long as the conversation is centred around specific behaviours that are familiar to that child, they are able to take part in it. Coia and Jardine Handley (2008), contributors to the intensive interaction literature, refer to that familiarity as comprising the child's 'cultural library', which other adults must seek to enter if there is to be any chance of real connection within the pair. Thus, the account of imitation that we are proposing here takes the novel step of bringing together the cognitive and intensive interaction literatures.

Primary health care workers' use of imitation

It will already be clear that imitative approaches hold considerable potential for children with ASD and for the parents, carers and professionals who care for and love them. It is accessible to everyone, costs very little to implement and results can be seen almost immediately. Indeed, it may be more appropriate to call the use of imitation an 'attitude', rather than a technique, for integrating its use into professional practice requires little more than an awareness of its effectiveness and a willingness to try it out. Where additional accounts of its outcomes are desired, recent texts (Nind and Hewitt 2001; Caldwell 2006, 2007; Zeedyk 2008) provide rich illustrations.

Imitation has the capacity to be used in a variety of situations with a variety of individuals. The main underlying principles of imitation – child led, focused on the interest of the child and validating – form the basis of any effective communicative exchange. This means that regardless of the extent to which imitation is applied (i.e. in subtle ways such as mirroring facial expression and posture or in overt ways such as imitation of actions, gestures and vocalizations), it has the potential to be effective in promoting social interaction between children with ASD and the people in their lives. This makes it a suitable approach for children who are highly verbal as well as for those who are not. Interestingly, it also makes the principles entirely suited to children and adults who are in no way 'autistic'. All of us are more comfortable in a relationship where we are confident that our partner is interested in us and is validating our experience. The intentional use of imitation just provides a more explicit way of achieving that for children whom care staff can find difficult to reach.

In terms of the cost effectiveness of such an approach, imitation requires minimal training and few additional resources and is therefore accessible for a wide variety of staff. Barriers that are frequently encountered, such as lack of finance or staff time, are less likely here. With initial training, ongoing monitoring and informed supervision, this approach can be used in everyday situations with a wide variety of individuals.

Summary

As the rate of ASD increases, so too does the need for high quality care and intervention. In line with this is a need for information about the ways in which ASD affects children and about how best to safeguard and promote wellbeing. The detail-driven nature of information processing in ASD, underpinned by sensory difficulties, results in a wide range of social and communicative problems. This forces many individuals to live a life of social withdrawal and isolation, which is regrettable for any human being, whatever their 'condition'. The use of imitation provides a means of quickly overcoming these barriers. It invites the child into a conversational world that is safe and interesting for them. Combining an understanding of how psychological, social and sensory information is processed with an effective approach to communication ensures that we are best placed to safeguard and support the wellbeing of children with ASD.

Chapter Eight

Communication, Behaviour and Child Protection

James Law and Leila Mackie

Introduction

Communication skills and behaviour are likely to be elements in the management of the child who has been maltreated. In the first instance the child's communication development may be one of the first markers that the child is not happy. Although children may be slow to speak for a number of reasons, a withdrawn sullen child should always be a concern for practitioners. Interestingly, it is often easier to engage with parents who may be reluctant to talk about a child's behaviour to discuss their child's communication development. This can then act as a conduit for discussion about other matters concerning development, for example, due to feeding, toileting or sleeping. They may all be markers of an underlying neuro-developmental condition or they may be related to mistreatment, but the important factor is that the child's speech and language skills may act as a way in to discussion of other matters.

Communication can also be a good way in engaging parents in the management of their child, because helping a child talk more is usually a positive experience for all concerned. Communication can also be a useful way of monitoring change in the child, as improved circumstances are often reflected in the child wanting to speak more. Finally, communication skills may be one of the best ways of judging how well a child is likely to cope with the experience of abuse or neglect, those with better communication skills tending to manage better over time (Lynch and Roberts 1982).

The chapter is organized in five sections. In the first we provide some definitions of key concepts together with some illustrations of the issues that arise with relation to communication and child protection across childhood. We then go on to look at evidence for the interaction between behaviour and communication across the lifespan and then focus on the emerging understanding of the link between communication and the impact of neglect. Much attention is paid to the very young child, but clearly these issues do not go away and we focus on the particular challenges associated with the middle school child. There is then a discussion of extreme cases, the feral child and examples of cases that have received media attention in the UK. We conclude with discussion of the behaviour–communication link and its knock-on effect on intervention.

Definitions and illustrations

In this section we provide some definitions of what we mean by communication, emotional and behavioural difficulties and by abuse and neglect.

Communication

Many children experience some kind of difficulty with their ability to communicate. These children may have difficulty with their *language*, that is, their ability to understand spoken language (receptive language skills) and/or their ability to formulate their ideas into words and sentences to express themselves (expressive language skills). They may also have difficulty with their *speech*, i.e. perceiving and discriminating the sounds that make up words or, in their expressive language, using these speech sounds correctly. Their difficulties could also lie in communicating effectively in social contexts, often referred to as *pragmatic* language or social communication skills. A child may have limitations in one or more of these areas and such difficulties now are known routinely as 'speech, language and communication needs' (SLCN). In some cases, such difficulties can be part of more general learning difficulties and in others such limitations exist yet 'the factors usually accompanying language learning problems – such as hearing impairment, low non-verbal intelligence test scores and neurological damage – are not evident' (Leonard 1998, p.1). These children are sometimes referred to as having a 'specific language impairment'. While there is widely recognized to be a heritable element to the development of communications skills it is increasingly obvious that the nature of the communication environment in which the child grows up has an impact on their performance.

Emotional and behavioural difficulties

The International Classification of Diseases (ICD-10) is the official system of classification of child psychiatric disorders in Britain, though the American

Psychiatric Association's (1994) Diagnostic and Statistical Manual of Mental Disorders (DSM-IV) classification (American Psychiatric Association 1994) is also used in the UK as well as in the USA and is similar. ICD-10 classifications for emotional and behavioural disorders (EBD) with onset usually occurring in childhood or adolescence are subdivided into the following categories:

- hyperkinetic disorders – including attention deficit hyperactivity disorder (ADHD)

- conduct disorders

- mixed disorders of conduct and emotions

- emotional disorders – e.g. separation anxiety, social anxiety, phobic anxiety

- disorders of social functioning – selective mutism, attachment disorders

- tic disorders

- other disorders.

Some authors suggest that there is a clear distinction to be drawn between internalizing and externalizing disorders, those that represent neurotic and emotional difficulties on the one hand and those with active behaviour difficulties on the other.

Abuse and neglect

The term 'child maltreatment' is used to describe all forms of abuse and neglect. Abuse is generally defined as being physical, sexual or emotional and is separated into acts of omission (things not done to children, i.e. neglect) and commission (things done to children). All definitions have at least three aspects: the action responsible; the person responsible; and the impact on the individual (Cawson *et al.* 1995). It can be very difficult to distinguish between abuse and neglect and other sources of less than optimal parenting, for example as a result of social disadvantage. There can be considerable differences in the expectations about the treatment of children based on culture and generations.

There follow three case histories which give some idea of the practical implications of the interaction between communication, behaviour and the environment in which the child grows up.

Case 1: Shawn

Shawn was seen by his health visitor for a routine check when he was 29 months of age. The health visitor had not been able to visit the family for a long time and his parents never brought him to the clinic. At the check-up he presented as an undernourished, withdrawn child who did not readily interact and who seemed from parental report and observation to not be communicating at all. This led to a referral to speech and language therapy and Shawn was assessed as having the communication skills of a one-year-old. His health visitor was sufficiently concerned to draw in the family social worker. This referral led to concerns of both abuse and neglect and resulted in the child being fostered. During this period, Shawn now aged three, was seen on regular occasions by a speech and language therapist and it was recorded that he responded well to his new environment and particularly to the other children in the foster family. He started to speak more readily and was generally far more responsive and engaged, and he started to understand much more of what was being said to him. After six months in foster care Shawn went back to his own family with a condition of continued involvement with speech and language therapy and he was seen at fairly regular intervals for another six months. Within a month he had started to become sullen and withdrawn and his communication faltered. It was not that he lost the skills he had acquired, but he did not continue to develop at the same rate as his peers and he just seemed to withdraw and opt out of situations where he needed to communicate.

Case 2: Ryan

Ryan was eight years old and his behaviour at school was becoming increasingly difficult for the school. Ryan's school attendance was poor, with no contact made from home. School was aware of 'family issues' going on and his dad moving in and out of the family home. Ryan had a sister at the same school, who was also increasingly not at school or late. Both children were unkempt and a member of staff had seen them both out late playing on the streets on their own on a few occasions. Comments from Ryan's sister raised concerns among school staff that they may be witnessing some domestic abuse. Social workers were involved and there were meetings between school and social work and educational psychology and his mother to monitor his progress. Following each meeting his attendance improved for a while and then tailed off. When Ryan did come in he was increasingly far behind his peers in academic work; it was difficult to determine the extent this was due to his absences. He was getting input from the school's Support for Learning (SfL) teacher where he worked hard, enjoying the adult attention in the small group and one-to-one setting, but he still struggled a lot with literacy. In class he did not seem motivated and often would act the clown, enjoying the responses this got from his peers. He needed constant reminding to pay attention and often appeared not to understand what he had been asked to do. Other children in the class were wary of him because his play tended to be rough, unpredictable and generally immature.

Case 3: Alex

Alex was in his first year at secondary school and very socially isolated. He received input from Support for Learning for his literacy skills and had annual review meetings to monitor his progress, however his parents did not attend review meetings and rarely contacted the school. Reports indicated that he did not know how to mix with others and was often at the edge of groups at break times. He sometimes got very angry and could unexpectedly lash out at others without provocation and therefore some of the other pupils were wary of him.

With his school work subject teachers reported him to be lazy and lacking motivation, with the need for constant reminders to listen and pay attention. However, as he was quiet in class often the teacher's attention was focused on more troublesome pupils. In group discussions his contributions in class were often irrelevant and he was easily led by other boys in his class and teased as a result. He had been actively bullied by a group of three boys who enjoyed getting a reaction from him. He was concerned about appearing different and he often refused the help of learning assistants in class for fear of the attention that it brought him. However, he did come to the 'safe haven' of the Support for Learning Department for two periods a week for literacy work and often stayed there over lunch time and other times when his classmates would be in the playground. He increasingly seemed to hang around there at the end of the school day, unwilling to go home. This began to cause concern to school staff and towards the end of his school he started disclosing issues of concern at home to a trusted teacher, who started taking appropriate action.

Evidence for the interaction between behaviour, emotional development and communication across the lifespan

The link between communication and emotional and behavioural difficulties (EBD)

The relationship between emotional development, behaviour and communication is now widely recognized in the literature. Children who are referred for professional help because they are anxious or aggressive commonly have poor communication skills (Cantwell and Baker 1987; Cohen et al. 1998a; Cohen et al. 1998b; Nelson, Benner and Cheney 2005; Ripley and Yuill 2005; Vallance, Im and Cohen 1999). There is also evidence for high levels of under-reporting of communication difficulties in children with EBD. Cohen et al. (1998a) found that of 380 children aged between 7 and 14 years, consecutively referred to psychiatric services, 40 per cent had a language impairment that had not been identified previously. But the reverse is also true, children identified with SLCN often have associated difficulties with their behaviour in class (Beitchman et al. 2001; Conti-Ramsden and Botting 2000, 2004; Lindsay and Dockrell 2000; Redmond and Rice 1998) especially if they have difficulties with their understanding of verbal language (Toppleberg and Shapiro 2000). Estimates of the proportion of children who have co-existing communication difficulties and EBD vary between 40 to over 90 per cent (Benner, Nelson and Epstein 2002). Furthermore children with SLCN have been shown to be three times more likely to be bullied in primary school (Knox and Conti-Ramsden 2007).

Why should communication skills on the one hand and behaviour on the other be linked? Does one cause the other or are there underlying difficulties which cause both? There are a number of plausible routes by which they coexist and different routes will operate for different individuals with different profiles and different individual circumstances. It is a truism to say that the child's early experiences play a role in accounting for subsequent performance. We know that a positive, affectionate and consistent interactive bond from a very early age between the main caregiver(s) and baby leads to secure *attachment* and is important for the development of communication and thinking skills and their emotional understanding (Bowlby 1997; Gerhart 2004). Secure attachments require the caregiver to respond to their child in a predictable and comforting way. As the child grows older their security and supported development allows them to gradually become more independent and self-confident away from their caregivers. Conversely, poor attachment, or *attachment disorder*, may occur for a number of reasons, but generally because the child's need for safety, security and trust are either not met or ignored (Bowlby 1997; Cross 2005). This may be due to caregivers having mental health issues.

Maternal depression has been found to severely affect the formation of a secure attachment (Lyons-Ruth *et al.* 1990) and has been linked to poor communication development in the child. Drug or alcohol addiction can also severely affect the ability to provide the consistent and comforting interactions required for secure attachment (Eiden, Edwards and Leonard 2002). Likewise families with multiple stressors and perhaps chaotic lifestyles can have an impact on the parents' ability to interact actively and positively with their children.

In the example of Case 1, Shawn, his lack of communication skills at the health visitor check was the most obvious problem that raised her concerns. In his case it was found that his mother was depressed and both parents had periods of substance abuse. Shawn was not receiving the necessary quality or quantity of interactions with his parents to develop a secure attachment. Unfortunately, though his parents received help for their drug addictions and his mother's mental health while he was in foster care, on his return these attachment issues in combination with other family stressors were not resolved.

Poor attachment contributes to problems with the development of communication and thinking skills and emotional literacy with a resulting impact on behaviour and emotional wellbeing (Cross 2005; Erickson and Egeland 1987; Gerhart 2004). Furthermore, insecure attachment can affect a child's ability to form attachments with others beyond their main caregivers as they get older and into adulthood. It can also have an impact on their own ability to form secure attachments with their children when they in turn become parents. Parental involvement continues to have a major effect on their child's learning over the preschool period. Parent-led activities such as creating opportunities to play with friends, reading, talking together and learning about negotiating and reasoning all have a major effect on the child's learning, communication and emotional development in to the school years.

There is increasing evidence that extremely negative environments can have an effect on the child's neurological development (Glaser 2000). In the first two years there is dramatic overproduction of dendrites followed by pruning due to lack of use. During this period of plasticity the determination of which synaptic connections will persist is environmentally regulated – 'neurons that fire together wire together'. The adult plays an instrumental role in modulating the infant's level of arousal, affect and behaviour. But similarly excess stress for the child has an adverse effect. Exposure to excess levels of cortisol can have a dramatic impact on the hippocampus and this in turn affects memory which is intricately linked to the development of language. Thus the link between poor communication skills on the one hand and both behaviour and mistreatment on the other is reasonably well-established (Allen and Oliver 1982; Coster and Cicchetti 1993; Culp *et al.* 1991; Fox, Long and Langlois 1988; Law and Conway 1992). This is particularly true for the child who has been neglected and where there is evidence of 'psychologically unavailable parenting' (Erickson and Egeland 1987) although care has to be taken that differences in performance are really associated with negative environments and cannot be attributed simply to differences associated with social disadvantage more broadly.

The challenge of the middle school child

Much of the emphasis in the literature and indeed the discussion above focuses on the preschool child. There are many very good reasons for this especially when it comes to prevention and early identification of communication difficulties, poor behaviour and indeed maltreatment. But of course the problems do not simply go away when the child goes into primary school. Indeed they probably become exacerbated as the pressures for the child to conform in school increase and the parents' role decreases as the child starts to define themselves in terms of their peer group.

Academic challenges

By middle primary the majority of children have reasonably fluent reading and writing skills, and oral and written language increasingly become the tools children are expected to use to access information and demonstrate what they have learned. For a child who has been raised in a confusing and chaotic home and therefore may be poorly attached and may have difficulties communicating their needs effectively, the whole classroom environment potentially presents a series of challenges. On the one hand there is the need to listen, comprehend and respond to the teacher's explanations, directions and questions, and the reading comprehension and expressive writing demands of worksheets and textbook activities. On the other hand there is a need to perform appropriately in class and with peers. The two are obviously related. Poor communication is often construed as lack of compliance and a problem in behaviour, and this in turn can lead to a spiral of negative associations for the teacher in the classroom. Indeed a high number of children that have been excluded from school have been shown to have SLCN (Gilmour *et al.* 2005; Ripley and Yuill 2005).

Current educational practice puts emphasis on the importance of group work. This method allows children to develop their negotiation and co-operation skills as well as conversational skills such as taking turns, listening to and considering the viewpoint of others, accepting constructive criticism, clarifying ideas. Though all very important skills, the development of which is highly beneficial for all children, this can be very challenging for children with SLCN. It is likely that these children will opt out of such activities and become observers, as was the case with our third case, Alex or alternatively may start acting up and playing the clown, as our second case, Ryan did. Again, as our case examples illustrate, such behaviour may be seen as work avoidance, reluctance, laziness or low motivation. It is only too easy to see the surface behavioural problems and not see the underlying communication issues that may be in part contributing (Cohen and Lipsett 1991).

Additionally, there is a high incidence of literacy difficulties in children with SLCN (Catts and Kamhi 2005) as illustrated with both Ryan and Alex. In particular, children with receptive language difficulties are at high risk of reading comprehension difficulties due to their verbal language limitations (Simkin and Conti-Ramsden 2006). Furthermore they are at a higher risk of text decoding and spelling deficits due to the phonological impairment that often is part of their presentation (Snowling and Hayiou-Thomas 2006). It is known that many children with EBD have literacy difficulties (Farrell, Critchley and Mills 1999). Due to the high under-identification of SLCN in this group (Cohen *et al.* 1998b; Cohen and Lipsett 1991; Toppleberg and Shapiro 2000), it follows that some of these children like Alex and Ryan, who are seen to be poor readers actually have *unidentified* receptive language difficulties that will also be contributing to their difficulties.

Moreover, these children may have difficulty following the rules of the classroom. This is especially likely if they have pragmatic language or social communication difficulties, as in Alex's case. As well as the clearer rules such as putting your hand up to ask a question, children are expected to know expectations such as when they can take a turn in class discussion and when and how to make requests, ask questions and ask for clarification. Teachers have high expectations that children should be able to understand these often 'unwritten rules' and children who fail to understand these expectations become increasingly obvious as they proceed through primary school. A child who is not understanding may therefore seem odd to his or her peers, as well as possibly resulting in being at the receiving end of disciplinary measures. With Alex it was found that throughout his primary school years he had often 'got it wrong' understanding these 'rules' so by upper primary to secondary he was increasingly inclined to opt out and retreat into his own thoughts as much as possible. This perhaps made it more difficult for professionals involved with him quickly to recognize and tease out the signs that there was cause for concern at home too.

Social challenges

Socially, both in and out of school, the important role of peer acceptance and friendship has also been frequently emphasized in the literature, both for scaffolding cognitive and social skills development and for emotional wellbeing (Asher and Gazelle 1999; Hartup 1995). In the middle school years children's friendships start to change so that play becomes less physical and verbal skills are increasingly placed in higher esteem. In order to be part of the group children need to become increasingly competent in understanding the non-literal language of jokes, puns, slang and ambiguous references.

Many of the underlying verbal and interaction skills required to form and maintain successful friendships have been found to be problematic for children with SLCN and for those with emotional and behavioural difficulties. Studies have shown that children with SLCN are generally less able than their typically developing peers to negotiate (Brinton, Fujiki and Highbee 1998), co-operate (Brinton, Fujiki and McKee 1998), access and participate in an ongoing interaction (Brinton *et al.* 1997; Liiva and Cleave 2005), resolve conflicts (Stevens and Bliss 1995) and to recognize and understand the emotions of others (Spackman, Fujiki and Brinton 2006). Not surprisingly, considering these difficulties with the underlying skills, a lack of friendships has also been reported in children with SLCN (Asher and Gazelle 1999; Durkin and Conti-Ramsden 2007; Fujiki *et al.* 1999).

Furthermore, in typical development, friendships allow many opportunities to learn, practice and enhance these underlying interpersonal and friendship skills. Children with SLCN, like Ryan, Alex and potentially Shawn are therefore in different ways at risk of getting caught in a negative cycle as their difficulty forming friendships excludes them from such opportunities, thereby widening gaps in ability and resulting in further disadvantage for these children. It is perhaps only to be expected that it becomes increasingly difficult for these children to interact in a positive way. The isolation resulting from rejection from their peers is likely to affect their psychological wellbeing and could result in behavioural difficulties (Cross 2005; Gallagher 1999; Redmond and Rice 1998).

Increasing self-awareness

Moreover, at this age children start to develop more of a sense of self and are increasingly likely to be aware of the differences between themselves and others, including a growing awareness of their limitations – both social and academic. This was increasingly becoming an issue for Alex who was desperate to fit in with everyone else. For a child with SLCN who is likely to find many class activities and social interaction generally very challenging, behavioural and/or emotional issues may arise due to frustration and the affect on self-esteem and self-confidence (Cross 2005).

Extreme neglect and the feral child

In the preceding sections we have focused on the research literature rather than the experiences of individual children. Very few of the stories of the individual children are ever told except to social workers, doctors and therapists. This is probably as it should be, given the nature of the experiences. Nevertheless, there has developed a parallel interest in the development of children who have experienced extraordinary early environments. There is a long history much of which would probably be better described as literary rather than scientific although there are examples where the details would appear to be better described rather than apocryphal (Newton 2002). Probably the most famous case is the wild boy of Aveyron (Itard 1932) but more recently we have seen extensive coverage of Genie, a child who had been effectively incarcerated up until the age of 13 (Rymer 1993). The focus of many of these discussions has been the attempts to teach the children in question to speak. One of the most extraordinary cases is Kaspar Hauser, mute when he was first identified in his late teens but able to discourse with philosophers in a matter of years (von Feuerbach 1832). These stories that go back to antiquity proved to be a particular fascination to those in the rationalist 18th century when the nature of humanity was a source of fascination, but feral children have continued to be of concern ever since. In terms of clinical practice, if children who have been neglected are identified early enough, as long as they do not have other developmental difficulties, they will develop language well enough (Skuse 1987). Those who are not identified until later are much less likely to do so and Genie is an example of this. Identified at 13 when she was barely using any words, her vocabulary improved, but she never really progressed to using grammar despite extensive teaching.

A recent illustration of this type of discussion is the case of Edik which has been reported by the first author and became a part of the Channel 4/Discovery documentary (Law 2002). Edik, a boy recently identified in an orphanage in the Ukraine aged six, had spent a period of two or three years up until he was four years of age living rough, at least part of the time with dogs. There is some uncertainty over the details of the story but the substance of it was corroborated by a number of independent witnesses, social workers, a paediatrician and a local teacher. His mother had learning difficulties and was not able to look after her five children effectively. She left them alone in a flat for weeks and months at a time. They lived off scraps from the local markets and Edik left the flat to spend the greater part of his time running with stray dogs on the estate in the derelict port on the Black Sea where they lived.

On arrival at the orphanage aged four years, Edik had severe skin and chest infections which persisted for six months. He was severely malnourished and fed directly from the plate with a licking movement that could not be emulated by either children or adults. It took him three months to feed properly and he continued for a long time to gorge himself to the point of vomiting. He was reported to run like a dog and his play was restricted to the very physical patterns seen with dogs. He would only jump and roll on and mount the other children. When not engaged in this type of physical activity he would rush around in the orphanage garden on his own, banging his head on the wall if he was forced to come in doors. He could not play with the other children and certainly showed no signs of knowing what to do with toys. Although he was not constantly aggressive to the other children, they tended to avoid him because he had the habit of lashing out unexpectedly. On arrival he was reported to have no words and seemed to understand no language addressed to him. Edik learned the routine in the orphanage in the first few months and had begun to talk after six months, although he continued to find it difficult to relate to the other children. His language started to take off until by the time his language was formally assessed he was found to have a vocabulary of at least 370 words, to have started to combine words into short sentences and his verbal comprehension was approximately equivalent to that of a three-year-old.

It is clear that the dominant feature of this child's experience is one of severe neglect (Trickett and McBride-Chang 1995). In fact he was responding like children who have been identified and transferred to more nurturing care earlier in their lives such as the Kulochova twins and Isabelle (Skuse 1984). Although extreme cases of neglect and abuse remain relatively rare, it is important to acknowledge that when the final reports have been written, examining the implications for services, concern about communication skills is identified as an important feature (The Bridge Child Care Consultancy Service 1995).

The implications of the behaviour/communication link for practice

All social workers, health visitors and teachers will encounter children with poor communication skills and depending on the circumstances, these may well have resulted from negative experiences in early childhood. Similarly speech and language therapists working with children are likely to encounter abuse and neglect. In some cases they will be informed of this. In others, they will be the one who first becomes aware of it either because of unusual communication behaviours or patterns in the case history, or because the child specifically 'discloses' to the speech and language therapist. In either case the speech and language therapist has a duty to pass on the information using appropriate local procedures.

In many cases children with SLCN should be construed as a 'vulnerable' group, and there is evidence that vulnerable groups (learning disabilities, deaf etc.) may be more prone to abuse. For example Petersilia (2000) found that children with any kind of disability are more than twice as likely as non-disabled children to be physically abused and almost twice as likely to be sexually abused. This includes children with SLCN. They also report a high probability for crimes to be repeated over time as those who victimize people with disabilities come to regard them as easy prey. Furthermore Petersilia reports that crimes against people with disabilities are less likely to be followed up and where they are, sentences are lighter.

How speech and language therapy can contribute

Speech and language therapists are frequently part of school-based education teams either by actually being attached to a particular school or special class or by providing an outreach service, possibly in collaboration with other specialist peripatetic professionals. Speech and language therapists within schools target ways to reduce the many social and academic challenges described above. Such communication targets are much more likely to be achieved in close collaboration with education professionals, health professionals (for example occupational therapists) and families so that skills learned in groups or individual sessions are carried through to everyday settings including the home.

In the complex presentations of children with child protection issues, there needs to be more awareness and consideration among all professionals involved that behavioural and emotional issues all too often go hand in hand with SLCN. The combined expertise in the form of integrated services and multi-disciplinary teamwork is considered to be the most effective for these children. We need to develop services to make them more holistic and allow us to fully include assessment and management of their potential communication limitations also (Benner *et al.* 2002; Cross 2005; Law and Garrett 2004; Law and Plunkett, in press).

Although speech and language therapy services are variable across the UK, generally there is still very limited speech and language therapy input into service for children with EBD or children who have been abused and neglected. In a major study of the provision of services to children with speech and language needs in England and Wales (Law *et al.* 2000) it was demonstrated that negligible levels of resources are allocated to meet the speech, language and communication needs of children if they are classified as having EBD. The same is true for children who fall within the remit of child protection agencies and it is hardly surprising that there is so little understanding of the impact of poor communication skills.

Within multi-disciplinary teams working with children who have suffered or are at risk of abuse or neglect, the speech and language therapist can contribute to the management in the following ways. First, they can provide training for other professionals in the team to increase awareness of the signs that there may be an underlying language/communication difficulty and therefore that assessment by a speech and language therapist is appropriate. Training could also include general strategies to adapt their communication style to maximize the success of their interactions with these children.

Second, they can carry out assessment of language and communication skills. Many of the interventions targeting the emotional and behavioural issues of these children are talking therapies and therefore if the child has difficulties expressing themselves due to language limitations and/or difficulties understanding this will unavoidably limit the amount they are able to gain from these. If the professionals involved have more information about how to adjust and support their intervention to allow for the child's communication limitations from information gathered in the speech and language therapist assessment, then this will increase the likelihood that the child will make progress with these interventions.

Finally, direct intervention focusing on developing the child's communication skills may be appropriate and can be delivered by the speech and language therapist. Close collaboration with a multi-professional team and parents allows targets to be carried over into the home and other everyday settings.

Summary

It is clear now that emotional and behavioural difficulties are associated closely with communication problems of one sort or another and this is of considerable importance to all those delivering services both for children who have been abused and neglected and for those who are referred initially for speech and language therapy. Of course, we need to be extremely careful in assuming causal links between the two. As we have seen, it is reasonable to assume that in some cases poor behaviour and emotional vulnerability in the child may have their roots in poor attachment and that limited or negative interactions may also affect the child's early language learning. But this is not necessarily true. For example children who are neuro-developmentally immature will also exhibit limited communication skills and many apparently behavioural symptoms such as slow toileting skills, attention difficulties etc. Nevertheless, neglect in particular is a powerful force limiting the child's experience and instilling negative attitudes to interaction, communication and the formation of relationships more generally. Key to this issue is awareness on the part of all those providing services to these children and their families that poor behaviour and communication go hand in hand. So, on the one hand, assessment for one without acknowledgement of the other is an incomplete assessment which may well have a bearing on the overall management of the case. On the other hand, this awareness has the potential to enhance the way in which a given case is handled and provide those closest to the child with some clear messages which counterbalance the cycle of negativity which so often accompanies such cases.

Chapter Nine

Protection Through Emotional Responsiveness

Barbara Juen and Florian Juen

Introduction

Almost any mental disorder in adolescence and adulthood can be associated with difficulty in experiencing and dealing with emotions and relationships. Therefore the most efficient way to help our children is to provide an emotionally responsive environment in which they can explore emotionality in a somewhat 'protected' and secure interactive system. Experiencing and regulating emotions is both the process and the result of this highly interactive learning procedure in various types of dyadic and even triadic settings throughout the first years of life (mother–child, father–child, peer group, child–teacher, mother–father–child and others).

Maladaptive learning processes within these systems can result in difficulties for parents, teachers, children themselves and society as a whole (Denham *et al.* 2002). Of course not all offenders are the result of maladaptive childhood processes, but a huge number of these various mental health problems could have been prevented by experiencing emotional responsiveness throughout childhood. Almost all of these problems are related to a lack of capacity of establishing and maintaining relationships. The need for prevention therefore seems to be extremely important. One of the crucial parts of a child's safe development is the availability of caregivers who are emotionally available and sensitive (Fonagy 1999). We argue that one of the most protective efforts for healthy child development is preventive assistance for parents who need it. This offers children a crucial base for their emotional and thus social and moral development from the beginning. In this chapter we would like to outline the impact of emotional availability of at least one caregiver on reducing the risk of developmental disorders, preventing mental disorders and thus protecting children in the way of offering a healthy base for development, especially in difficult and traumatizing environments. It will be seen that even highly stressful and traumatic events and experiences can be dealt with as long as the capacity to experience and regulate accompanied emotions has been learned in a functioning emotionally responsive relationship.

Attachment and the human interactive mind

Experiences made in one's life are represented within the inner world of the individual and have social meaning. Along some other relevant influences, this 'experience-based mental representational system' and the accompanying structure is crucial for humans' individuality and thus co-responsible for all behavioural outcomes in both a positive and negative sense. Of course there is no one-to-one imaging of single events. It is rather a dynamic result of a chain of emotionally relevant patterns experienced throughout life. Information about inner psychological processes and their origins should thus lead to a better understanding of mental dynamics and processes underlying problematic interactive behaviour like aggression and anxiety in children (Warren, Emde and Sroufe 2000).

Human beings are highly socially oriented. Attachment theory offers a framework to explain these processes. From the very beginning of life babies seek social stimuli. Humans need to experience their caregivers as trustworthy and responsive so that they can be relied upon to serve as a secure base that can be trusted in when they are in need. This is necessary in order for infants and children to explore their environment (Bowlby 1969). Attachment behaviour is a child's capacity to send signals to adults in order to provoke care-giving behaviour. Depending on the adult's reaction to these signals a child will keep or modify those attachment behaviour patters in order to reach 'the best' they can get. Children should experience their care-giving adults as a source of nutrition, protection and consolation. Soon these experiences are internalized and stored as expectations of what kind of reaction will follow. These representations determine behavioural outcomes towards self and others. Depending on the kind of expectations, Mary Ainsworth (1985) differentiated between several kinds of attachment styles following Bowlby's model. In order to observe reactions of children to separation and reunion she developed a standardized setting called the 'strange situation'. Based on these observations she described three different attachment styles:

- *Secure attachment:* A securely attached child at age 8–12 months reacts with distress when separated from the caregiver, but can be consoled by the caregiver rather easily and within a short period of time if the separation does not last very long.

- *Insecure ambivalent attachment:* An insecurely ambivalent attached child reacts with distress to the separation, but cannot be easily consoled afterwards showing ambivalent behaviour (insecure ambivalent).

- *Insecure avoidant attachment:* An insecurely avoidant attached child does not react with overt distress at all and therefore shows no need to be consoled afterwards (insecure avoidant). Ambivalent behaviour means switching rapidly from seeking contact to rejecting the mother.

Some years later Mary Main (1995) described a fourth style that she called *disorganized attachment:* A disorganized attachment style is expressed in the lack of a consistent strategy to separation and reunion (even ambivalent or avoidant behaviour is a strategy). These children may react in a very aggressive or even absurd way, like approaching the caregiver backwards or freezing a position suddenly.

All of these behaviour types seem to be driven by 'inner psychic models' that develop and form out of early interactive experiences with caregivers. This assumption is widely reported and the attachment-based concept of 'Inner Working Models' is one of the most established models to underpin this postulation. The internalization of experiences in early childhood interaction lead to representations of self, of others and of interactions (Fonagy 1999; George and Solomon 1996; Spangler 1999). This integration process is strongly influenced by early interaction processes between child and caregivers (Fonagy 1994; Papousek, Schieche and Wurmser 2004; Patrick *et al.* 1994). Thus, early experiences gain lifelong relevance (Dozier, Stovall and Albus 1999; Zimmermann *et al.* 2000). The internalization of these repeated interactive experiences with caregivers leads to expectations of others' reactions towards interpersonal signals (Bowlby 1969; Bretherton, Ridgeway and Cassidy 1990). Behavioural problems can be considered as regulation strategies for children who have not experienced effectiveness of their 'normal' behavioural strategies. Moreover this exploration of emotionality within a protected relationship develops resources for coping with stressful events such as trauma.

In the first years of life children can be described in short as being dependent and flexible. They need caregivers' reaction or response, and depending on the nature of this reaction or response they can adapt their strategy. Both are highly necessary to grow up and survive.

Attachment and exposure to traumatic experience

The term resilience refers to patterns of positive adaptation in the context of situations that threaten life or development (Masten and Gewirtz 2006). Factors promoting resilience can be internal as well as external. Masten (2001, 2004) mentions the following factors as especially important for children: relation to competent and sensitive caring adults, relation to peers, problem-solving skills, self-regulation skills, self-efficacy, belief in a meaning of life, hope, socio-economic resources and a stimulating social context. Most of these factors are established or learned from early childhood onwards in an interactive emotion-based system. The adaptive functions that may help children to cope with adverse events are highly based on attachment relationships as described above, on a learning and problem-solving system (a human brain in good working order); on a mastery motivation system, self-control or self-regulating capacity, as well as a social-control or social-regulatory capacity.

In the face of trauma, caregivers are a secure base as well as a barometer for danger, reassurance and hope. According to Masten and Gewirtz (2006) preparing a large population for any kind of major threat requires a developmental perspective. The same is true for prevention in the face of violence and abuse within the family system. Strengthening caregivers in their everyday interaction with their children is one of the most important factors within the prevention of trauma. Building capacity (human, social, organizational) is seen as important as fostering development of healthy adaptive systems and plans for mobilizing, supporting and restoring adaptive systems (Masten and Gewirtz 2006). In our view (Juen *et al.* 2007), attachment theory can provide a good framework for prevention of trauma as well as for the prevention of violence. Trauma Type I (single trauma) as opposed to Trauma Type II (chronic trauma) is defined as a life-threatening, usually uncontrollable, event beyond the scope of ordinary human experience that often occurs rather unpredictably. Psychosocial care after single traumatic events includes meeting victims' material, social and psychological needs, while at the same time recognizing that all people have a vital role to play in social and community structures, and no matter how vulnerable, they still have resources to offer in terms of knowledge, skills and experience (IFRC 2003).

Children's different view of the world and their different ways of coping with stressful events are often surprising to adults and can be used as a guidance and resource in themselves. In dealing with children after stressful events we should nevertheless be aware of our own emotional reactions and their possible negative effects on the child: one of our common reactions to children's trauma is our wish to protect them from any knowledge about stressful matters such as death, illness and violence. However, our impulse to protect children is double-edged: on the one hand this longing leads us to protect the child from being overwhelmed by negative emotions. This urge to protect the child could be very helpful because it takes the child's vulnerability into account. On the other hand our wish to protect the child may lead us to inhibit the child's understanding about what has happened to him/her and others, and may produce fears within the child and hinder the process of coping with the event – thus it helps 'us' to regulate our arousal.

Another common reaction is our wish to deny the traumatic nature of the child's experience. This may lead us to a denial of children's needs after critical events. We may believe that children cope amazingly well with the events if we do not see any signs of negative emotions in them. For example they may play as if nothing had happened. Therefore it is of utmost importance that we are able to recognize children's resources without neglecting their special needs. Our recognition of children's very special way of coping should be very useful in helping children to cope with adverse circumstances in their own way instead of expecting them to do so in an adult manner. Thus, on the one hand we should be able to acknowledge the special vulnerability of children and on the other hand we should be able to be aware of their special way of coping with negative events.

Having experienced chronic trauma such as sexual or physical abuse, a child may have much more severe difficulties with coping than with problems that stem from a single traumatic event. The age of the child, the duration of the trauma and the lack of a good enough caregiver, all influence the child's ability to cope. A further problem is that many of these chronic traumas occur within the family unit, thus these traumas are often named 'attachment traumas'. Not only do they happen within the attachment system, they also threaten and harm the child's attachment system as a whole. Attachment traumas cause untold difficulties for children. For adults who are confronted with children suffering from attachment trauma it is highly important to know that they have to offer the 'lost' secure base, before the child will be able to cope with the traumatic experience. Therefore it is crucial to first understand the nature and origin of the child's basic comfort-seeking behaviours or lack of such, as well as their various efforts to regulate negative emotions.

It should also be considered that children don't express emotions in the same way as adults and that consequently in order to understand them properly it is very important to listen and observe very carefully. Listening to what children say, both in words and through their non-verbal behaviour, is essential in order to gain knowledge about their feeling states. Children can be observed rather easily while talking to them or while they are playing.

In children it is normal that they experience difficulties using their capacities (including their ability to express and regulate emotions) within difficult stressful situations. Emotional capacities have to be learned in a highly interactive process throughout the first years of life. Moreover in case of stressful events it is important to talk with parents and other adults who know the child in order to find out whether the child has changed in a significant way since exposure. Children suffer from symptoms of acute stress disorder (intrusions, hyper-arousal, avoidance and dissociation) the same as adults, but these symptoms are often expressed in a child-like manner. A child's most dominating fear after a stressful experience is that he or she will be left alone. Therefore, it is common for children to become more 'clinging' and to rebel against the absence of their usual caregivers. The experience of reliable and sensitive reactions to attachment behaviour during the first years of life influences the quality of regulation of stressful events later on. Children's fear and anxiety may also cause them to act much younger than their developmental age and thus provoke care-giving behaviour. They may show regressive behaviour such as bedwetting, thumb-sucking and being very clingy or afraid of strangers more than usual. What is important is that these behaviour patterns are rather untypical for the specific child. Children's reactions and their ways of coping depend on many factors, such as age, gender, culture and other aspects of the context. One of the most important factors influencing coping skills and reactions are the child's age and developmental stage. Often children's play activities may involve exposure to aspects of the event(s).

Coping with adverse circumstances

Following death and critical events, usual roles and daily routines will often be lost. Several difficulties may influence parents' ways of caring for their children and can disrupt their normal growth and development. It is common for people to look to others for guidance about how to react in a situation. This is especially true for children. Younger children in particular look at parents and other family members for clues as to how they should react. Consequently a good way to helping a child is through helping the parents. Familiar daily routines and normality give the child a feeling of security and control. Attendance at school and playing with other children helps them to continue with the familiar aspects of their life. It is exactly these routines that are affected in reaction to trauma. As parents are often not able to keep or provide the necessary routines, teachers may be important resources for traumatized children. For children a closer tie, including more physical contact than usual, not sleeping alone, having the light on etc. could be essential. This is of course more difficult when an attachment relationship is not close and sensitive even in the absence of a stressful threat.

Children are also often confused about the facts and their feelings. They need reliable caregivers to give structure within facts and feelings. This is only possible within a secure attachment system. Listening to children's questions carefully can help clarify what they understand and what they need to hear. When children have lost a loved one, they often need information about what has happened and why it has happened in order to rebuild their basic assumptions about their world and themselves (Janoff-Bulman 1989). Talking to children about trauma-related matters may seem very difficult because we are all reluctant to traumatize the child further by confronting them with facts with which they cannot cope. This fear is not completely unreasonable. Confronting the child with too many facts may be problematic. To find the right amount of information is important – sensitivity is needed to fit the child's needs. The best way to avoid both of these problems is to let yourself be guided by the child's own questions and to listen carefully to the child's narration and body language.

Rituals also are a very important means of coping with adverse circumstances. They help us understand and regulate our negative emotions. Furthermore they give us a sense of belonging and community. In every culture rituals are a very important part of mourning. They help us to say goodbye to the deceased person, but they also tell us when it is time to go on with our lives. For children simple rituals may be a great help to cope with the events. Participating in adult rituals is also very important for children. Writing letters, drawing pictures or bringing presents to significant places (the grave, place of death, a place where one has been happy together etc.) are rituals that help children cope with loss. Memorials and anniversaries show us that remembrance is an important task in the process of mourning. Children often need assistance with this task. Often children are told that when a person has died it is important that we remember this person together. In order to help children to remember we can use memory boxes. In these boxes we can put things that once belonged to the deceased person as well as letters we wrote to them (Goldman 2000; Mankell 2004).

In dealing with a stressful experience, one has to be able to both confront oneself and gain emotional distance to the experience (Sroufe 1996). Caregivers should be very careful not to confront the child without their consent. They should always ask the child if he or she wants to go to the funeral, talk about the deceased person, etc. Furthermore it is of utmost importance that caregivers observe the child's reactions to confrontation carefully and provide opportunities to gain distance if necessary. Finally a very important aspect of emotion regulation in the face of stressful experiences is the opportunity to experience accompanying positive emotions. In dealing with bereaved or traumatized children we sometimes forget about positive feelings. In order to recover, children need to gain distance from what has happened to them. We therefore need to help them to have fun and feel good as often as possible.

Disturbing the attachment system – chronic trauma

Physical and sexual abuse of children occurs all over the world. However, children who have physical or mental disabilities or learning difficulties (also as a consequence of isolation) are at greater risk of being abused than others. Most often violence is wielded by family members, which consequently leads to disruption of attachment capabilities in the children as well as other developmental deficits. Children are vulnerable because they are less powerful and more naïve. Adults have many opportunities to abuse children by virtue of their more powerful positions. Sexual abuse is one form of chronic traumatization that may lead to severe disturbances in a child's development. As in any trauma it is crucial to provide protection and safety for the child immediately. Furthermore it seems to be very important to avoid further traumatizing the child by acting without his or her consent. As in any other traumatic situation we should try to understand the child's point of view and inform them about every step of action. If ever there is the possibility do not act without the child's knowledge and consent. If child abuse is suspected, the most important steps to be taken are the following:

(A) Acknowledge the child's situation and feelings. Access support and help: then report.

(C) Carefully listen to what the child says. Comfort the child; ensure the child is safe.

(T) Take notes: document what the child says and what is observed (Fairholm and Juen 2008).

Sexual or physical abuse is a long-term trauma in most cases and may affect the child's development in many ways. First of all, self-development may be severely disturbed. The child may have difficulties feeling her own body. When asked about how she feels she may say 'empty' or 'I do not feel anything'. At the same time, the child may have a very low self-esteem. He may think the abuse is his fault. The child may also be prone to negative relationship experiences because he is not able to differentiate between 'friendly–unfriendly', 'safe–dangerous', 'good–bad' etc. (e.g.Wolfe, Sas and Wekerle 1994). In helping children who have experienced long-term physical and/or sexual abuse one has to take into account that first of all the child has to build up resources before it may be possible to face the stressful experiences.

In these cases the development of a trusting relationship with the child may take a very long time.

As a first step one has to assist the child to build up positive self-esteem and learn to regulate and tolerate positive as well as negative feelings. It is also very important to help the children to recognize 'triggers' of their stressful experiences (that are permanently present in their everyday life) and acquire strategies that help to minimize them. Thinking or talking about the trauma, understanding what has happened and learning to tolerate the emotions associated with remembering the trauma may not be possible for a very long time, if ever. Some of these children will remain vulnerable for their whole lives. Others will be prone to aggressive and violent behaviour because they lack the ability to regulate the negative emotional effects, trying instead to establish control via aggression towards self and/or others.

Attachment theory and the prevention of trauma

Attachment theory in our view holds great promises as a framework for (primary) prevention and early intervention of trauma, and in the strengthening of resilience. The earlier prevention starts the more fundamental it is. With 'attachment focused' preventive work it could be possible not only to help children develop important regulation capabilities that can help them regulate stressful situations, it can also be possible to prevent trauma itself by assisting caregivers to be responsive and sensitive. Abuse is often an extreme result of a circle of maladaptive regulation in which positive interactive experiences for both child and caregiver are more and more unlikely. Abuse is usually not an affective reaction to a single event but the result of a process in which the system is overwhelmed. Enabling and facilitating social competence, high self-esteem and secure attachment in the child is likely to create the conditions for relationships that are based on mutual recognition and respect (Svanberg 1998).

A secure attachment organization may provide a substantial buffer against distress as children learn to make sense of a complex environment and to communicate in a highly interactive process. One of the crucial efforts in early life is to build up an internalized representational world that helps us to understand our own behaviour, as well as the behaviour of others, as meaningful. According to his concept of mentalization and his 'playing with reality' theory, Peter Fonagy and colleagues illustrate the meaning of this reflective approach to the self and the process of achievement within the early attachment relationship (Fonagy et al. 2002). Mentalization is defined as the unconscious attempt to interpret others' feelings, thoughts and wishes. If the child has good enough caregivers he or she develops the ability to consciously interpret others' mental states which is named reflective functioning (Fonagy *et al.* 2002). This theoretical background may help us to understand problems in early development that can potentially lead to aggressive and violent behaviour in preschool children or to antisocial and delinquent behaviour in adulthood. As Tremblay states, the best age to predict antisocial behaviour is around five (Tremblay *et al.* 1999), which illustrates clearly the necessity of such an (attachment related) understanding.

It seems that many of the violent movements and individual aggressive acts of the last decades, which appear to have become more frequent in everyday life, have their origins in early childhood (Gauthier 2003). Bowlby (1973) mentioned the importance of the close links that anger and anxiety have with separation and loss of an attachment figure. Early interactive experiences of separation and loss have high impact on our developing representational system. Separation and loss means instability of the self-system, especially in early childhood, which leads to higher arousal for increasing protection by retraction (anxiety) or higher tension (anger). Talking to prisoners who were arrested due to various outcomes of antisocial behaviour, ranging from assault to murder, we almost systematically come to talk about their childhoods with a great majority of these individuals reporting that they grew up in a traumatic environment where they had been repeatedly violated and brutalized. Our task is to change these traumatic environments in early childhood in order to protect and assist children in their subsequent development. Children can't simply choose their environment, instead always having to take it as it is. Environment-based prevention that can offer sensitive and reliable relationships, is the real task that has to be achieved.

In our opinion, psychological and behavioural problems, as well as personality disorders, cannot be understood without tracing their developmental origins to the very first years of life. Our basic argument is to regard difficult behavioural outcomes as a result of a dynamic mental process caused by any kind of insecure, chaotic or traumatizing family environment in early childhood. In the development of these inner processes affects and their regulation play a major role. We assume that according to the attachment background of a child the experience of affects and the capacity to regulate them differs (e.g. Fonagy *et al.* 2002). Hence it is not primarily the behaviour we are interested in but the role of underlying dysfunctional affects and their relevance to specific attachment experiences of children.

The role of primary health care practitioners

As stated, children have to be observed carefully in order to understand their state of mind as well as their capacities to cope with stressful situations. In recognizing children in need of support and protection, the primary health care systems play a very important role. According to Fairholm and Juen (2008) there can be many different signs of child abuse. Each child is unique and each form of violence can impact a child in a unique way. Nevertheless there are some common physical indicators of abuse, neglect and violence such as bed-wetting, hurting oneself, problems with speech, e.g. stuttering, poor physical development or poor health, eating disorders or physical injuries. There can also be behavioural signs, which may include low self-esteem, sleeping disorders, problematic behaviour like lying, stealing and aggression, or behavioural extremes such as being extremely compliant, passive or extremely demanding in ways untypical for this specific child. Other signs in behaviour may be withdrawal, depression, lack of trust or sexualized behaviour.

A child who is being abused or neglected also often displays emotional signs, such as a sense of powerlessness, betrayal or despair, sadness, shame, isolation, anger, worry or stigmatization. Any of these attitudes may express a child's need for protection. Family violence is defined as actions that result in physical, sexual or emotional harm to any person in the family. The risk of family violence is moreover closely linked to alcoholism, substance abuse, lack of anger management and a belief that violence is an acceptable way of problem solving. Emotional abuse is defined as constant attacks on a child's self-esteem, psychologically destructive behaviour by a person in a position of power, authority or trust. Often physical and emotional abuses come together. Emotional abuse may be carried out by rejecting or ignoring the child but also by degrading the child through insults or criticism, or terrorizing him through the use of threats etc. Physical abuse is usually connected to physical punishment or is often confused with discipline. If you see a child who often experiences accidents you should take a closer look at the kinds of injuries the child presents. Children who experience normal accidents in everyday activity often have wounds in areas such as the forehead, knees and elbows. Children who are physically abused, however, often have bruises or cuts in unusual or unexpected areas such as their back, face and side of the head, buttocks, upper thighs, lower legs and lower abdomen. If child abuse is suspected you should act immediately as stated above.

However, the primary health care system may do more than providing protection where it is needed. It is also a very important source of prevention. By carefully observing families' capacities to provide a safe and trusting environment, and by supporting attachment systems in a sensitive and culturally appropriate manner, primary carers may be an important resource for children as well as their caregivers. In our experience it is of utmost importance that professionals in this field are able to build up a co-operative and trusting relationship with parents. Support for children can be given best by supporting the attachment system as a whole and not simply focusing on the child alone. We assume that even if there are exceptions to the rule, in general caregivers want to support their children, not to harm them, even if they seem to be unable to do so in an appropriate way. By forming a 'working alliance' with the caregivers that is based on the common aim of protecting and supporting the child, much more can be achieved than by working without or even against the caregiver.

Caregivers' resistance or lack of interest in co-operation with the helpers often results from feelings of helplessness, shame and/or guilt. If the primary health care system clearly aims to support the caregiver in fulfilling his or her role as a parent without accusing or devaluating them, it may be even more successful in providing the kind of prevention that is needed. Prevention in a psychological sense is a type of support for emotional development. As already stated, severe threat activates a regulation strategy for protecting the self (physical and psychological). We need our emotional system to appraise the meaning of stimuli for ourselves. This is true for children as well as for their caregivers. In our opinion we all have to consider prevention across the whole lifespan of the individual.

A review by Yoshikawa (1995) clearly illustrates that the most effective prevention focuses on very early family and early educational support. Also Svanberg (1998) reports clear benefits of early and prenatal involvement and even reports high economic benefits for the health care system with such an approach. The earlier prevention starts, the more effective it is. Finally we argue that preventive work should focus on the attachment system as a whole, start early and last for a longer time. Preventive work should also be appropriate to the needs of specific age groups, always focusing on the retrieval of resources that have not been fully developed. This predominantly psychological task needs to be accompanied by socio-economic and socio-political provision that focuses on the reduction of key contributory factors such as poverty, unemployment and low education. In our view, in order to find a solution you have to take several approaches. With one single approach you won't reach the goal.

Chapter Ten

Assessment and Interventions for Child Trauma and Abuse

Jacqueline Feather and Kevin Ronan

Introduction

Children who present to primary health practitioners may have a history of trauma that is a significant, but perhaps undetected, factor in their physical health presentation. Traumatic events may range from a single incident experienced by a child who has had an otherwise uneventful childhood, such as an accident or natural disaster, to chronic abuse and neglect. In the latter case, a growing body of research has emerged internationally that clearly demonstrates many types of abuse and violence witnessed and experienced by children are not unique or singular experiences (Saunders 2003). It is not uncommon for children to have experienced a number of forms of abuse or violence on multiple occasions (Finkelhor *et al.* 2005). In addition, whether having experienced a single incident of trauma or multiple abuse and violence, some children may demonstrate resilience whereas others exhibit long-lasting effects. For these children, referral for treatment is imperative. To ensure best outcomes for this most vulnerable population, health care practitioners need to (1) be aware of the range of trauma presentations in children; (2) make or refer for assessments of trauma and abuse history, current risk and treatment needs; (3) refer for evidence-based treatment targeted to specific identified concerns; (4) monitor treatment progress and outcomes. This chapter aims to support this process for primary health care practitioners by providing information and guidelines, including working with parents, caregivers and therapists.

Trauma presentations in children

Recognition of the impact of traumatic events on children has lagged behind the recognition of the effects on adults (Davis and Siegel 2000). Lenore Terr, a pioneer in the field as a result of her studies of the children of Chowchilla,[4] described prominent characteristics that distinguish the traumas of childhood: thought suppression, sleep problems, exaggerated startle responses, developmental regressions, fear of the mundane, deliberate avoidances, panic, irritability and hypervigilance (Terr 1979). Terr considered four characteristics to be common to most cases of childhood trauma: (1) strongly visualized or otherwise repeatedly perceived memories; (2) repetitive behaviours; (3) trauma specific fears; and (4) changed attitudes about people, aspects of life and the future. Terr distinguishes between Type I trauma, resulting from one event and Type II resulting from long-standing or repeated ordeals. Type I is thought to be characterized by intrusive recollections and Type II by denial, numbing and dissociation (Terr 1991).

Only relatively recently has it been acknowledged that children may develop post-traumatic stress disorder (PTSD) as a result of traumatic events in childhood. PTSD as a diagnostic entity was not related to children and adolescents until the publication of DSM-III-R (American Psychiatric Association 1987). Current criteria for PTSD in DSM-IV-TR (American Psychiatric Association 2000) make some acknowledgement of the differential experience of trauma for children. For example, instead of intense fear, helplessness, or horror, children may exhibit agitated or disorganized behaviour. Nightmares may be more general; for example, about monsters or threats to self and others, not just specifically about the traumatic event itself. Children may engage in traumatic play, involving repetitive acting out of the trauma. Also, sexually abusive traumatic events may include developmentally inappropriate experiences, without threatened or actual violence or injury. In other respects, PTSD in children and adolescents is similar to PTSD in adults, including the cardinal symptoms of re-experiencing, avoidance and increased physiological arousal (Davis and Siegel 2000). PTSD is now widely recognized in children, with effects on neurobiological, psychological and social development.

There is considerable evidence to suggest that traumatic experiences as a child can have a profound effect on the developing brain (Nemeroff 2004). Biological and neuropsychological models explain the problems of traumatized children as efforts to minimize objective threat and regulate emotional distress. The overactivation of neural pathways (e.g., via experiencing a traumatic event) and/or deprivation of sensory stimuli (e.g., via disrupted attachment, neglect)

---

4   A group of children who were kidnapped and buried in a school bus in Chowchilla, California.

may lead to a persistent pattern of hyperarousal or dissociation (Perry *et al.* 1995). This can lead to a child being constantly 'on edge' and feeling very easily threatened. Disruptions to cognitive functioning including attention and abstract reasoning/executive function have been found (Beers and De Bellis 2002). Memory disturbances such as amnesia, fragmentation of memories and non-verbal, involuntary intrusions such as images, sounds, smells, bodily sensations may also occur (van der Kolk 2005).

Practitioners need to be aware that there are limitations to the diagnostic category of PTSD for children and adolescents. The current DSM-IV-TR does not adequately describe trauma-related syndromes observed in children, especially from deliberately inflicted trauma such as abuse (Perry *et al.* 1995). Severely traumatized children with dramatic symptoms of physiological hyperarousal and cognitive dysfunctions may not meet diagnostic criteria for PTSD and may display symptoms of other diagnostic categories as well, such as externalizing, affective, dissociative and borderline personality features. Chronic PTSD in maltreated children has been associated with helplessness, guilt, hyperaroused physical reactions, avoidance, disturbances in memory and information processing, negative abuse related attributions and a coping style that is more avoidant and less approach-based (Cohen and Mannarino 1996; Linning and Kearney 2004). Co-morbid psychological disturbance, in particular other anxiety disorders and depression, as well as related problems are common for abused children with PTSD (Linning and Kearney 2004).

In addition, trauma appears to be a necessary, but insufficient, cause of PTSD in children, with many factors modifying the response to trauma (McFarlane and Yehuda 2000). The aetiology and course of PTSD in childhood is likely to be a complex function of developmental stage, prior experiences and temperament, parent and family functioning, subsequent coping and reactions to secondary adversity (Pynoos 1994; Ronan and Johnson 2005). In fact, a simplistic, linear view of PTSD (i.e. traumatic event = PTSD) will under-estimate its complexity and lead to simplistic or incomplete treatment plans.

While the concept of PTSD is useful in that it provides an orientating framework for understanding, studying and treating the trauma in children, it needs to be kept in mind that the diagnostic complications can also hinder research and clinical practice with traumatized children (Perry *et al.* 1995; Terr 1991). The experience and understanding of trauma in children differs from that of adults and care must be taken in applying conceptualizations which explain the symptoms and causes of PTSD in adults to children (Pandit and Shah 2000).

Prevalence

Population studies that have examined rates of exposure to traumatic events and PTSD in children and adolescents indicate that 15–43 per cent of girls and 14–43 per cent of boys have experienced at least one traumatic event in their lifetime; of these, 3–15 per cent of girls and 1–6 per cent of boys could be diagnosed with PTSD (Cuffe *et al.* 1998; Giacona *et al.* 1995). Other studies have reported the types of traumatic events experienced by young people, including abuse and interpersonal violence. Lifetime prevalence data from the United Kingdom (UK), United States (USA) and New Zealand show remarkable consistency in the figures for sexual abuse (10%, mostly female) and familial physical abuse (7–9%) (Cawson *et al.* 2000; Fergusson, Horwood and Lynskey 1996; Fergusson and Lynskey 1997; Finkelhor 1994; Millichamp, Martin and Langley 2006). The UK and USA studies found that at least 20 per cent of young people had experienced non-family physical assault or bullying (Cawson *et al.* 2000; Finkelhor and Dziuba-Leatherman 1994). However, the UK study found that children were most at risk in their own family and that overall they were much more at risk from physical abuse and emotional abuse than of sexual abuse. Emotional abuse included witnessing frequent violence between parents, being regularly humiliated, or told by their parents that they wished them dead or never born and serious physical neglect at home, including being left without food or having to fend for themselves because parents were absent or had drug or alcohol problems. Those from the worst off socio-economic strata were more likely to have been maltreated. However, even in the professional and managerial class, 4 per cent of respondents reported being severely physically abused. Almost no children had reported the abuse to the police, social services, teachers or other professionals. These prevalence figures provide a benchmark for practitioners in primary health care settings. Importantly, findings here are a salient reminder that young people are likely not to disclose traumatic experiences, particularly those that occur within their family homes.

Children in populations at-risk for emotional and behavioural problems have much higher rates of PTSD and other child mental health problems. Children and youth in the child protection/child welfare and youth justice systems are particularly vulnerable. Recent research in the USA has shown that nearly half of children aged 2 to 14 years with completed child welfare investigations had clinically significant emotional or behavioural problems (Burns *et al.* 2004). Studies have documented the prevalence of PTSD in abused children between 6.9 per cent and 67.3 per cent depending on the nature of the abuse (Ackerman *et al.* 1998; Deblinger *et al.* 1989; Dubner and Motta 1999; Famularo *et al.* 1994; Linning and Kearney 2004; McCloskey and Walker 1999). Overall, prevalence of PTSD is generally reported for about a third of abused children. Histories of any type of abuse can be associated with elevated symptoms, while multiple abuse more likely portends the development of PTSD (Naar-King *et al.* 2002). Of children exposed to domestic violence, tentative findings indicate that those who are solely witnesses may be somewhat less at risk of developing symptoms (about 20%) than those who are targets of physical abuse (about 40%), but children who report being both a witness and a target are highly at risk of developing PTSD (up to 100%) (McCloskey and Walker 1999). There is some evidence that sexual abuse results in higher levels of PTSD compared to physical abuse (Dubner and Motta 1999; Runyon and Kenny 2002). Children who have been jointly physically and sexually abused appear to be at greater risk for psychiatric disturbance, including PTSD (Ackerman *et al.* 1998).

Assessment

In order to assess for child trauma, particularly trauma from abuse, it is necessary to be cognizant of the range of signs, symptoms and sequelae. This section is intended to provide primary health practitioners with the symptoms and behaviours that research has found to be associated with child trauma, including child abuse trauma. It is important to bear in mind that some symptoms may be misinterpreted and others may be masked, for example, physical health complaints and cognitive processes that contribute to anxiety and trauma responses. Symptom identification in this area must be considered in conjunction with developmental, individual and contextual factors in order to understand what symptoms may mean. That is, symptoms in isolation, particularly those that might be developmentally appropriate (e.g., young children having nightmares), are less likely to point to problems in this area than a convergence of signs and symptoms. In other words, a holistic approach to assessment screening is recommended.

Unlike other child physical or mental health problems that are characterized by a distinct group of symptoms, traumatic experiences in childhood result in a wide range of manifestations. As introduced earlier, identification of trauma in children is further confounded by reporting difficulties. Children and adolescents may be reluctant to reveal symptoms or abuse based on the avoidant aspects of anxiety and PTSD, coupled with emotional responses and social motives such as guilt, shame, or a desire to maintain family relationships (Friedrich 2002). Younger children have cognitive features that may limit their ability to report on symptoms and experiences (Hewitt 1999). In addition, different types of trauma may result in particular sets of symptoms, and multiple trauma presentations may add further complexity. In order to assess whether a child may be experiencing trauma symptoms, checklists of signs and symptoms should be coupled with an assessment of risk and protective factors.

Risk and protective factors

Risk and protective factors may exacerbate or ameliorate the impact of traumatic events on children. These factors may be considered within three frameworks crucial for working with children and adolescents: developmental, individual and family and other contextual factors.

DEVELOPMENTAL

Symptoms and behaviour can vary according to the age at which the trauma occurred, and may wax and wane with development (Cicchetti and Rogosch 2002). Mindful of significant individual differences in presentation, there may be age-specific features for some symptoms. Due to the relative immaturity of their developing nervous system, younger children may be more vulnerable to PTSD and to the impact of traumatic experiences on brain development (Nemeroff 2004). This is likely to be mediated by cognitive processes. The cognitive processes typical of younger children give them less capacity to protect themselves (Famularo et al. 1994). Younger children are less able to organize events into a system that can be managed emotionally and they may re-enact their trauma repetitively through play (Terr 1991). Exposure to violence has been linked to emotional dysregulation in young children (Osofsky 1995). This inability to modulate the expression of affect in proportion to what a situation calls for can lead to subsequent difficulties, including overcontrolled affect (e.g., depression) and undercontrolled problems (e.g., behaviour problems) (Gross 1998). In adolescents, risk-taking behaviours may exacerbate problems, while protective factors such as positive peer group characteristics, school climate, other adult support and family may ameliorate the negative effects of abuse (Perkins and Jones 2004).

INDIVIDUAL

Clearly, not all children develop PTSD or evidence trauma symptoms. Protective factors may include older age and male gender. Younger children and girls have been found to be more likely than older children and boys to develop PTSD (Pfefferbaum et al. 1999; Pfefferbaum et al. 2000). Individual perceptions and coping skills also appear to influence symptom development. Some children's perception about living in unsafe circumstances may lead to depression and anxiety or behaviour problems (Buckner, Beardslee and Bassuk 2004), whereas it may not for other children (McMillan, Zuravin and Rideout 1995). The chance of a child developing PTSD as a result of trauma may be reduced by effective coping skills (Deblinger, Steer and Lippmann 1999). Notwithstanding a child's individual responses, a child's safety and wellbeing is inevitably dependent on contextual factors.

FAMILY/CONTEXTUAL

Children who are in situations where the cumulative effects of multiple risk factors outweigh protective resources are more susceptible to short- and long-term social, cognitive and psychological problems (Iwaniec, Larkin and Higgins 2006). Risk factors that may increase the likelihood of a child developing PTSD include severity and chronicity and, in the case of interpersonal violence, victimization by more than one perpetrator or someone close to them and coercion used to maintain secrecy (Browne and Finkelhor 1986; Davis and Siegel 2000; Linning and Kearney 2004). Family factors that increase risk for PTSD include lower socio-economic status, higher stress, poorer maternal mental health and more extensive family drug and alcohol use (Linning and Kearney 2004; Shipman, Rossman and West 1999). Parents in at-risk families tend to be less interactive, supportive and nurturing, and exhibit more aggression, negative affect, psychopathology, marital conflict and poorer parenting skills (Deblinger *et al.* 1999; McFarlane and Yehuda 2000). Children and adolescents with greater family support (e.g., warmth and affection, use of positive discipline, effective monitoring and supervision) and less parental distress demonstrate lower levels of PTSD (Deblinger *et al.* 1999; Pynoos *et al.* 1987).

In the case of child maltreatment, while the experience of abuse may predict psychopathology, childhood family variables may be better predictors of adjustment (Higgins and McCabe 2003). This is particularly relevant for recovery, because abused children who develop PTSD may have more psychological risk factors. The multiple risk factors frequently present in the environments of abused and neglected children limit conclusions about the specificity of effects. Children may be symptomatic if their family context is chaotic and distressing, or characterized by parental violence or the use of coercive discipline practices, even if they have not been directly physically or sexually abused (Allan, Kashani and Reid 1998). Severity of effects can be related to qualitative features of the parent–child relationship, such as interpersonal sensitivity and affective tone (Zielinski and Bradshaw 2006). Child outcomes may vary depending on the relationship between the child and the perpetrator (Putnam 2003). Abused and traumatized children may exhibit disrupted attachments with their parents or caregivers (Rogosch, Cicchetti and Aber 1995). The child's living circumstances, such as removal from home and multiple care-giving transitions may increase the risk for subsequent problems (Herrenkohl, Herrenkohl and Egolf 2003). Consequently, contextual factors not only influence the incidence of maltreatment, but may also moderate its developmental effects (Zielinski and Bradshaw 2006).

Wider contextual factors may also impact on a child's trauma experience. Culture may influence a traumatized child's mode of symptom expression and may shape the salience of the event and how it is responded to by other members of the culture (Cicchetti and Rogosch 2002). Legal and medical processes (e.g., intrusive practices) may re-trigger and exacerbate problems whereas other processes (e.g., sensitive questioning and good 'bedside' manner) may help. In other words, how we interact with children as practitioners matters.

Sequelae

Children and adolescents may develop trauma symptomatology as a result of single-incident trauma such as a motor vehicle accident or natural disaster. These symptoms may be more straightforward for primary health care practitioners to identify, as they tend to manifest following the event. If symptoms occur within one month, this is recognized as acute stress, which may or may not ameliorate with time and appropriate support. If symptoms continue beyond one month, then post-traumatic stress assessment and treatment should be considered. For children experiencing interpersonal violence and abuse, the symptom picture will generally be less clear. Reviews of research related to physical abuse, sexual abuse and child witnesses to domestic violence have found that these traumas not only vary in severity, frequency and duration, but they are modified by a range of variables, and there is no symptom picture that characterizes all abused children (Kitzmann *et al.* 2003; Putnam 2003). However, research has identified some symptom patterns associated with different abuse types. Table 10.1 has been designed to facilitate the identification of symptoms and behaviours that research has shown to be associated with particular traumatic experiences.

Table 10.1 Child symptoms and behaviours associated with traumatic experiences: single- and multiple-incident trauma, including natural disasters, accidents, health-related

Various symptom patterns linked to the major symptom criteria of acute stress disorder or post-traumatic stress disorder, including re-experiencing (e.g., nightmares, repetitive play), hyperarousal, avoidance/numbing (e.g., excessive 'daydreaming'.

In many cases and in the absence of deaths, ongoing injury, life threat, ongoing risk for more incidents, parental distress, secondary stressors (e.g., family stress), symptoms tend to reduce with time, support, resumption of normal routines.

In the event that symptoms continue to carry on past a few months, or there are multiple incidents, assessment and possible intervention is warranted.

Table 10.1 cont.

Interpersonal violence

Sexual abuse

- Commonly reported indicators include fear, sleep problems, anxiety, depression, anger, aggression, sexually inappropriate behaviour, cognitive distortions such as guilt and shame.
- Those who report intercourse have increased risk for deprssion and suicide attempts in adolescence (Fergusson, Horwood and Lynskey 1996).
- In a sample of non-clinically referred children, 63% met criteria for at least one psychiatric diagnosis and 30% met criteria for two or more, including 21% with PTSD (McLeer, Dixon and Henry 1998).

Physical abuse

- Interpersonal difficulties including insecure patterns of attachment and peer relationships.
- Aggression and behavioural problems.
- Cognitive and academic impairment.
- Suicidal and risk-taking behaviour.
- Trauma-related emotional problems such as anger, guilt, shame and psychological problems including depression, anxiety, PTSD, conduct disorder, attention deficit/hyperactivity disorder (ADHD) and substance abuse.
- Approximately 8% have current diagnoses of major depressive disorder (MDD); 6.9–42% meet criteria for PTSD (Deblinger *et al.*, 1989; Dubner and Motta 1999; McCloskey and Walker 1999).

Witnessing domestic violence

- The majority of child witnesses to DV (63%) show poorer outcomes compared to the average child (Kitzmann *et al.* 2003). Outcomes worsen with the amount and severity of the violence.
- Externalizing problems including aggression and conduct disorders and internalizing problems such as withdrawal, depression and anxiety and trauma symptoms through to diagnosable PTSD (McCloskey and Walker 1999).
- Younger children are more likely to exhibit somatic complaints and experience greater distress.
- Increased risk of physical abuse, emotional/psychological abuse and neglect.

Emotional abuse

- Emotional instability, social impairment, learning difficulties, physical health problems, internalizing and externalizing behaviours, suicidality and psychiatric diagnoses.
- Verbal abuse and emotional neglect have negative effects on children's feelings and ideas about enjoyment of living, purpose in life and prospects and expectations for the future.
- Hostile verbal abuse is similar to physical abuse in the negative impact on children and psychologically unavailable care-taking may be the most devastating of all maltreatment forms.
- A recent study found emotional abuse (including that perpetrated by family *and* peers, including bullying) was the strongest predictor of the severity of PTSD symptoms in a sample of adolescent inpatients with a reported history of a range of abuse types (Sullivan, Lipschitz and Grilo 2006).

Neglect

- Neglect is an act or omission that results in impaired physical functioning, injury, or development.
- Neglectful supervision or abandonment can impact on attachment security and emotional, social and cognitive development.
- Failure to be given the necessities of life can cause physical growth delays, adverse brain development and other neuropsychological outcomes.

Multiple abuse

- More susceptible to short- and long-term social, cognitive and psychological problems (Iwaniec *et al.*, 2006).
- Witnessing violence and/or psychological abuse predicts anxious/depressed problems; child psychological and physical abuse together predict aggressive behaviour.

Treatment

Therapists who treat child trauma should be able to describe a coherent theoretical rationale and the research evidence upon which their therapy approach is based. In addition, we feel it is quite important for treatment practitioners to be able to demonstrate the effectiveness of their own approach through the use of simple evaluation techniques (e.g., Feather and Ronan 2006; Ronan and Johnston 2005). The theoretical and research literature elucidates the mechanisms that explain the impact of traumatic experiences on physical, cognitive, emotional and behavioural features, and evidence-based treatments that ameliorate these effects. The following section provides a brief summary of the theory and research that has contributed to the current models of child trauma treatment, in order to assist primary health care practitioners to communicate with therapists and make appropriate referrals for children and families.

Theoretical models and treatment outcome research

The trauma model that has its roots in psychoanalysis and psychodynamic theories emphasizes the importance of the therapeutic relationship for healing and the use of expressive therapies for facilitating trauma processing. Likewise, cognitive behavioural therapy (CBT) approaches highlight the importance of a collaborative therapeutic relationship, as well as use of creative applications of the model, particularly when working with children (Kendall *et al.* 1992). These ideas underpin the ultimate aim of the therapist and child (and parent/caregivers) working together with a range of modalities to alleviate symptoms and enhance coping such that the child will think, feel and behave differently in the present and the future, beyond the experience and effects of abuse.

Models of clinical practice in the field of child trauma and abuse have a tradition of integrating a number of theoretical approaches and perspectives (Macdonald, Lambie and Simmonds 1995). These practical process-based models of therapy are derived from various frameworks including systems theory, attachment theory, family therapy, narrative therapy, and may be informed by developmental, feminist and empowerment perspectives. The social and cultural context of the abuse is taken into account; for example, with regard to ensuring social support and planning for safety. CBT techniques are often utilized to deal with negative effects of abuse such as unhelpful behaviours, emotions, beliefs or physical symptoms.

Behavioural models provide a clearly delineated rationale for the analysis of variables maintaining trauma symptoms and for treatment elements including anxiety management, social modelling, practice and use of exposure to treat trauma. Cognitive models provide a rationale for cognitive restructuring methods such as 'coping self-talk' and gradual imaginal and *in vivo* exposure techniques that enable integration of trauma memories as a coherent whole that can be assimilated. More recent cognitive approaches, such as cognitive science and memory theories, provide a rationale for verbal as well as non-verbal trauma processing modalities, in order to address both explicit and implicit memories. Neurobiological theories reinforce the need to address physiological responses to trauma, such as hyperarousal and dissociation, as well as emotional, cognitive and behavioural reactions. Constructivist narrative approaches seem particularly applicable to children, with an emphasis not only on resolving past trauma, but also on creating a new narrative for life.

In addition, it is evident from theory and research that contextual factors play a significant role in how traumatic effects play out in a person's life. Therapists working with children and families should take account of developmental age and stage, attachment and family relationships, cultural world views, support systems, treatment needs of the parents themselves and the involvement of other professionals and agencies. Clearly, therapy should be planned and conducted within the context of an ecological approach. Local models of clinical practice that have been developed to cater for particular social and cultural needs may be combined with evidence-based approaches from elsewhere to ensure best outcomes for traumatized children and their families (Murupaenga, Feather and Berking 2004).

Child treatment outcome research has lagged behind that of adults. Adult outcome literature provides a rationale for focused assessment, agreement on therapy goals and tailoring therapy to the problems identified. These ideas are echoed in overall recommendations for child treatment (Cohen, Berliner and Mannarino 2003). For child trauma, initial support has been found for the usefulness of anxiety management techniques, systematic desensitization and gradual exposure approaches (e.g. Farrell, Haines and Davies 1998; Saigh 1987). For abuse-related trauma, phase-based approaches are generally rec- ommended, with a focus on symptom reduction and stabilization, trauma-processing and life integration (Briere and Scott 2006), including with children (Deblinger and Heflin 1996). Trauma-related attachment problems may be addressed by the therapist providing a secure base from which both children and caregivers can explore new ways of relating (Pearce and Pezzot-Pearce 1994).

To date, child and adolescent treatment outcome research findings have supported CBT in particular to be efficacious over a range of child problems. Notably, efficacy and effectiveness studies support the usefulness of CBT for anxiety disordered children (Barrett *et al.* 2001; Kendall 1994), and TF-CBT (trauma-focused CBT) for children with PTSD from sexual abuse (Cohen and Mannarino 1997; Deblinger *et al.* 1999) and physical abuse (Feather and Ronan 2004, 2006). TF-CBT treatment outcome research has extended this protocol to community clinic settings and multiple-abuse with good results (Cohen *et al.* 2004; Feather and Ronan 2006). TF-CBT is designed for children and adolescents from about nine years of age, who are developmen- tally able to manage the cognitive elements of the approach.

Younger children and those who have trauma histories that are early and long-standing may have a lack of words to convey thoughts and emotions and an inability to differentiate self from non-self (Perry *et al.* 1995). These children are likely to benefit from expressive approaches that use play as a basis for psychotherapy. These approaches have received less research atten- tion, but are widely used clinically to address abuse and trauma in children. Play therapy models have been found to help children make sense of experi- ences of trauma and abuse (Cattanach 1992). Release play therapy for 3–10 year old children with PTSD has shown positive and promising clinical results (Kaduson 2006). The usefulness of art therapy techniques such as drawings of self and family, life maps and clay work for children with trauma and abuse histories has been documented (Gil 2006; Kaduson and Schaefer 2004). Empirical evidence shows that sandplay therapy can reduce presenting symptoms and increase insight and understanding in children who have been abused (Grubbs 1994) and exposed to violence (Parson 1997) by enabling children to play out traumatic situations in consecutive sand trays.

Child trauma researchers have found that in clinical settings treatment may extend to as many as 40 or more sessions depending on the needs of the child and the complexity of the case (Deblinger and Heflin 1996). However, research on briefer therapy protocols, including for child abuse trauma, indicate that in many cases far fewer sessions can produce clinically significant change (Cohen et al. 2004). Specific factors affecting treatment outcome include the severity, chronicity and type of trauma experienced, as well as age of exposure, current age and stage of development and parent/caregiver involvement (Feather and Ronan 2006). Importantly, the literature suggests that treatment protocols need to be developmentally appropriate to the child, encompass parent/caregiver psychoeducation and facilitate caregiver support of the child's therapy (Cohen, Mannarino and Deblinger 2006; Deblinger and Heflin 1996).

Treatment illustration

To illustrate an evidence-based treatment for child trauma, a TF-CBT treatment programme will be presented (Feather and Ronan 2006). It was developed in a local clinical setting for multiply-abused 9–15 year old children with PTSD. The programme is set out in a 16-session format, with regular scheduled parent/caregiver sessions. The treatment sessions are described in a manual which is designed to be flexible to cater for the range of issues which may present and to be adaptable to different developmental stages (Feather and Ronan 2004). An introduction to the manual provides a rationale for the treatment elements.

To summarize the approach here, the treatment is phased, with each phase emphasizing important elements identified in the theoretical and empirical literature, complemented with aspects from local clinical practice: *Phase 1* focuses on developing the therapeutic relationship and psychosocial strengthening, including relationships with parent/caregivers and social support. *Phase 2* is derived from the efficacious CBT programme for anxiety disordered children developed by Kendall and colleagues (Kendall et al. 1990) and helps the child develop coping skills based on a four-step coping template, 'The STAR Plan'. *Phase 3* is based on a gradual exposure procedure for processing and resolving trauma, derived from behavioural and cognitive models and utilizing expressive therapy modalities such as sand-play and art therapy. *Phase 4* provides a transition to life beyond therapy; any issues that are so far unresolved are addressed, a narrative emphasis is incorporated to help the child to create a new future to step into, and relapse prevention is covered. Booster sessions are offered if required.

The treatment manual is designed to be used flexibly. For example, some children may not need all sessions, or may cover therapy elements more quickly, whereas others may take longer to work through the sessions and/or require booster sessions, depending on their characteristics and context. The consistent therapy session structure enables the process of therapy to be more predictable and allows for frequent summaries and opportunities for feedback from the child. The emphasis on collaborative empiricism enables the therapist and child to form hypotheses or ideas about what might help him manage his symptoms and feel better. The child tests these in and out of the sessions, reviewing progress week by week. In this way, the therapy is designed to facilitate the generalization of in-session therapeutic change to everyday situations that the child encounters, to ensure better outcomes and reduce relapse.

A key consideration in treating PTSD as opposed to anxiety is that anxiety is typically about current and future threat whereas PTSD, while an anxiety disorder, also has much to do with a past event(s). Children who have PTSD are processing trauma and/or its sequelae in a way that often involves not only ongoing distress but also ongoing reminders (Ehlers and Clark 2000). Hence, the aim of a treatment programme for PTSD needs to be to help children develop skills to manage their symptoms and to process trauma so that it is seen as a time-limited past event(s) that can be managed effectively by the child and his family/caregivers, coupled with a focus on current and future concerns. A CBT approach holds that gradual exposure is an optimal strategy for reducing PTSD symptoms (Kendall *et al.* 1992). This can be achieved in a number of ways, including using creative media to create a trauma narrative and desensitization to trauma triggers in a safe therapeutic environment (Yule, Smith and Perrin 2005). The therapist helps the child to learn that he can approach his fears and not experience the feared consequences, leading to an overall reduction in anxiety and trauma symptoms in everyday life.

Adapting a treatment for abused children involves special considerations. Child abuse invariably affects the relationships children have with their family members and means the involvement of helping professionals in the child's life. Many children who come to the attention of child protection services are placed in care to ensure their safety, including a number of children who have been treated with this protocol. Removal from parents adds another layer of trauma for these children and necessitates forming new relationships with caregivers and addressing attachment-related concerns. Abuse-informed issues are incorporated in the treatment, such as psychoeducation about abuse and personal safety, and emotional processing of guilt, blame, anger, separation, grief and loss, as recommended in practice guidelines (Saunders, Berliner and Hanson 2004). Finally, the inclusion of parents or caregivers in interventions is recommended to help the child generalize gains to their everyday lives following therapy.

The TF-CBT protocol has been evaluated using a single-case design research approach, as recommended and employed by clinical researchers for the initial testing of a new manualized treatment protocol (Kane and Kendall 1989; Kazdin 2000). Results have been promising in reducing PTSD symptoms and increasing coping in a group of clinically referred children with diagnosed PTSD who represent a range of trauma and abuse presentations and cultural world views (Feather and Ronan 2006; Feather *et al.* 2007). This research may provide a template for other clinicians who seek to provide evidence-based treatment in their own local clinical settings.

A couple of final reminders for health practitioners:

1. If a screening suggests trauma and/or abuse, referral to a trusted therapist is warranted for assessment and possible treatment.

2. Those therapists who might be most trusted would have some of the following attributes:

   a. They would welcome questions about their practice.

   b. They would have information on their overall approach, including supportive research findings, how long they have been using the approach and with how many clients, their training and experience and so forth (see Table 10.1 for more information).

   c. They would show a willingness to:

      • include parents/caregivers in the assessment and intervention

      • use evidence-supported assessment and intervention practice

      • monitor progress of their interventions and share that information with clients and referring health practitioners.

Part 3

Strategic Interventions in and Beyond Primary Health Care

Chapter Eleven

Proactive in Protection: A Public Health Approach to Child Protection

Lindsay Ferguson

Introduction

This chapter describes a public health approach that uses proactive, organization-wide ways to protect children. A public health approach has the potential to improve the efficacy of responses to children's and families' needs for support and/or protection. The needs of children and how policies and public services address these needs are also described. Lazenbatt and Freeman (2006) suggest that the statistics regarding child physical abuse in the UK justify it being regarded as a public health issue across socio-economic groups.

A public health approach revitalizes and strengthens the health service commitment to preventing children coming to harm by embedding it in everyday business. Theoretically, this contrasts with traditional child protection systems, where once a potential need for child protection has been identified, it becomes someone else's responsibility. It allows for the realization of the concept of meeting the needs of a child by sharing the care; as opposed to referring or handing over the case to another agency. This approach means that children and families get the support they need much more quickly than they do now, as they wait for under-resourced statutory services to respond, as high risk cases take priority. There are illustrations of how this could change the way we work. As argued by Spencer and Baldwin (2005), this kind of approach can help to shift the balance from highly individualized and reactive responses, to one where interlinked services respond proactively in keeping children safe from harm.

The needs of children for support and/or protection

The need for a proactive and integrated approach to safeguard children in primary care is well known. In the UK, 7 per cent of children have been reported as suffering serious physical abuse by a parent or carer (Cawson *et al.* 2000) and two children under 15 years die from abuse or neglect each week (Department of Health 2003a). Public services respond to tens of thousands of suspected and actual abuse or neglect cases. Between 2006 and 2007, 56,199 children were referred to the Scottish Children's Reporter Administration, which is responsible for securing the protection of children who offend or are offended against. This represents 6.1 per cent of Scotland's children (SCRA 2007). The vast majority of these children (44,629 children) were referred on care and protection (non-offence) grounds. A total of 11,960 referrals were made to child protection services, i.e. police and social work departments (Scottish Executive 2007); 2593 (68%) children's names were put on the Child Protection Register (2.8 per 1000 population aged 0–16 years) and 49 per cent of the children named on the Child Protection Register were under the category of neglect.

The changing focus of public sector responses to children in need for support and/or protection

In 2002, a national audit of child protection services was carried out which looked at over 180 cases where children had been subjects of child protection procedures. The report's title '*It's Everyone's Job to Make Sure I'm Alright*' was a quote from one of the children whose case was examined. One of the major conclusions in the report was that children were not always getting the help they needed when they needed it. In some cases children felt no safer after having been through the child protection system (Scottish Executive 2002).

Outcomes of similar investigations conducted over the course of recent years have changed the perceived challenges related to safeguarding children. In the not too distant past children who were identified as suffering from abuse were registered on the Child Protection Register in Scotland under one of the following categories:

- physical abuse
- sexual abuse
- emotional abuse
- neglect
- failure to thrive.

This abuse-focused labelling then made way to a classification approach emphasizing perilous characteristics in the children's immediate social network. Categories now focused on parental behaviours and mental states:

- cyclical abuse
- substance misuse
- domestic violence
- parental mental ill-health
- parental learning or physical disability.

Today, professionals and policies tend to frame challenges in safeguarding children in broader societal issues:

- violence, criminal and gender-based
- societal stressors, poverty
- sexualization of children
- child pornography and internet risk
- inadequate or protectionist parenting
- young carers
- asylum seekers and trafficked children
- migrant workforce
- unhealthy and dangerous environments.

Challenges for the National Health Service

The reports of inspection of child protection services that have taken place since 2007 are available on Her Majesty's Inspectorate of Education homepage (HMIE 2007) and have indicated that particular issues for health services are:

- health care workers have not been involved consistently
- information sharing not reliable
- staffing issues in some areas
- risk assessment, care planning and decision making generally poor
- record keeping and use of chronologies of significant events, health factors, etc., needs improvement
- longer-term sustained interventions required
- roles need clarification.

It is clear that for some time various health care professionals have struggled with role definition (Appleton 1996) and with meeting expectations (Crisp and Lister 2004). A study reported in *Growing Support* (Scottish Executive 2003d) found practitioners across agencies agreed on what makes children and families vulnerable, but there was less agreement on when they should intervene. No single group accepted the main responsibility for enabling the most vulnerable families to engage positively with universal services. Health services were therefore forced to rethink their strategies and to develop new approaches to safeguarding children in primary health care and beyond.

The Health Service's response to meeting children's safeguarding needs

These gradual shifts in focus have resulted in the safeguarding of children being framed more and more as a public health concern. Many of the issues that are now perceived to be central to the safeguarding of children are central to primary health care provision in general. Indeed, under the Children (Scotland) Act 1995, health care professionals are obliged to co-operate with local authorities (i.e. social care) who hold the statutory duty to protect children. Of course, this should be done in the most effective way possible. Various steps have already been taken within the health care sector to accommodate this fresh take on safeguarding children. Key among these steps was the development of professionals' capacities and capabilities and the provision of guidelines and protocols.

Key health professionals involved in safeguarding children

In Scotland the health service is organized into 14 health boards which provide services in the acute and community sectors. Each one has a Child Health Commissioner (Scottish Executive 2003c) whose role is crucial in the strategic planning of all health and integrated services for children including child protection (see Chapter 12).

Over the last decade, health boards have developed child protection services and now there is a growing workforce of child protection nurses across Scotland. Some areas have given midwives, mental health and emergency care nurses a special role in child protection, and in others GPs and dentists have taken a lead role. In the larger urban areas, link public health nurses have been recruited who continue to carry caseloads while supporting their colleagues with child protection cases.

In Scotland, public health nurses (health visitors and school nurses) take a lead role in child protection. They have developed skills and enhanced their roles in working with children and families suffering violence, abuse and neglect. Specialist nurses who have postgraduate qualifications in childcare and protection provide training and support to the workforce. They work closely with designated lead clinicians and lead executive officers for child protection in each NHS board and with members of multi-agency Child Protection Committees in each local authority area.

Guidelines, protocols and policies

In general, health policy in Scotland promotes health improvement and wellbeing rather than treating disease (Scottish Government 2007a). A preventative child-centred approach (Scottish Executive 2007a) was chosen addressing childhood illness and the circumstances that children and young people live in that affect their long-term health prospects. It promotes inter-agency working and integrated services, and demands that all organizations involved in providing services collaborate with Local Safeguarding Children Boards to provide the support for children to fulfil their potential in terms of health and general wellbeing. A series of guidelines, policies and protocols reflect this development.

Guidelines for health care workers in NHS Scotland in responding to domestic abuse

Scottish Executive (2003a) brought a necessary focus on working with families where abuse was suspected. It emphasized the need for a proactive approach, using open-questioning methods and adopting a non-judgemental approach. Unfortunately, it was not accompanied by an implementation or monitoring process to ensure compliance with the recommendations. However, through local domestic abuse strategy groups, emphasis has been put on the need for training for all practitioners in the identification of children suffering from the impact of domestic abuse and on various multi-agency initiatives to share information and plan effective interventions. Concern about the consequences of parental drug and alcohol abuse for children also led to concentrated action across the disciplines.

Protocols for practice have been developed to follow the recommendations of *Getting Our Priorities Right* (Scottish Executive 2003b), which defines key practice points for health practitioners working with families in which substance misuse is a problem. *Hidden Harm – the Next Steps* (Scottish Executive 2006b) sets out actions being carried forward to reduce the risk of harm caused by parental substance misuse. These protocols are being audited as part of multi-agency self-evaluation, expected to play an integral role in organizational quality assurance systems in preparation for multi-agency inspections. These inspections were introduced as part of the Child Protection Reform Programme. This programme produced a Children's Charter and A Framework for Standards for Child Care and Protection against which services can be measured (Scottish Executive 2004a).

Implementation of Health for All Children (Scottish Executive 2003f) provides a system of screening, surveillance and health promotion for all children, but also identifies the need to target the most vulnerable. The focus is on prevention and early intervention, working with other agencies and agreeing shared measurable outcomes for families and their children. Soon after birth the needs of every child and family are to be assessed and a care programme appropriate to their needs set up, which may be defined as core, additional or intensive, relating to their needs. There have been difficulties in the implementation of this scheme. In some areas the numbers of cases requiring a high level of care are overwhelming the providers of universal services. Many of these are children require a multi-agency response, further stretching available resources.

Getting it Right for Every Child (GIRFEC) (Scottish Executive 2005a) is a major national policy, with a whole systems approach across all services that help children at all stages of need and not just those who need protection. The vision for all children being that they become successful learners, confident individuals, effective contributors and responsible citizens. To do this they need to be:

- safe
- healthy
- achieving
- nurtured
- active
- responsible and respected
- included.

This policy involves the devolvement of a substantial degree of decision making to frontline practitioners within an organization. It relies on universal services (health and education services) providing support, anticipatory care and early intervention for children and families so that social workers can concentrate on their statutory duties. The health service has an important role in this as a provider of universal and specialist services.

In England, a similar approach has been adopted under the *Every Child Matters, Change for Children* initiative (Department for Education and Skills 2004a). The aim of this approach being for every child to have the support they need to:

- be healthy
- stay safe
- enjoy and achieve
- make a positive contribution
- achieve economic wellbeing.

Community involvement in safeguarding children

Empowering and enabling health care professionals, however, is only one part of improving support and protection for children. It is equally important to revitalize communities to work with agencies to reduce child abuse and neglect (Pecora, Wittaker and Maluccio 2006). Various examples of the benefit of community involvement have already been made public. For instance, the *NEWPIN project* (Pound and Mills 1985) provides intensive parent education in a whole-community approach that puts child protection in the hands of individuals, families, communities and government jointly. Another project, *Neighbourhood Mapping For Children's Safety*, was carried out in Craigmillar, Edinburgh where it was suggested that child protection strategies are more effective when the needs of the community and the nature of harm children can suffer in that community are fully understood (Nelson and Baldwin 2004).

Other initiatives involve the private and voluntary sectors supported by health practitioners, as described by Davies (2004), who argues that professional child protection responses can be informed by using the intelligence available through the establishment of community networks of responsible adults. This approach was supported by Lord Laming (2003), whose opinion was that the 'eyes and ears' of the community should be used more where children may be known to be in need.

The coming together of agencies and communities to provide easily accessible services for all the people living in the community regardless of their social status is important in the fight to raise children out of poverty. Some studies suggest that there are strong links between poverty and child abuse in relation to adults drifting in to poverty as a result of an abusive childhood. However, this is a complicated process influenced by, among other factors, family circumstances, lack of nurturing and neglect (Frederick and Goddard 2007).

When any person is concerned about the welfare of a child in Scotland they can refer to the police who have Child Protection Teams in place. This is most likely to happen in an emergency. Alternatively, the person can refer to the local authority social work department. Whatever the source of the referral, the case would be discussed and investigations would be carried out. In an emergency, a legal order may be sought to remove the child to a place of safety or a multi-agency child protection case conference may be called where decisions can be made as to whether the child's name should be put on the Child Protection Register (an alert system that allows for information to be shared across organizations on a need to know basis) and under what category. A child protection plan must be agreed and a lead person named to co-ordinate the work to reduce or remove any risk to the child.

However, it is also possible for anyone to refer a child to the Children's Reporter in the area, whose responsibility is to make enquires and decide if 'Compulsory Measures of Supervision' (Children (Scotland) Act) are required. If this is the case, a Children's Panel is convened presided over by trained lay people. The result of this can be an application to a Sheriff's Court for an order, which would carry conditions such as where the child should live. A child would be subject to this order for up to 12 months, with regular reviews and possible renewal. These processes can run concurrently when a child is at serious risk. The multi-agency team working with such cases may include practitioners from statutory and non-statutory agencies.

A public health approach to protecting children

A public health approach focuses on the whole population, not just the diagnosis and treatment of disease, seeing the importance of prevention and early intervention at primary, secondary and tertiary levels. An example of this is where domestic abuse is regarded as a public health issue and has led to routine enquiry of all women who attend health services in parts of the United States of America as to whether this is an issue for them (Landenburger, Campbell and Rodriguez 2004). This has raised awareness in the health service and in the general public, allowing for earlier intervention.

The three levels of prevention can be applied to protecting the health and wellbeing of children (Sidebotham 2003). They also fit into the framework already in place for child health screening and surveillance. This is illustrated in a continuum of care as shown in Figure 11.1, which shows the range of inputs for children at present which can be used to review children's wellbeing and needs for support or protection. The continuum of care is not necessarily a purely sequential process. The entry point to secondary or tertiary prevention

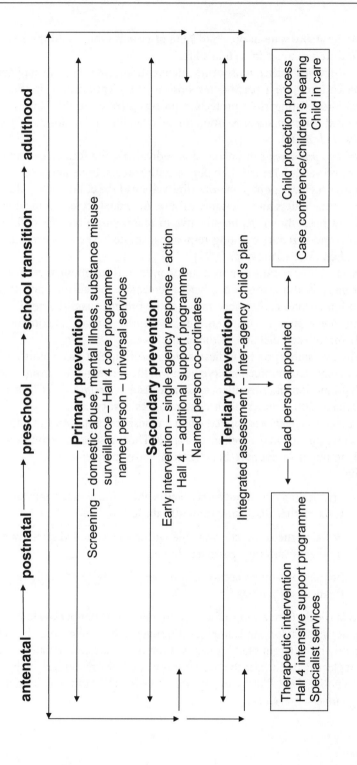

Figure 11.1 Continuum of care for children and families to improve or maintain health and wellbeing to optimize outcomes for children

may occur at any time in the child's life or even pre-birth and the level may vary at different times in a child's life.

As discussed earlier, most of the interventions carried out to support and protect children are a reactive response to the identification of abuse and referral into existing child protection processes (Keys 2007). However, it is recognized that primary prevention can help families to care for their children (Pecora *et al.* 2006).

Primary prevention can be aimed at individuals, families or communities. Primary prevention for children begins with antenatal care and screening for circumstances that might jeopardize the welfare of the child, such as domestic abuse, mental illness and substance misuse. Antenatal screening for domestic abuse has been shown to be effective in identifying potential child abuse pre-birth and to reduce the long-term impact of domestic violence and abuse on children (McFarlane *et al.* 1992)

Primary prevention opportunities continue throughout the child's life with family health assessments, health screening and surveillance. Primary prevention enables early interventions to be provided and the need for secondary prevention to be identified, with the aim of maximizing the well-being of each member of the family.

The assessment process indicates the level of support each family requires. Families requiring minimal intervention would receive the core programme of health promotion and surveillance, as prescribed in *Health for All Children* (Hall and Elliman 2003), unless their circumstances change.

Secondary prevention is applied when it is suspected that stresses within the family may impact on the welfare of a child. Those assessed as requiring additional or intensive support benefit from early interventions, which could include:

- practical advice about safety tactics and information about services for a mother disclosing domestic abuse

- utilizing the resources available within the extended family when a mother is suffering postnatal depression

- helping parents to access debt or benefits advice when there are financial difficulties.

This is particularly relevant to the need to reduce the number of children suffering neglect. Taylor and Daniel (2005) suggest that neglect may be defined differently by different practitioners. Children who are emotionally or physically neglected, or both (as the two logically interlink), rarely seek help; others need to notice them. This is an important role for all health practitioners providing universal services.

Tertiary prevention is required when an assessment of need indicates thera-peutic, educational or social input is needed for the child and/or family to help them regain and maintain an optimal level of health and wellbeing. Via an integrated assessment of need for children a child's plan is agreed and a lead professional is identified with the appropriate skills, knowledge and compe-tencies to facilitate measures to meet the child's needs. In very complex cases when the child's health needs are a priority, the lead professional is likely to be a health care professional.

A public health approach towards safeguarding of children

The approach proposed here builds on the concepts of primary, secondary and tertiary prevention. It also suggests a structure that makes effective use of health service resources. It aims at building capability and capacity across the workforce to share the care and protection of children through the application of public health approaches as described above.

The proposed approach (Figure 11.2) is based on principles of children's rights, empowerment of children and families and enablement of the workforce. It is supported by two conceptual structures, accountability and support. It promotes clear lines of accountability within health and across other agencies in terms of working together. In order to facilitate the taking and monitoring of accountabilities it also supports professionals in the form of training, supervision and effective management at all levels.

The approach is based on the premise that anyone can notice children who are not growing up in safety and can act effectively to safeguard children if they are enabled to do so through training and support from their commu-nity. Sidebotham (2003) suggests that the signs of abuse can be 'easily recog-nized by either professionals or lay persons and could be used to trigger further investigation and action' (p.42).

This approach is enabling. Frontline practitioners support families to meet their own needs and facilitate their access to specialist services. Practitioners in universal services provide the preventative and anticipatory care for families and use all the resources available to them to meet the needs of families and only share the care with statutory agencies (social work) when they can no longer meet all the needs.

Operationalization

The practical application of such an approach is dependent on three inter-woven factors:

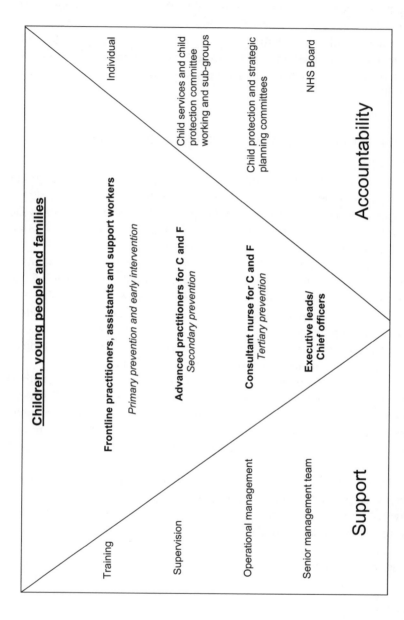

Figure 11.2. A model for working with children and families for Health Boards

1. The centre of the triangle is the skilled workforce of frontline, advanced and consultant practitioners who are enabled to support children and families by the empowering and committed ethos of the organization.

2. Practical support for the workforce in the form of:

   • robust education and training programme at pre- and post-registration levels on family functioning, risk assessment and decision making in practice

   • strong management and management systems

   • support and clinical supervision.

3. Clear lines of accountability throughout the organization and the inter-agency structures.

Workforce

The literature suggests that health practitioners have a role in the identification of children and families in need of support and/or protection, from primary prevention through to therapeutic intervention. This approach relies on the development of consultant and advanced practitioners as described in the *Career Framework for Health* (Scottish Executive 2006c). An integrated assessment is becoming the normal process for a child whose needs require the involvement of more than one agency. If specific health needs are identified, the advanced practitioner supports the practitioner identified as the lead professional, or in complex cases might fulfil that role of lead professional. The consultant practitioner advises strategic multi-agency forums such as child protection committees, domestic abuse strategy groups and drug and alcohol action teams. Working with service managers, the practitioner would be responsible for ensuring a structure is in place for support and supervision and that there are clear lines of accountability.

Training and education

Research suggests that some health professionals are reluctant to become involved in protecting children because of possible repercussions (Hall and Elliman 2003), or are inhibited by hierarchical structures and disapproval of senior colleagues (Nayda 2004). Some staff are unable to act appropriately because of their lack of experience; for example, student nurses may not have the skills to respond appropriately to children's needs (Jackson 2005) so need to be supported in practice.

To develop practice a structured programme of training is required. This can be provided through existing training programmes, making them available to a wider audience. This could include all health staff working with children, young people and families in children's or adult services.

It is sometimes assumed that inter-agency training is more effective in improving multi-agency working, however assessment of the impact of these programmes is still quite crude and requires more development. Murphy (2004, p.139) states that, 'Inter-agency training is a central contributor to the creation and maintenance of inter-agency collaboration' and he recommends the use of the standards proposed by Shardlow *et al.* (2004). These are a basis for the design of such programmes although Taylor and Daniel (2006) do recognize that to 'link educational standards to operational standards is highly complex' (p.181).

Lines of accountability

It is essential that health practitioners and managers understand where their boundaries of responsibility and accountability lie in protecting children. This should be clearly stated in job descriptions. All health and social care workers are accountable to the public and professionally to their employers. Multi-agency teams, however, require practitioners to be accountable jointly to children and families, alongside their colleagues in other agencies.

Supervision

Marcellus (2005) argues that practitioners working with families must be able to reflect on their practice and acknowledge ethical dilemmas. They need to have an understanding of the complexity of family functioning and dynamics to enable them to intervene at the earliest opportunity to prevent the child's circumstances deteriorating. They also need to have an understanding of the impact their interventions.

A structure of supervision, support and advice should be in place to enable and facilitate practitioners at all levels to make decisions on the best way to meet the needs of children and families. The process of supervision should enable practitioners to demonstrate positive outcomes in their work with children and families through good-quality assessment, care plans and evaluation. A supervisory relationship should be negotiated and agreed by all parties to support effective supervision and reflective practice (Fowler and Chevannes

1998). This process should be linked to performance management and quality assurance processes to demonstrate practitioners' fitness for practice.

Working with families where there is violence and abuse can be highly emotive and requires practitioners to reflect on their own attitudes to family violence and abuse, and to understand how they can facilitate positive change for children and families (Landenburger *et al.* 2004). It is essential that practitioners are supported in order to develop the confidence and competence to fulfil their roles in this most challenging area of work. In a study of 20 serious case reviews Brandon, Dodsworth and Rumball (2005) identified that practitioners were more able to use their professional discretion when they received good support, supervision and training.

Management

It is essential that all managers are committed to the ethos of rights-based enabling care and receive appropriate training along with practitioners. Managers should oversee the workload, workforce and performance of practitioners in acute and community services. Primary health care organizations should have structures in place to include all services, such as dentists, pharmacists and GPs, in these processes.

Protection of children and young people must be embedded in quality assurance, clinical governance and performance management processes. Practitioners must be engaged in self-evaluation systems and inspections for child protection, working to meet the quality indicators set out in guidance such as the *Quality Improvement Framework for Children and Young People and Their Families* (Scottish Executive 2006d).

Inter-agency working

The need for adequate resources and effective inter-agency working are emphasized by Lazenbatt and Freeman (2006), who suggest that health practitioners: 'should become accountable and not fear the challenge to historical working practices by crossing traditional boundaries' (p.232). Although health practitioners are to be encouraged to intervene early where a child may suffer harm, in many cases they cannot do this alone as they either do not have the skills, knowledge and competencies or statutory powers. They therefore need to work collaboratively with other practitioners in statutory or voluntary agencies (Charles and Stevenson 1991).

Statham (2004) suggests that a multi-agency holistic approach should be used, with strong links between services for children and adults. The following three examples demonstrate how a public health approach could work:

1. A two-year-old girl whose mother has learning disabilities has delayed development in communication and social skills. She is referred to a speech and language therapist. Through therapy, the communication skills of the parents and child are improved and attachment is enhanced. Thus, the child is more likely to reach her potential.

2. A community nurse visits a patient to dress a leg ulcer. The patient tells her that she is worried about her daughter, who she suspects is being abused by her partner. She also fears for the safety of her grandchildren. The nurse gives information regarding available services. She also offers to meet the daughter and give her a chance to talk about the situation. She makes plans, as appropriate, as well as informing other practitioners involved with the family. If the risk to the children appears to be high she also refers them to the child protection services.

3. The play area on a housing estate is subject to vandalism. This discourages parents from allowing their children to play there. A parent complains to a public health nurse about the situation. This leads to a community meeting taking place and a plan being agreed, which enables the parents to write to the local authority and engage with elected officials to seek a solution.

Despite its potential, however, it is generally accepted that there are organizational and professional barriers to effective inter-agency working (Murphy 2004) and 'the best forms of co-ordination tend to occur where inter-agency working is embedded in strong networks of informal relationships' (Howarth and Morrison 1999, p.110). It is important to establish multi-agency agreement on formal processes and networks that facilitate collaborative working for the benefit of children and families. This is especially important in establishing clear, effective communication and information-sharing systems. Inter-agency working is enhanced through inter-agency training and by practitioners' participation in the work of child protection committees.

Conclusion

The impact of domestic abuse on children is well recognized in the literature and all health practitioners need to realize their potential to contribute to the needs for support or protection of children and families (Crisp and Lister Green 2006). Primary health care professionals, particularly, need to acknowledge that family violence should be considered a public health issue that is integral to their work (Landenburger *et al.* 2004).

Taking a public health approach has the potential to make a considerable difference to the safeguarding of children (Spencer and Baldwin 2005). To date, public health nurses take the brunt of the responsibility for protecting children in the health service. However, many other practitioners are involved and have good working relationships with children and families. One of them may be the most appropriate professional to lead on the work with a family or community to reduce risk to children.

There is considerable evidence to suggest that a shift from reactive to proactive responses to children's needs could be achieved by applying public health approaches. Barlow (2006) recognizes the need to shift from child protection to family support and improved parenting and that it should focus on the needs of individuals, families and communities. Crisp and Lister (2004) suggest that 'public health approaches will be considered to be an integral component of a truly comprehensive child protection service' (p.662).

A public health approach stimulates a new way of thinking that establishes the safeguarding of children as a mainstream health service issue. It facilitates the effective utilization of the whole health workforce to provide services for children and families. Health care professionals are trained to use holistic ecological approaches within a cultural sensitive ethos. All practitioners play a role in assessing the needs of their patients and clients in the context of their social circumstances and the community in which they live.

Chapter Twelve

The Role of the Child Health Commissioner in Safeguarding Children

Caroline Selkirk

Introduction

This chapter will outline the role of the Child Health Commissioner. It describes in detail the key components of the role and explains how it contributes to safeguarding children and young people by making sure that their agenda is prominent in the strategic plans of public sector organizations, which provide care within primary care settings. The discussion of the Child Health Commissioner's roles and responsibilities also includes an overview of measures to monitor and assess children and young people's services.

Following the introduction of the Child Health Commissioner's role and remit the use of a collaborative commissioning model will be promoted. A cyclical process to collaborative commissioning will be illustrated along with examples of resources relevant to each stage within the cycle. The collaborative commissioning cycle not only includes the processes up to the point of approval of plans and strategies but also their implementation. Importantly, it recommends the use of rapid cycle change or test of change, rather than a big bang approach.

The role of the Child Health Commissioner

The role of Child Health Commissioner in Scotland was first described in 1998 in the Acute Services Review report, which recommended that Health Boards should have a designated commissioner of services for children and that a useful dialogue between commissioners and professionals could be developed in a multi-professional forum (Scottish Office 1998).

Soon after the introduction of Child Health Commissioners, the Child Health Support Group published a position paper promoting strategy, leadership, planning, prioritization and targeting and service delivery as the key elements required to deliver a combined and integrated child health service (Child Health Support Group 2001).

In 2004, the Scottish Child Health Commissioners' Group (2004) refreshed and expanded the remit of the Child Health Commissioner to align them with the key elements suggested by the Child Health Support Group. The job description of Child Health Commissioners featured the following key roles and responsibilities: strategic planning, advising, joint working, monitoring and quality assurance and involvement. An additional heading, commissioning, has been added in this chapter. The latter was added to emphasize this key element of the Commissioner's role.

Consequently, the Child Health Commissioner contributes to the safeguarding of children by making sure there is a robust strategy in place, which identifies the needs of children and young people, advises the NHS Board on how it can improve outcomes for children, works closely with a wide range of partners in order to improve services for children, monitors progress against agreed targets, monitors the quality of service and makes sure that children and their families are involved in decisions about their care and the planning of services to improve their life chances.

The Commissioner's five key roles and responsibilities are discussed in more detail in the next section.

Strategic planning

It is the responsibility of the Child Health Commissioner to ensure that there is a health care strategy for children and young people living within the Board[5] area or receiving services from the Board. Social care providers in Scotland are required to produce a similar document (Scottish Executive 2004b) in conjunction with local partners including health, police and the voluntary sector. The relevant section of a Board's child health strategy should be reflected in this plan and indeed will often have been developed within the local partnership. This approach encourages local services and agencies to work together using their different skills and resources collectively in order to improve outcomes for children.

There are a number of aspects of children's services which are best planned at Health Board level. These will include most aspects of secondary care services such as inpatient paediatrics, child and adolescent inpatient and

---

5   Board refers to Health Board, an administrative unit within NHS Scotland.

day care and specialist services such as those provided for children with complex needs.

Scotland's population of five million requires that some services be provided at a regional or national level. Paediatrics and child health has a relatively small workforce and it is therefore important to plan well in advance for retirement of key staff. A key clinician retiring in one of the larger centres can affect the pattern of service for children across the whole of Scotland, resulting in children needing to travel further for services and in some cases as far as England.

It is for this reason that the Child Health Commissioner needs to develop a strong national network and be involved in the debate about national planning of services. In this role, commissioners have to address three key questions:

- How can we retain as many services as possible in the local community?

- How can we support other Boards to provide services for their residents?

- How do we work with the tertiary services to facilitate treatment or provide shared care, where children have to travel for a service?

Advising

The Child Health Commissioner has an independent advisory role to the NHS Board members on all aspects of children's services. This includes providing advice on proposed changes to services and resources and making recommendations about the prioritization of proposals within the Child Health Strategy. In order to be able to do this effectively the Child Health Commissioner needs to have robust and extensive networks and be well informed about the pressures facing the local service as well as the emerging political and strategic context.

In order to understand the local service the Child Health Commissioner needs to maintain an ongoing dialogue with local clinicians about how the service is performing, what developments need to take place and how to encourage the service to take a longer-term view of service planning.

Joint working

Improving health outcomes for children and young people is an inter-agency endeavour. It is only by health care professionals working together with children, young people and their families, local authorities (education, social work, criminal justice, housing), the voluntary sector, police, local businesses, local communities that children's overall life circumstances will be improved.

Most agencies recognize the importance of consistent high quality parenting and indeed across health care, local authorities and voluntary agencies staff are working with parents and carers to develop strong parenting skills. However, to be successful it is important that all agencies are using evidence-based programmes and intervention models. While this seems an obvious observation, to make this happen with every family requires agencies to work together to agree the most appropriate evidence-based model for a family and then for every service provider to use that model. Establishing this consistency across professions and disciplines in areas like child protection, sexual health, substance misuse, parenting, children with complex needs, child and adolescent mental health, etc. is difficult.

The challenge of joint working is agreeing joint objectives and outcomes and performance managing these on a multi-agency basis. The CitiStat model (Perez and Rushing 2007) described later in this section provides a model for joint accountability. This model is entirely consistent with the Council for Virginia's Future (Virginia Future Forum 2007) model, which influenced the development of 'Scotland Preforms', promoted within local authorities in Scotland. The Council for Virginia's Future is described in the Scottish National Party's (Scottish Nationalist Party 2007) manifesto as allowing cross-party and non-party engagement in developing achievable goals and includes executive statements. It sets out a clear vision for each department and agency and offers a measurable way to ensure delivery of priorities.

Monitoring and quality assurance

The Child Health Commissioner has a specific role to monitor the quality of local child health services. This can be undertaken by formal review, analysis of progress against an action plan, analysis of complaints, audit visit to services and listening to the views of patients and staff. There is little value in writing a brilliant child health strategy if there are no mechanisms in place to ensure that the service changes which have been commissioned are delivered.

The commissioning cycle described later in this chapter looks at improvement methodology, behaviour change and performance monitoring in more detail. Below is an overview of selected monitoring and quality assurance tools.

QUARTERLY MONITORING OF CHILD HEALTH STRATEGY

The recommendations in child health strategy must be monitored on a regular basis. Once a quarter is a useful frequency, as this allows sufficient time in which to expect progress, but not so long that problems around delivery go unaddressed. If recommendations have been written clearly and ideally as measures for improvement, it will be possible to produce run charts showing progress over time, for example, a run chart of waiting times for CAMHS (Child and Adolescent Mental Health Service) by month. Some areas will not be easy to measure on such a frequent basis, such as teenage pregnancy or alcohol consumption by young people. These are often produced annually by national organizations or specific data collection projects. In these cases it is important that the Child Health Commissioner takes greater note of the input measures, such as the number of sexual health clinics or drop-in sessions available for young people and their geographical distribution. Like adults, young people will use services which they trust and are easy to access. In many areas of Scotland rurality can make this particularly challenging.

SELF-ASSESSMENT TOOLS

The self-assessment is a tool used by most external inspection agencies to provide information in advance of their visit. This is a tool that allows the Child Health Commissioner and providers of local services an opportunity to review their ongoing performance, identify areas for improvement and take action. This activity should not be reserved as preparation for external visits, but as a measure of good practice on an ongoing basis.

SERVICE VISITS

The Patient Safety Leadership Walk Rounds (Frankel *et al.* 2003) advocated by the patient safety initiative is a good way of 'being seen and seeing' the service. Staff and patients usually welcome the opportunity to talk to senior staff about the service.

Service visits consist of senior strategic staff conducting regular visits to different areas of the service. They are an opportunity to meet with local and available frontline staff and inquire about a wide range of areas such as complaints, pressures on the service, patient safety, near misses and what circumstances and behaviours led to adverse events (Frankel *et al.* 2003).

AUDIT

Most large organizations have an internal audit department. Staff with expertise in audit make a valuable contribution to monitoring by checking compliance and consistency with policies and strategies. It is important to maintain consistency and quality of patient records. This not only assists in terms of patient safety – a clear record of what treatment has been given, at what time and with what outcome – but also to support the safety of children and child protection by driving up the quality of recorded information so that when relevant information is shared with social work colleagues about children who are on the child protection register or where there is cause for concern. Finally, in some cases these records will be required by the Courts as evidence in the prosecution of individuals who may have harmed a child.

PERFORMANCE MANAGEMENT AND IMPROVEMENT

TayStat is the implementation in NHS Tayside of CitiStat (Office of Chief Researcher 2006), a performance management and improvement methodology developed for the public sector in Baltimore, Maryland, USA. The pilot was evaluated by the Office of the Chief Researcher and found to be beneficial. A leaflet produced by NHS Tayside (Taylor and Selkirk 2007) describes the process in detail and is summarized within the following text.

A TayStat meeting consists of a TayStat Panel who address questions to the respondents. The respondents are the Chief Executive and Officers from the Board. The Panel are the Chairman and non-executive members of the Board. The questions may arise from the analysis of the Scrutiny Report or from the briefing note, which summarizes performance for key performance indicators against agreed targets or as trends. Questions may also relate to the content of actions carried forward from previous meetings.

The respondent may call upon supporting officers to provide detail in the response to the question. The response should not describe the problem but outline the action being taken to resolve the problem. The result of the consequent discussion is then documented as clear actions with timescales. Such actions are relentlessly followed-up at subsequent meetings until a satisfactory resolution of the problem is achieved.

The key benefits of this system are (Taylor and Selkirk 2007):

- robust scrutiny of performance
- clear accountability
- challenging culture
- sound data quality
- sound performance data
- explicit ownership/understanding
- whole-systems approach

- data linked to decisions
- focus on taking prompt and appropriate action
- preventing problems spiralling out of control
- fast resolution of issues
- explicit links between data, performance and actions agreed
- ensuring that the actions have the desired effect without adversely affecting other parts of the system
- improved service delivery
- improved health and health services for patients.

COMPLAINTS AND ROOT CAUSE ANALYSIS

The regular reviewing of complaints and records of root cause analysis are useful indicators of the quality of service. By reviewing complaints by category it is possible to identify recurrent complaints about the same or similar issues. Root cause analysis identifies issues both in terms of individual practice and systems problems.

As a Child Health Commissioner, it is important to identify where the system contributes to a poor patient experience – e.g. the building in which the service is provided is not fit for purpose or the process is unnecessarily cumbersome. 'Lean thinking' has made a significant contribution to this problem (Institute for Healthcare Improvement 2005). Processes often evolve over time with additional steps and practices being added without old and unhelpful steps being discarded. It is not uncommon when using 'lean' methodology to discover that it is possible to make the journey for the child easier and with fewer steps and to also release resources, which can be redirected to provide a greater level of service and address unmet need.

A GUIDE TO BEST PRACTICE AND INTERVENTIONS

It is often useful to produce a guide to best practice and interventions to support the Child Health Strategy. This should set out clearly the evidence base which supports your recommendations. A guide to best practice should set out the evidence for the key interventions which could be used to deliver improvement and evaluate their effectiveness and make recommendations regarding which interventions the organization should implement (see Box 12.1). The clinician's guide to applying the ten high impact changes (NHS Modernization Agency 2005) provides an excellent example of a guide to best practice and effective interventions.

This ensures that everyone understands the evidence base, can access more detail if they require it and, importantly when implementing key worker standards, that service providers are clear that their service will be judged against the Complex Care Network United Kingdom key worker standards.

Box 12.1 Key workers for children with complex needs

When considering the introduction of key workers for children with complex needs, service providers should consult the work carried out by the University of York Social Policy Research Unit and in particular an article *Care Coordination and Key Worker Services for Disabled Children in the UK* (Greco, Sloper and Barton 2004). Also, they should be referred to the key worker standards published by the Care Co-ordination Network UK (Care Co-ordination Network 2004).

Involvement

In order to create a strong collaborative commissioning cycle it is important to increase the level of involvement from children, young people and their families in the discussion about improving services to better meet their needs. It is also vital to create a climate where there are strong clinical leaders who are working and advocating for improvements in services for children and young people. Those wishing to make significant improvements in life chances for children must not only look at access to health and social services but also housing, employment, educational opportunities and building strong communities that value and support children. Therefore to be successful we must have excellent working relationships and joint objectives with key partners including local authorities, the voluntary sector, colleges, universities and local businesses.

There are a number of vehicles that can be used to gather the views of children, young people and their families. These include:

- *Existing groups.* Schools councils, young peoples groups, community projects already working with young people, IT links and young people's websites, e.g. cool2talk or Dialogue Youth, Scottish Youth Parliament, parent-teacher groups.

- *Additional opportunities.* Direct contact with children using health services, e.g. interviews done by child protection, Her Majesty's Inspectorate of Education (HMIE) visits.

- *Surveys.* Patient satisfaction surveys, annual general practice (GP, family physicians) surveys: all GP practices are part of a scheme called the Quality Outcomes Framework (QOF). This requires them to have an annual review of patient experience.

- *Workers already working with children, young people and their families.* Improving the health of children is a multi-agency endeavour. Partners include: local authorities, universities, the voluntary sector and where appropriate the private sector.

A strong involvement culture will see not only the involvement of children, young people and their families, but managers and clinical staff who welcome and actively seek participation from the public. Managed Clinical Networks (Scottish Executive 2007b) have provided one mechanism to encourage this dialogue but Open Space events also provide opportunities for engagement.

Commissioning

Commissioning is the process through which organizations such as NHS Boards arrange for appropriate services to be provided for its population (NHS Tayside Board 2007). Services are commissioned from the service delivery part of its organization or, where appropriate, from another service provider. This will typically be through an annual commissioning plan, strategy, service level agreement or other contract. This model can be used by other public sector organizations and also for multi-agency commissioning.

The commissioning process must provide opportunities for children and their families, the public, clinicians, managers and key partners to influence the Board's commissioning plan. A commissioning plan needs to be based on an understanding of the problem and describe the outcome that needs to be achieved.

It is the role of the Child Health Commissioner to commission the services for the local population. In NHS Tayside this will be for 83,000 children under 18 years of age, living within three local authority areas.[6] This includes commissioning activities that will deliver government targets, e.g. ensuring that 80 per cent of all three- to five-year-old children are registered with an NHS dentist by 2010/11 (Scottish Government 2007a). It is the

---

6   Administrative units of regional governments; data provided by Phyllis Easton NHS Tayside.

responsibility of the commissioner to deliver effective services, which can be shown to result in the desired improvement.

Experience has shown that a collaborative commissioning approach is best suited to achieve effective service delivery and desired results.

Collaborative commissioning

The collaborative commissioning approach provides a framework for commissioning services. The aim of collaborative commissioning is to continually improve patient care and patient experience through an active and positive collaboration between patients, clinicians and managers where we work together to solve problems and deliver innovative solutions (NHS Tayside Board 2007). It describes how and when to involve children, young people and their families, clinicians, managers and partners in the commissioning process. The collaborative commissioning model is designed to influence commissioning plans in NHS Boards and other public sector organizations.

It is not and should not be confused with a consensus model. It is possible for different stakeholders to hold different views. What is important is that they have all had an opportunity to influence the strategy and their views will be available to the decision-making body when they come to agree promises or recommendations for changes in service provision.

Collaborative commissioning is not about moving commissioning power from one group to another. It is the responsibility of strategic managers to lead and manage a process that brings together views from all the stakeholders in an ongoing debate about what and how services should be provided (Selkirk 2007). However, it also requires strong citizen leadership, strong clinical ownership and leadership and robust management and commissioning expertise.

Collaborative commissioning is best conceived as a cyclical process. The following section describes each stage of this cycle in detail (Figure 12.1).

STAGE 1: CONSIDER CLINICAL EVIDENCE, HEALTH POLICY AND BEST PRACTICE, ECONOMIC APPRAISAL, FORECASTING AND CAPACITY

There are a wide range of organizations and publications, which provide an evidence base for clinical practice within health services. These include the National Institute for Clinical Excellence (NICE), the Scottish Intercollegiate Guidelines Network (SIGN), academic and medical journals and quality standards published by Quality Improvement Scotland (QIS). There are also a range of best practice documents (NHS Modernization Agency 2005). Health policy is set out in documents such as *Better Health Better Care: An Action Plan.*

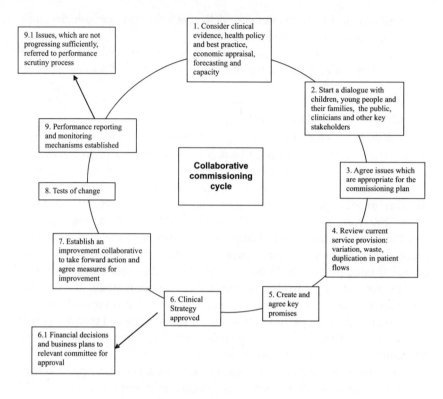

Figure 12.1 Collaborative commissioning cycle

Reproduced with permission from A Template for Child Health Services within Unified Board Areas, Child Health Support Group, Scotish Executive, May 2001.

It is important in strategic planning terms to plan for the service required in the future and not simply to think about the current problems and pressure on today's service. A population profile, for example, is a vital requirement of any child health strategy (Evans and Stoddart 1994). A good forecasting and capacity plan will make adjustments for a growing population with increased health care needs. It needs to focus on number of children and burden of disease, number of staff and skills and competencies required to meet the projected demand, capital programmes which will ensure suitable premises are available and are of suitable size and appropriateness of the client group and budget requirements to fund the agreed capacity.

STAGE 2: START A DIALOGUE WITH CHILDREN, YOUNG PEOPLE AND THEIR FAMILIES, THE PUBLIC, CLINICIANS AND OTHER KEY STAKEHOLDERS

Stage 2 sets out a range of ways in which services can enter into and improve dialogue with children, young people and their families as well as clinical staff and partner agencies. 'Better Health Better Care' has introduced the concept of a 'Mutual NHS'. This policy direction is intended to 'strengthen public ownership of the NHS by improving rights to participate, embed patient experience information in the performance management of the NHS and strengthen collaboration and an integrated approach to service improvement' (Scottish Government 2007b, p.5).

Increasingly, young people are demonstrating that they wish to and are more than capable of taking a very active part in the design of services. Pupil councils in schools, the Scottish Youth Parliament, Dialogue Youth run by local authorities, Young Scot and numerous other groups all provide an easy way for commissioners to fully engage with young people.

STAGE 3: AGREE ISSUES WHICH ARE APPROPRIATE FOR THE COMMISSIONING PLAN

In the course of any discussion about improving services it is likely that a number of simple practical suggestions which do not require to be commissioned will be offered, for example: 'Can you provide simple information about the clinic appointment I am going to attend and what I can expect to happen?

Commissioning decisions should relate to large significant changes or when significant funding is involved, e.g. reducing the level of inpatient care on a site, asking for funding to expand the child and adolescent mental health service or setting out an expect outcome which must be provided at all sites, e.g. implementing *Health for all Children* (Scottish Executive 2005b) screening.

STAGE 4: REVIEW CURRENT SERVICE PROVISION: VARIATION, WASTE, DUPLICATION IN PATIENT FLOWS

In looking at the current provision of services the Child Health Commissioner and the service provider need to be able to identify and address:

- variation in practice including referrals and outcomes
- practice, which is potentially harmful to patients, e.g. infection, errors in drug administration
- activities which result in waste, e.g. the same test being done by both general practice and the secondary care provider when

sharing the results of the first test would have sufficed. LEAN thinking is an excellent tool for identifying and reducing waste (Institute for Healthcare Improvement 2005; Ohno 1988).

Further information on each of these areas as wells as tools and techniques can be found on www.ihi.org. The service can also monitor its performance through a range of mechanisms, some of which were illustrated earlier in this chapter.

STAGE 5: CREATE AND AGREE KEY PROMISES

In commissioning services it is vital to be clear about the outcomes to be delivered. These include patient-focused objectives. In essence these are SMART (specific, measurable, achievable, realistic, timed) objectives that describe the benefit to patients. This means that in asking a Board to sign up to and often provide substantial resources for service change the service in turn is agreeing to deliver promises to patients.

Feedback from patients and clinicians needs to be considered and reflected in a commissioning plan. The commissioner then describes a number of measures for judgement. The service providers will have a number of measures for improvement, which support service change.

STAGE 6: CLINICAL STRATEGY APPROVED

All Boards must have in place strong financial systems of governance. It is vital that the financial implications of the proposed clinical strategy are both accounted for and understood.

STAGE 7: ESTABLISH AN IMPROVEMENT COLLABORATIVE TO TAKE FORWARD ACTION AND AGREE MEASURES FOR IMPROVEMENT

At this stage of the cycle it is helpful to consider the use of an established model for improvement of care delivery and outcomes. Details of such a model for improvement can be found on www.improvingnhstayside.co.uk or www.ihi.org. The Improvement Guide (Langley et al. 1996) is another such guide, setting out three important questions that individuals, groups and planners should ask themselves when planning improvements in the delivery of services. These measures can then be used to monitor performance against outcomes and measures:

1. What change can we make that will result in improvement? (CHANGES). This involves describing the changes you are planning to make which will result in the improvement you want to achieve.

2. What are we trying to accomplish? (AIM). To answer this question it is helpful to be clear about what the problem is and what we want to achieve. For example, some children are unable to access the child and adolescent mental health service within a reasonable timescale.

3. How will we know that a change is an improvement? (MEASURES). This involves describing what success will look like in a way which is measurable. The key question is 'How good by when?' (Langley *et al.* 1996).

It is usually helpful to set out a trajectory from where the service is now to where it needs to be. This is unlikely to be a straight line but one where we see improvement as the result of planned intervention, e.g. recruitment of additional staff. Improvement is achieved by working together using the Plan-Do-Study-Act model to undertake small steps of change in order to achieve the desired improvement (Langley *et al.* 1996).

STAGE 8: TESTS OF CHANGE

Tests of change (Langley *et al.* 1996) are where a change is tried out on one day with one person and then modified on the basis of what is learned. This same change is then tested with three and subsequently five people. This allows change to be made in a low risk fashion (see www.improvingnhstayside.co.uk for more detailed information).

STAGE 9: PERFORMANCE REPORTING AND MONITORING
MECHANISMS ESTABLISHED

All systems should have in place a strong scrutiny model which identifies areas where performance is not on trajectory or waiting times for services are increasing. Such a system will ask for an improvement plan which will set out proposed actions together with clear measures for improvement which have a timescale.

Conclusion

The main remit of a Child Health Commissioner is to make sure that services for children are delivered consistently, coherently and effectively. In order to achieve these aims an effective Child Health Commissioner needs to develop a range of skills and competencies. These include strategic thinking, ability to deal with complex issues, people management skills including an ability to deal with conflict and good understanding of child health, excellent networking ability. Moreover, the Child Health Commissioner needs to be able to assure the organization about the quality of services it provides. This is done by monitoring and assigning services, identifying areas for improvement and making proposals for improvement, in services for children young people and their families.

The collaborative commissioning approach described enables and empowers the Commissioners to build and develop services based on sound evidence, best practice and the monitoring of local services. Yet, not only formal evidence is considered; an important part of collaborative commissioning is to gather information from professionals, carers and the public, including children. The Child Health Commissioner's remit is to gather formal and informal types of evidence and establish effective communication between senior officers of the health, social services, education, criminal justice and police and voluntary agencies to ensure an integrated child health service for the local population. If successful, the Child Health Commissioner is at the centre of all issues relating to children's services.

Chapter Thirteen

Child Death Review

Catherine Powell

Introduction

In the United Kingdom (UK), as in many other parts of the developed world, the death of a child or young person is a rare,[7] but highly significant, event that will have a major impact on families, professionals and communities. Clearly, some deaths, such as those from life-limiting conditions, may be expected. Many others, however, such as those from accidents, maltreatment or conditions that are not usually fatal, will be classified as 'unexpected'. Of particular concern, is the fact that there are notable geographical and socio-economic variations in childhood death rates (Edwards *et al.* 2006; Fleming *et al.* 2004). Deaths in childhood inevitably raise questions about the presence of 'avoidable' or 'preventable' factors. Such factors may relate to a range of issues such as physical safety, earlier identification of risk of maltreatment, or more timely and appropriate health care. While these features are often readily identifiable in the case of unexpected deaths, it is increasingly accepted that deaths from 'natural causes' may also have modifiable contributory factors (Bunting and Reid 2005; Covington, Foster and Rich 2005).

In acknowledgement of the 'sentinel' importance (Jenny and Isaac 2006) of the death of a child or young person and the potential to learn lessons for child health and safety, the practice of systematically reviewing *all* childhood deaths is being introduced within the UK. New multi-agency child death review processes aim to seek an understanding of why a child or young person has died, to use this information to gain insight into the individual death and to ensure that any messages for prevention and the future safety and protection

---

7   The Department for Children, Schools and Families (DCSF) provide an information sheet which usefully outlines contemporary patterns and causes of child deaths. This notes that there are some 5000 deaths of children under 15 years of age and 1000 of those aged 15–19 years in the UK each year (Department for Children, Schools and Families 2008a).

of children are fed into policy, legislation and practice. A range of practitioners working in primary health care settings may be asked to contribute to the child death review process.

Drawing on the literature from countries that have established child death review processes, the statutory guidance in England (HM Government 2006) and recently published reports that have informed the development of child death review processes in the UK (CEMACH 2008; Sidebotham *et al.* 2008), as well as novice personal experience of child death review, this chapter aims to update and support primary and community care practitioners in making a full and meaningful contribution. Importantly, the chapter highlights the benefits of child death review processes, which can be summarized as: improving multi-agency working; more effective identification of suspicious cases; a decrease in inadequate death certificates; a better understanding of the causes of child death and the move to a public health approach to the prevention of all child deaths, including those from maltreatment.

Child death review: messages from the literature

Multi-agency and multi-disciplinary child death (fatality) review teams have been established in the United States (USA) and elsewhere for some 20 years. Initially these teams were developed because of professional concerns about under-reporting of deaths from child maltreatment. However, they have evolved over time to encompass review of all childhood deaths with a focus on the identification of preventable factors and the development of evidence-based interventions to prevent future deaths. Examples of outcomes from child death review team work include safe-sleeping campaigns, shaken baby and sudden infant death prevention, use of smoke detectors, fencing of swimming pools, bicycle and vehicle safety, improved access to health care provision for vulnerable families, immunization campaigns and improved bereavement and support to grieving families (Bunting and Reid 2005; Durfee, Tilton Durfee and West 2002; Rimza *et al.* 2002). While the majority of child deaths are 'entirely non-suspicious' (Fox 2008), explicit discussion of the possibility of child maltreatment remains central because of continuing widespread concerns about under-ascertainment. In addition, as Jenny and Isaac (2006) note, deaths where emotional abuse or neglect were contributory factors are rarely defined as such, neither, they argue, are deaths of young people from suicide or extreme risk-taking that can follow earlier abuse or neglect.

A crucial factor in the success of child death review teams is that they are made up of individuals from a range of agencies who are able to contribute a wealth of health and social information to discussion of individual cases. As Jenny and Isaac (2006) comment:

The most important aspect of CDRT [Child Death Review Teams] is to have people from the various disciplines involved with child health and safety participate and share knowledge and information. (p.268)

Guidance on best practice from the US National MCH Center for Child Death Review[8] reflects the need for membership to include those from public health, paediatrics, primary health care, social care, the police service, emergency services, the medical examiner or coroner and the 'District Attorney'. The benefit of having additional *ad hoc* members to discuss specific issues is also noted. As discussed next, a similar approach to multi-agency membership is being taken within the UK, although in England the accountability rests with the Local Safeguarding Children Board (LSCB), rather than those who may have more diverse individual responsibilities for child health and welfare. In addition to the multi-agency format, it is important that child death review team members are in positions of sufficient seniority to influence programme and policy development that addresses emergent 'preventability factors' to improve children and young people's health and wellbeing and to prevent future child deaths. Experience from the USA suggests that the process of multi-agency child death review also helps to improve inter-agency working more generally by 'building bridges' between different agencies with resultant improved communication and joint working in everyday practice.

Although there are important differences in the scope of their work (including a regional focus, a strong health bias and the anonymization of cases), a recently published report from CEMACH (2008), discusses the findings of regional child death reviews undertaken in England, Wales and Northern Ireland. Here the deaths of children aged 28 days to 18 years were subject to detailed analysis and panel discussion. Recommendations from the study include the need to ensure that health professionals, including those working in primary health care, are skilled in recognizing and meeting the needs of a sick child; better access to child and adolescent mental health services (CAMHS) for those at risk of self-harm; the follow-up of children who are not brought to appointments and better immunization coverage. Importantly, the study was supportive of the usefulness of in-depth child death review and has been influential in informing the systematic reviews being adopted within the UK.

---

8   www.childdeathreview.org/home.htm

The development of child death review in the UK

The implementation of child death review processes became a mandatory requirement for LSCBs in England on 1 April 2008 (HM Government 2006). This chapter will focus on developments in England, although it is understood that Wales, Scotland and Northern Ireland are planning similar processes.

Background

The requirement for LSCBs to establish child death review processes is outlined in Chapter 7 of the statutory guidance on safeguarding children *Working Together to Safeguard Children* (HM Government 2006). This obligation, which is enshrined in the Children Act 2004, builds on earlier proposals to set up child death reviews as part of the government's overarching *Every Child Matters* response to Lord Laming's inquiry into the death of Victoria Climbié (HM Government 2004; Laming 2003). The proposals for child death review also encompass the principles from Baroness Kennedy's report concerning good practice in reviewing sudden and unexpected deaths in infants (Royal College of Paediatrics and Child Health 2004). However, in contrast to the latter's focus on infants and unexpected deaths, the new child death review processes are applicable to *all* children aged 0–18 years (excluding stillbirths). Furthermore, while developments in other countries have been somewhat *ad hoc*, often relying on local champions and goodwill, the new statutory requirements for England are recognized to:

> set the scene for England to become the first country in the world to have national standards and procedures for the investigation and management of unexpected child deaths and for reviewing all child deaths. (Sidebotham *et al.* 2008, p.11)

Purpose

The overall aim of child death review processes is to understand why children die and to put in place interventions to improve child safety and welfare and to prevent future deaths. As has been noted, this includes a consideration of any child protection concerns. LSCBs are thus required to collect and analyse information about each death of a child normally resident in their area with a view to identifying: any cases that may require further investigation including the need for a Serious Case Review;[9] any concern about the health and safety of children in the area and any wider public health or safety concerns that arise from a particular death, or pattern of deaths in the area. LSCBs are also

---

9   As per Chapter 8 of *Working Together* (HM Government 2006).

required to put in place procedures to ensure that there is a co-ordinated response to an unexpected death. Unexpected death in childhood is widely defined as 'the death of a child that was not anticipated as a significant possibility 24 hours before the death, or where there was a similarly unexpected collapse leading to, or precipitating the events that led to the death' (HM Government 2008, p.156). Two processes, the 'Rapid Response' (for unexpected deaths) and the 'Child Death Overview Panel' (for all deaths), are outlined in the guidance (HM Government 2006) and described next.

Rapid Response

The Rapid Response is best explained as a multi-agency approach to gathering information that supports the investigation of a sudden unexpected death in a child and, importantly, also supports the family. There are three phases to the Rapid Response (although these may overlap) and these are described as: the immediate response; the early response; and the later response (Department for Children, Schools and Families 2008b).

The immediate response concerns the first two to three hours after a child's death. This will normally involve the transfer of the child to an emergency department. Following cessation of any resuscitation attempts and confirmation of death, arrangements will be made for a 'joint investigation' that involves the police, social care, the coroner and the lead paediatrician for sudden unexpected deaths. Ideally, a comprehensive health and social history will be gathered jointly by a police officer and a paediatrician while the family are in the department. There will also be the need to examine the child and to gather material for pathological examination. It is anticipated that local joint protocols will be developed and utilized to help to guide practitioners in information gathering, examination and the taking of samples from the dead child.

The next phase of the Rapid Response is the 'early response' and this takes place over the next 24–48 hours. It will include arranging an autopsy (post-mortem examination) and the setting up of a multi-agency planning and information-sharing meeting. General practitioners, midwives, health visitors and school nurses may be invited to attend this meeting specifically to contribute background information on the child and family's health and social circumstances. In some cases the planning meeting will be followed by a joint visit to the place where the child died (especially if this is at home). This 'scene examination' will involve the investigating police officer and a health care professional, who may be a paediatrician, health visitor or specially trained nurse. The general practitioner may also be in attendance. The purpose of the home visit is to provide an 'holistic evaluation' (Royal College of Paediatrics and Child Health 2008) of the circumstances of the child's death and to facilitate bereavement care and support to the family. Although the Rapid Response is a new process and therefore has not yet been subject to comprehensive evaluation, evidence from one area that had previously established a similar model of working was that parents reported the joint home visit as being 'helpful rather than intrusive' (Fleming et al. 2004).

The 'later response' phase of the Rapid Response, which will take place over the next three to four months, concentrates on completion of the investigation, the findings of the coroner's inquest, a final case discussion and feedback to the family. If, at any time, there are concerns that child maltreatment has been a previously unidentified contributory factor to the child's death, then police and social care undertake enquiries and the case may be subject to a Serious Case Review. The final case discussion and report will, in turn, feed into the review of all child deaths that is undertaken by the second of the new processes: the Child Death Overview Panel.

The Child Death Overview Panel

In England each LSCB is now expected to establish a multi-agency and multi-disciplinary Child Death Overview Panel. However, because the guidance in Chapter 7 of *Working Together* (HM Government 2006) suggests that panels need to serve a population of 500,000 or more, LSCBs may collaborate with neighbouring authorities to form joint panels. As noted above, the primary purpose of the panels is to review all deaths of children who are normally resident in the area and to use the learning to improve child health and safety and prevent future deaths. While it is expected that any deaths that may be considered to be 'suspicious' will already be known to the relevant authorities, the Child Death Overview Panel also gives professionals an opportunity to recommend further statutory child protection inquiries and/or that a Serious Case Review be undertaken. It is anticipated that panels will 'meet regularly' (typically monthly) to gain an overview of the childhood deaths that have been notified to them and to discuss a number of selected cases in some depth. The success of their endeavours rests on the provision of background case information by those working with the child and family and in the large majority of cases this will include contributions by primary health care professionals.

In common with best practice identified elsewhere, the membership of the Child Death Review Panel should be multi-disciplinary. In evaluating the experiences of 'Early Starters' i.e. nine authorities who had already established child death review teams and processes prior to the statutory requirements,

Sidebotham *et al.* (2008) conclude that as a *minimum* panels membership should comprise:

- Public Health.
- Paediatrics (incorporating both hospital and community based child health services).
- Specialist Community Public Health Nursing (Health Visitors and School Nursing).
- Children's Social Care.
- Police.

My own experience in a recently established Child Death Overview Panel, which embraces the population from four LSCB areas, is that in addition to that membership, there are representatives from education and the ambulance service and further representation by rota of each of the four LSCB managers. Sidebotham *et al.* (2008) recognize that the above 'core' membership may be supplemented by additional members where they may add particular additional information or expertise. These may, for example, include further health representatives from midwifery, primary health care or child or adult mental health services as well as those from the coronary service, bereavement support organizations or other emergency services (e.g. traffic police, coast-guard, fire service).

The successful functioning of a Child Death Overview Panel rests with having good chairing arrangements and high quality administrative support. As Sidebotham *et al.* (2008) note, the Chair should be the LSCB Chair or their representative and should be independent to services provided directly to children, young people and their families. The administrator or 'co-ordinator', who may be supported by additional clerical help, is the 'lynchpin' who ensures smooth and effective running of the panel. This role is critical in ensuring that the information-gathering processes are initiated and completed so that when the panel meets the members have all the information they need to ensure that the objectives of the process are met through informed debate and analysis. The three-stage process of initial notification, more detailed information gathering and analysis by the panel is now described.

It is important that Child Death Overview Panels are informed of all the deaths of children and young people in their area. Thus the first stage of the process is the 'notification' to the panel's administrator that a child has died. It is expected that this will happen within one working day of the death. Responsibility for notification rests with the agencies involved in the death; this may be the emergency department or hospital, or it may be the general practitioner, or other primary health care practitioners such as children's community nurses. Children's hospices may also initiate notifications to the panel; here deaths are likely to be those that are classified as 'expected'. Parents should be informed of the requirement for all childhood deaths to be notified to the local Child Death Overview Panel and many areas are developing parental information leaflets that provide further information on the new review process. Initial data collection via questionnaires to LSCBs for the 'early starter' study found that multiple sources of notification may be required in order that no deaths of children were missed and as much useful information as possible be gathered.

The aim of notification is to provide basic details of the dead child including their full demographic details, together with ethnicity and the names and relationship of family and household members. The referrer also needs to include as much detail about the death and subsequent management as they are able to at this early stage. This will take account of the date and time of death, the place of death, whether a death certificate has been issued (and any cause of death that has been specified) as well as circumstances leading to the notification. Details on the management of the death should ascertain whether the death was expected or unexpected, whether the coroner or registrar have been informed and details of any arrangements for a post-mortem. Finally, the names and contact details of professionals from other agencies who have been involved in the care of the child or family are included to assist with further information gathering, if required, for more in-depth review. A notification proforma is used to gather the information.

Members of the Child Death Overview Panel will be apprised of the deaths of all children in their local authority area. From the information available on the notification proforma a subset of the deaths will be selected for more in-depth review. It is expected that this will occur some four to six months after the death to allow for completion of inquiries, investigations and any inquest. For these cases practitioners will be asked to complete an 'Agency Report Form' which gathers narrative and quantitative information in relation to the child and the circumstances of their death. Work with the 'Early Starters' (Sidebotham et al. 2008) led to a suggestion that information could be gathered in four domains. Building on the 'Assessment Triangle' (Department of Health 2000) information is organized through consideration of factors relating to: the child; parenting capacity; the family and environment and the provision of services. Those completing the agency reports are also given the opportunity to raise any issues for discussion by the panel. As previously, parents will be informed of the decision to discuss their child's death and given an opportunity to provide information via the Chair (although they will not attend in person).

Information from agency reports will be collated and an Analysis Proforma completed following in-depth review at the Child Death Overview Panel meeting. Drawing on information on all four domains, the panel will work towards reaching a consensus as to identifiable contributory factors; the category of death (using a pre-determined hierarchical classification) and, crucially, categorize the 'preventability' of the death. The analysis proforma additionally provides the panel with an opportunity to document any issues identified in the review; any learning points; recommendations and the follow-up plans for the family. The recommendation from the 'Early Starter' study is that no more than three to five cases can be discussed in-depth at any one meeting.

The outcome of the work of the Child Death Overview Panel will be regular reporting to the LSCB, with subsequent activity focusing on the development of local policy and programmes in response to issues identified. Ultimately it is expected that the output from local Child Death Overview Panels will be collated and analysed regionally and nationally to inform initiatives that improve the health and safety of children and prevent future child deaths.

Discussion

Although the process of child death review will be new to most primary health care practitioners, it is suggested that its core purpose has much in common with the core attributes of safeguarding and indeed of health professional practice. I have summarized these elsewhere as: benefiting the health and wellbeing of individuals, families and communities; working in partnership with other agencies; health improvement and addressing inequalities (Powell 2007). Clearly, health professionals may already be aware of, or indeed contributing to, other forms of child mortality review and this has led some to question the new child death review processes. However, while such meetings may be complementary, a multi-agency review can alternatively offer an action-oriented richness of understanding about why children die. As one of the informants to the 'Early Starter' study proffered:

> The internal reviews that are already happening in many hospitals... and have been running for some time, but they have two very different, requirements. One is to have a bird's eye view of all deaths within the district and the other is part of the internal hospital governance arrangements and therefore different information needs to be provided for each setting; you can't necessarily use the same information for both. So getting people's heads clear around that, particularly when they've been in the habit of running mortality meetings whether that's intensivists or neonatologist or whole hospital

arrangements and shifting sideways and taking the emphasis off the medical bits and did the SHO get out of bed or did somebody write down the pulse rate, towards collecting wider information about, when did this mother book for antenatal care, or what do we know about father's drug use, really much more relevant. (Sidebotham *et al.* 2008, p.37)

It is, of course, too early to report extensively on the outcomes and success of child death review processes in England. However, the work undertaken with 'Early Starter' panels began to demonstrate the potential of undertaking reviews in the UK in that 'preventability factors' relating to factors in the child, parents or carers, the environment or services provided were identified in 17 out of 24 cases that were discussed at observed panel meetings. It is rewarding to see that evidence was also found of specific actions being taken as a result of the panel meetings; this included lobbying a member of the European Parliament for improvements in swimming pool safety, joint working between education and CAMHS to address risk of self-harm and improvements in local bereavement services. (Sidebotham *et al.* 2008).

Conclusions and the way forward

This chapter has outlined new statutory child death review processes in England: the Rapid Response and the Child Death Overview Panel. These build on the work of CEMACH and existing protocols on responding to sudden death in infancy developed in the UK, as well as the success of child death review teams in the USA and elsewhere. Practitioners working in primary health care settings have an important contribution to make in ensuring notification and reporting of child deaths and they may find it helpful to access the resources highlighted in this chapter.

In a recent editorial, Freemantle and Read (2008) broadly welcomed the introduction of child death review processes within the UK. They noted that such reviews must be rigorous and systematic and that when combined with appropriate epidemiological research may help to decrease child mortality. This is a view that I share; indeed I would go further and argue that child death review is one of the most promising child health initiatives of recent years. It is thus anticipated that child death review will be warmly embraced by primary health care practitioners as a process that will benefit families, professionals and communities and most importantly of all, the future health and safety of children.

Part 4

Safeguarding Challenges in the Primary Health Care Context

Chapter Fourteen

Parental Problem Drug Use

Anne Whittaker

Introduction

Primary health care has an important role in the care of children and families affected by parental problem drug use. This chapter focuses on the skills required to work effectively with drug-using parents. It aims to complement guidance on working with children and includes an overview of drug policy and drug treatment, the scale and nature of the problem, a framework for care and good practice and examples of harm reduction strategies and interventions. The chapter draws on evidence from impact and intervention studies on parental problem drug use, as well as qualitative research on drug-using parents and their families.

In order to clarify the scope of this chapter, 'problem drug use', 'drug dependence' and 'parental problem drug use' are defined in Box 14.1.

Box 14.1 Definitions

Problem drug use

The Advisory Council on the Misuse of Drugs (ACMD 2003) defines 'problem drug use' as any drug use which has serious negative consequences of a physical, psychological, social and interpersonal, financial or legal nature for users and those around them. Such drug use is normally heavy, with features of dependence and typically involves the use of one or more of the following drugs: opiates (e.g. heroin and methadone); benzodiazepines (e.g. diazepam); and stimulants (e.g. crack cocaine and amphetamines).

Drug dependence
'Drug dependence' is a syndrome and is defined in the International Statistical Classification of Diseases and Related Health Problems (10th revision ICD-10 criteria) as 'a cluster of behavioural, cognitive and physiological phenomena that develop after repeated substance use and typically includes a strong desire to take the drug, difficulties controlling its use, persisting in its use despite harmful consequences, a higher priority given to drug use than to other activities and obligations, increased tolerance and sometimes a physical withdrawal state'.

Parental problem drug use
Refers to any person with 'problem drug use' who acts as a father, mother, carer or guardian to a child. This includes biological and non-biological parents, resident and non-resident parents and parents who do not have legal parental responsibilities and rights.

The policy context

Safeguarding and promoting the welfare of children affected by parental problem drug use is a key objective of policy and practice (ACMD 2003). As well as understanding the policies and practices which govern the delivery of children's services and child protection practice, practitioners working with drug-using parents need to understand the policies, practices and evidence which underpins the treatment and care of problem drug users (Kroll and Taylor 2003).

Drug policy and drug treatment in the UK is based primarily upon a 'harm reduction' approach (Department of Health 2007b; Reuter and Stevens 2007). This approach seeks to prevent and minimize the health and social harms associated with problem drug use and aims to facilitate social reintegration. The UK Government's (HM Government 2008) ten-year drug strategy places child welfare, families and the treatment and care of drug-using parents at its heart, signalling a shift towards 'whole-family' approaches.

Drug treatment approaches

A variety of drug treatments have been found to be effective in reducing harm to individual drug users, their children, families and communities (Department of Health 2007b). These include: substitution maintenance therapy, psychosocial interventions, self-help and mutual aid approaches, contingency management, couple and family interventions.

Well-delivered methadone maintenance programmes provided within primary health care settings and specialist drug treatment centres have been shown consistently to reduce illicit drug use, high-risk injecting and sexual behaviours, offending behaviour, overdose risk, the spread of blood-borne viruses and to improve psychological and social functioning and the uptake of health care (WHO, UNODC and UNAIDS 2004). Drug treatment provided within primary health care can achieve outcomes equal to specialist drug treatment centres (Ashton 2008; Robertson 1998).

The scale of the problem

The precise number of children, parents and families affected by problem drug use is unknown. *Hidden Harm* (ACMD 2003) estimated that between 250,000 to 350,000 children in the UK have a problem drug-using parent. Over 50 per cent of drug-using parents report that their dependent children live elsewhere (ACMD 2003). Many children will live with their non-drug dependent parent (mostly mothers), some (about 5–10%) will be in local authority care and many others will live with kinship carers (family and friends). The circumstances of these children and the permanency of these living arrangements is uncertain, as is the level of involvement that non-resident drug-using parents (mostly fathers) have with their children. The nature and extent of kinship care has only recently been studied, but appears to be substantial (see Aldgate and McIntosh 2006; Farmer and Moyers 2005).

While drug-using mothers are far more likely than drug-using fathers to report living with their dependent children, it is important to remember that drug-using fathers outnumber drug-using mothers by 2:1 (ACMD 2003). Drug-using fathers are also more likely than drug-using mothers to be living with children who are not their own (and who they may not declare as 'dependent'). It is not known how many children live in families where one or both parents have a drug problem.

A gendered perspective

The research evidence on drug-using parents is overwhelmingly concerned with maternal drug use (ACMD 2003). Policy and practice guidance reflects this bias with a focus on strategies to improve the treatment and care of pregnant drug users and drug-using mothers. While this is understandable, the invisibility of drug-using fathers remains an ongoing concern (McMahon, Winkel and Rounsaville 2008; Scaife 2008; Templeton *et al.* 2006). Equal attention needs to be paid to the effects of paternal drug use and the parenting needs and parenting capacity of drug-using fathers.

Men are more likely than women to develop drug dependence, report high-risk drug-taking activity and to die from drug-related problems (EMCDDA 2006; Thom 2003). While drug treatment outcomes for men and women are similar (Best and Abdulrahim 2005), research suggests that differences exist between the way drug-using mothers and fathers utilize and benefit from services designed to help their children and family (Fals-Stewart, Fincham and Kelley 2004; Marsh and Cao 2005). Evidence also indicates that children are affected differently by maternal and paternal drug problems and when both parents use drugs (Hogan and Higgins 2001; Scaife 2008).

Child protection practice and 'family' support, are also highly gendered, with a focus on mothers and mothering (Daniel and Taylor 2001; Ghate, Shaw and Hazel 2000; Lloyd, O'Brien and Lewis 2003; Scourfield and Coffey 2002). Fathers are often ignored, both as a potential risk to the family and as a potential asset (Daniel and Taylor 2001; Guterman and Lee 2005). In cases of child maltreatment, 'mother blaming' is a well-recognized phenomenon, reflecting and reinforcing the notion that women are primarily responsible for the care and protection of children (Daniel and Taylor 2006). The censure, scrutiny and surveillance of drug-using mothers, especially pregnant drug users, is well documented (Boyd 1999; Klee, Jackson and Lewis 2002; Rosenbaum and Irwin 2000). When motherhood and fatherhood are considered within the context of child welfare practice and problem drug use, gender clearly matters.

The impact of parental problem drug use

Evidence on the negative effects of parental problem drug use on children and families is well established (see ACMD 2003; Cleaver, Unell and Aldgate 1999; Gorin 2004; Harbin and Murphy 2000; Kroll and Taylor 2003; Tunnard 2002; Velleman and Templeton 2007b). Poor parenting capacity, poor developmental outcomes for children and increased rates of child maltreatment have been widely reported. All aspects of children's development can be affected, from conception onwards. Children growing up with drug-using parents are also at greater risk of developing problems with substance use themselves (Velleman and Templeton 2007a).

On a cautionary note, much of the evidence is North American where drug trends, drug cultures and drug treatment are somewhat different to that found in the UK (ACMD 2003). Significant gaps in the literature on drugs in the family exist (Templeton *et al.* 2006), for example on ethnic minorities. The literature generally lacks an explicit theoretical basis and fails to provide an explanatory link between maternal and paternal drug use and specific child developmental outcomes (Hogan 1998). Findings are not universal. Studies show that outcomes for children (including those exposed to drugs *in-utero*) vary greatly and are multi-factorial (ACMD 2003). Problem drug use rarely presents in isolation and may not be the sole or primary cause of difficulties within the family.

Several studies have found no increased risks to children attributable to parental drug use alone (Smarsh-Hogan, Myers and Elswick 2006; Templeton *et al.* 2006). Even when drug use does impact on parenting capacity and family life, not all children are affected. Protective factors and resilience in children and families are important and can act as a 'buffer' against the effects of drug-related harm and child maltreatment (Velleman and Templeton 2007b).

Levels of vulnerability in children and parents also affect parenting practices and the likelihood of adverse outcomes (Kumpfer and Bluth 2004). Evidence on the social capital of drug users and drug-taking 'risk environments' highlights the importance of wider social, cultural, contextual and structural factors which shape the lives of drug users (see Ezard 2001; Pauly 2008; Rhodes 2002). Drug-related harm and drug dependence are disproportionately concentrated in the most socially disadvantaged areas and the most socially excluded populations (Reuter and Stevens 2007; Shaw, Egan and Gillespie 2007). Notwithstanding the effects of problem drug use *per se*, children and families living in these circumstances will have the worst outcomes and will require the most assistance (Cabinet Office 2007).

Overall, studies on parental problem drug use lend support for an 'ecological' approach (Sidebotham 2001), which sees child development and family functioning as a dynamic process, influenced by culture, communities, family and individual factors and the interplay between them. Rarely however, has this conceptual framework been applied to research on parental problem drug use.

Global effects of parental problem drug use

Parental problem drug use tends to have a global effect on the care-giving environment. Longstanding, severe and untreated drug problems are correlated positively with more severe financial hardship, homelessness, criminal convictions and incarceration, poor parental physical and mental health, parental conflict and domestic abuse, family breakdown, social rejection and isolation, poor parenting practices, poor child development, increased rates of child maltreatment (primarily neglect) and a greater likelihood that the drug-using parent no longer lives with their children (Locke and Newcomb 2003; Meier, Donmall and McElduff 2004; Ornoy, Michailevskaya and Lukashov 1996; Tunnard 2002).

Parenting capacity can be affected in a number of ways, depending on the parent's pattern of drug usage (including type, quantity, frequency), drug supply source (illicit or prescribed) and associated lifestyle (including criminal involvement, social networks and family support). Disrupted family routines and inadequate parenting are commonly associated with daily illicit drug use, injecting drug use and polydrug use – especially the use of cocaine/alcohol in addition to opiates (Street *et al.* 2004; Tunnard 2002). Dependent drug users, who rely on illicit supplies, tend to report difficulties with parenting because their daily life revolves around the procurement and consumption of drugs. Funding an illicit supply of drugs typically involves diverting family finances and/or offending behaviour (usually acquisitive crime or drug dealing). Fluctuating periods of intoxication and withdrawal affects the parent's behaviour and mental state, making consistent and safe parenting less likely. Problem drug use is associated with lower levels of involvement with children, less sensitive parenting, inadequate parental supervision of children, inadequate stimulation, low levels of parental involvement in children's education and less secure parent–infant attachments (Hogan 1998; McMahon *et al.* 2008; Tunnard 2002). Conversely, parents who are receiving effective drug treatment (e.g. methadone maintenance and psychosocial support) are far less likely to report such problems (Hogan and Higgins 2001). Their children may have outcomes comparable to children growing up in similar socio-economic circumstances (see for example Burns, O'Driscoll and Wason 1996; Street *et al.* 2004).

Children's views and experiences

Research which has explored children's perspectives, reveals the extent to which their lives can be affected by their parent's drug use and the kind of coping strategies they employ (see Bancroft *et al.* 2004; Barnard and Barlow 2003; Gorin 2004; Gruenert, Ratnam and Tsantefski 2004; Hogan and Higgins 2001). Children's accounts commonly reveal disrupted schooling and family routines, social isolation, emotional and physical neglect and powerful feelings of shame, fear, sadness, anger and loss. Children often express considerable worry about their parent's health and wellbeing and can fear for their safety. Their loyalty to the drug-using parent is often strong, and wider social and family ties are often pivotal in their lives. Secrecy and concealment is common on account of the illegality of drugs and the stigma which surrounds problem drug use. Children report being bystanders in the criminal activities of their parents, witnessing illicit drug-taking activities, being involved in violent incidents, low self-esteem and early initiation into substance use themselves. Some take on a 'parental role' and have unmet needs as young carers. Children's testimonies reveal that they are rarely the focus of assessment or service intervention (Gorin 2004).

Drug-using mothers' views and experiences

Qualitative research on pregnant drug users and drug-using mothers has explored their views and experiences of services, their parenting beliefs and practices, social capital, coping strategies and unique needs in relation to drug treatment and parenting (see Banwell and Bammer 2006; Hogan and Higgins 2001; Klee *et al.* 2002; Powis *et al.* 2000; Richter and Bammer 2000; Rosenbaum and Irwin 2000).

Drug-using mothers value motherhood and demonstrate that they are concerned about the welfare of their children (Klee *et al.* 2002). Pregnancy in particular, is seen as a 'window of opportunity' to engage drug-using women in drug treatment and other health and social care services (Department of Health 2007b). The drive to be a 'good' mother is often cited as a key reason to enter drug treatment and to participate in specialist parenting and child welfare programmes (Powis *et al.* 2000). Conversely, judgemental staff attitudes, punitive responses, shame and the fear of losing custody of their children can deter them from approaching services. Prevailing societal views of drug-using mothers, which are stereotypically derogatory, have a profound effect on their self-esteem, parenting confidence and level of social support (Banwell and Bammer 2006). Barriers to accessing and utilizing services include everyday family and household responsibilities, financial constraints, criminal justice issues and obligations to friends and family. Partners often exert a strong influence (both positive and negative) on the mother's drug-taking behaviour, mental health, parenting practices and service utilization (Klee et al. 2002).

Drug-using fathers' views and experiences

While there is a large body of evidence on the role of fathers in family life and their involvement in health and social care settings (see Burgess 2008), the voices of drug-using fathers on these matters have rarely been heard (Templeton *et al.* 2006).

In my own qualitative research study (Whittaker 2008), drug-dependent fathers living in Scotland, were asked to talk about fatherhood and family life and their involvement with services. Against a backdrop of severe disadvantage and social exclusion, the men portrayed fatherhood as a serious endeavour which brought a sense of purpose and meaning to their lives. For many, fatherhood represented a route out of problem drug use, a life of crime, poverty and an unpromising future. All the men described taking an active role in child-rearing and aimed to give their children 'a better life' than what they had themselves. Providing 'hands on' childcare was considered normal, desirable and indeed essential if the father was to establish a close 'bond' with his children, maintain a good relationship with his partner and remain in the home. All agreed that drug use could and did compromise fathering capacity and that fathers needed to employ a range of strategies to minimize the negative effects of paternal drug use on the family (e.g. getting 'stable' on methadone, staying out of prison, avoiding troublesome neighbourhoods and drug-using 'pals', staying away from children when intoxicated).

With regard to service involvement, the men reported contact with a wide range of professionals and services. Narratives however, revealed that they were mostly ignored, excluded, marginalized and problematized. The stigmatization, stereotyping and unequal treatment of drug users and drug-using fathers was, according to the men, an undisputed obstacle to parenting support. The men were acutely aware of being seen as inadequate parents and realized that professionals lacked interest in their parenting practices and the kind of relationship they had with their children. Almost none of the fathers spoke of family assessments or interventions that went beyond questions about their drug use and drug treatment plan. Fathers with non-drug-using partners appeared to be completely overlooked. The men's accounts revealed the extent to which they were peripheral to the child welfare and parenting agenda.

Despite the men's aspirations for being a 'good' father, they reported multiple barriers to involved fatherhood (both actual and potential). An impoverished upbringing, lack of educational qualifications, low employability, financial hardship, poor health and outstanding legal problems were the norm. Social environments were hazardous because of 'reputations' and normative 'male' behaviours which condoned involvement in crime, male-on-male violence and drug dealing. Relationships with partners and wider family members were important, but often contingent and fragile. Some men reported conflict with partners and domestic abuse that threatened their relationship and place in the home. Skills in childcare, confidence in parenting ability and the men's level of involvement with children varied considerably, depending on a myriad of factors. In most cases, the men's accounts indicated that drug use was not the most salient one. Consistent with an ecological perspective, the men's fathering capacity was shaped by a range of personal, relational, historical, cultural, contextual, economic and structural factors.

Other studies of drug-using fathers (see Hogan and Higgins 2001; Klee 1998; Klee *et al.* 2002; McMahon *et al.* 2007), also challenge simplistic notions of fathering on drugs and assumptions about their unconventional (and irresponsible) approach to fathering. Together they highlight the need to focus on and engage with drug-using men as fathers.

Framework for care

Inter-agency guidelines on protecting children living in families affected by parental problem drug use are now standard in most areas. These local frameworks need to be taken into account when delivering treatment and care to parents and children.

Inter-agency guidelines should include:

- Guiding principles on child protection and drug treatment.

- Standards on information sharing and confidentiality.

- Guidance on inter-agency working and the 'lead professional' role.

- A 'care pathway'.

- Guidance on the management of pregnant drug users and babies with neonatal abstinence syndrome (NAS).

- A focus on drug-using fathers (and expectant fathers) and the care that they should receive.

- A focus on drug-using mothers and the care that they should receive.

- Standards on family support and supporting kinship carers and other family members where appropriate.

- Screening and assessment tools.

- Proforma 'Family Support Plan' or 'Action Plan'.

- Tools and guidance on care plan 'reviews'.

- A concise summary of 'what works' in drug treatment, family support and child protection.

- Guidance on safeguarding children and links to child protection procedures.

The way inter-agency guidelines and 'partnership' working are operationalized varies greatly from one area to the next. Frequently, responsibility for devising an operational strategy falls to local service providers and frontline practitioners. Whatever the situation, it is advisable to have a robust strategy in place in order to minimize the chances of children 'slipping through the net'. This means agreeing, documenting and establishing routine information sharing and referral pathways, as well as systems for joint assessment, care planning and care management.

The care process

The care process with drug-using families should be the same as any other 'vulnerable' or 'at-risk' family who present with multiple and inter-related health and social care needs.

The care process or 'care pathway' involves four main stages:

1. Assessment.

2. Planning.

3. Service delivery.

4. Review.

There is an inherent assumption in policy documents that children living with drug-using parents are potentially 'in need' and possibly 'at risk' and that identification of parents and/or children should trigger an assessment of the mother and father's parenting capacity and the child/children's welfare (ACMD 2003; Cabinet Office 2008b).

Where there is a level of concern about the welfare or safety of a child, an inter-agency assessment should be undertaken and a 'lead professional' identified to co-ordinate the assessment process. An assessment of need and an assessment of risk may be required and the way the parent's drug-taking behaviour and lifestyle affects the child's development and social circumstances should be closely examined (see assessment guidance: Department of Health 2004; Scottish Executive 2003a).

Typically, additional services are required to help families manage and overcome their difficulties. Deciding how best to help a family usually involves an inter-professional meeting (with the parents) to plan a programme of care. Families 'in need' benefit from having an agreed family support plan or 'action plan', co-ordinated by a lead professional. Usually, but not always, the lead professional role will be undertaken by a health care professional who is closely involved with the family. When children are involved in the child protection system, social services take the lead. When all the children in the family are school age, both education and social services may be involved along with the GP, school nurse, educational psychology, specialist drug services and other young people's services.

Family support plans should address:

• The needs of each child and each family member (including non-resident parents and 'significant others' in the child's life).

• Standards of child care and developmental milestones to be achieved.

• What needs to be done to achieve desired outcomes for the children.

- Goals of treatment and care for each parent/carer.
- What is expected of the parents and what the parents can expect from services.
- The respective roles and responsibilities of professionals involved with the family.
- Timescales and a date for review.

Because of the fluctuating nature of problem drug use, it is important to re-assess 'need' and 'risk' at regular intervals. Having a 'contingency plan' is advisable should the child's needs fail to be met. Regular reviews of the family's care plan should include: a summary of the work undertaken in the review period and what progress has been made; a reassessment of the mother and father's parenting capacity and the child's health and development; standards of child welfare; the family's social circumstances (including social support) and the home care-giving environment. A strengths-based approach should identify and build on individual, family and environmental resources, the family's positive coping strategies (including harm/risk reduction strategies), positive parenting practices, co-operative relations between partners and positive involvement with extended family and services.

While the overall goal is to improve outcomes for families, what is in the best interests of the child should remain the central focus. At any time during the care process, if there is reasonable cause to suspect or believe that a child is at risk of harm, a child protection referral must be made.

Interventions

Drug treatment should be evidence based and in accordance with Department of Health (2007a,b) and NICE guidelines (2007a,b,c,d). Four domains should be addressed: drug and alcohol use; health (physical and mental); social circumstances and functioning; and criminal involvement (Department of Health 2007b).

The successful delivery of any type of drug treatment relies upon a 'therapeutic alliance' between service provider and drug user (Department of Health 2007b). Adversarial relationships, patronizing and judgemental attitudes, punitive approaches, coercion and enforced treatment are associated with poor attendance, poor compliance with treatment and treatment drop-out.

Evaluations of drug treatment identify various factors which are associated with superior outcomes (NTA 2004). These include:

- Fast and easy access to treatment.
- Goals of drug treatment matched to client preference.

- An empathic approach and positive ethos.

- Long duration of treatment programme.

- Flexible rather than rigid treatment regimes.

- Completion of treatment programme.

- High attendance.

- Retention in treatment.

Psychosocial interventions should always be included in drug treatment plans (NICE 2007c). Psychological therapies (e.g. motivational interviewing, relapse prevention, cognitive behaviour therapy, community reinforcement and contingency management) can help the drug user change their drug-taking behaviour and address co-existing problems such as anxiety, depression and post-traumatic stress disorder. Informal psychosocial interventions are also effective, e.g. self-help group such as Narcotics Anonymous (NA), support groups for families and carers, opportunistic brief interventions. Other 'wrap-around' services can include: housing assistance, welfare benefits and debt advice, training and employment schemes, legal advice, community-based recreational activities, childcare and so on.

There are several special issues to do with drug treatment which ought to be considered and, where appropriate, addressed with drug-using parents. Some of these are discussed next.

Safe storage of drugs in the home

Protecting children from accidental ingestion of drugs is vitally important (Department of Health 2007b). Discuss methods of storing illicit and prescribed drugs (and drug paraphernalia) in the home with all drug users and ensure that they understand how to respond if a child ingests drugs. Recommend that parents talk to their children about the dangers of taking medicine that is not meant for them.

Pregnancy

Problem drug use during pregnancy is associated with increased risks for mother and baby (Hepburn 2004; Johnstone 1998). Risks can be greatly reduced when good quality antenatal and postnatal care is provided, along with effective drug treatment (Department of Health 2007b). The greatest risks are associated with relapse, injecting drug use, heroin and cocaine use and failure to attend health and social care appointments. By contrast, methadone treatment for opiate-dependent women during pregnancy is more likely to result in continuity of care and improved obstetric and neonatal outcomes

(WHO *et al.* 2004). Pregnant women on methadone should not be pressurized into reducing or stopping their prescription. Some women may require an increased methadone dose during pregnancy in order to achieve stability (Department of Health 2007b). Some may be keen to reduce while pregnant; if appropriate, opiate detoxification can be undertaken with caution, usually during the mid-trimester (NICE 2007b). Methadone is not a contraindication for breastfeeding (Department of Health 2007b) and should be encouraged, except where the mother is HIV positive, injecting, using cocaine or crack, alcohol or high doses of benzodiazepines.

The effects of maternal drug use on the foetus and newborn baby are broadly similar and largely non-drug specific (see DrugScope 2005). The adverse effects of smoking during pregnancy are well documented (NICE 2008). Although there is uncertainty regarding a safe level of alcohol use during pregnancy, low levels (defined as 1–2 units once or twice a week) are not associated with harm to the unborn baby (NICE 2008). High maternal consumption of alcohol is associated with fetal alcohol syndrome and fetal alcohol spectrum disorder (BMA 2007b).

Neonatal abstinence syndrome

Neonatal abstinence syndrome (NAS or 'baby withdrawals') is well documented in infants born to women dependent on opiates and benzodiazepines (Johnstone 1998). Parents who have an infant with NAS often feel guilty, ashamed and 'to blame' for their baby's condition and may lack confidence in their parenting ability (DrugScope 2005). Caring for a baby with NAS can be extremely demanding and stressful and parents often need a lot of patience, support, reassurance and encouragement. This should be taken into account when devising a pre-birth family support plan or child protection plan.

Warn parents that babies with NAS can be 'hard to parent' for weeks or even months following birth. The infant may be difficult to feed, settle and console. Delayed growth and development may be evident during the first year and poor co-ordination and gaze may effect parent–infant interactions and attachment (Lloyd and Myserscough 2006). Mothers, fathers and other potential carers (e.g. kinship carers and foster carers) should be shown how to care for a baby with NAS using supportive comfort measures and carer–infant interaction techniques (French *et al.* 1998).

Domestic abuse

Parental conflict, separation and domestic abuse are associated with problem drug (and alcohol) use and increased rates of child maltreatment (Cleaver *et al.*

1999; Humphreys, Thiara and Regan 2005). Risks to children are increased when problem drug use and domestic abuse co-exist (Brandon *et al.* 2008).

Problem drug use does not cause domestic abuse, but can be a contributing factor, e.g. poor impulse control, agitation with intoxication and withdrawals (BMA 2007a). Other factors associated with an increased risk of domestic abuse include: childhood history of abuse and exposure to family violence, low educational attainment, unemployment, financial hardship, lack of housing, social isolation, poor physical and mental health, and pregnancy (Barnish 2004). Parental conflict and domestic abuse can trigger relapse and domestic abuse can escalate following separation. Both victims and perpetrators of domestic abuse commonly report substance use.

Intervening and providing support for children and families is crucial (Mullender 2004). Appropriate services may include individual and groupwork for the children, mediation or relationship counselling for the couple, anger management and domestic abuse perpetrator programmes, advocacy and family system-centred interventions, although the evidence base for the effectiveness of these interventions is limited (Ramsay, Rivas and Feder 2005).

Family support

Under the broad heading of 'family support', this section briefly considers interventions which aim to improve relationships within the family, parenting skills and family functioning.

While the concept and practice of 'family support' is somewhat contentious (see Featherstone 2006; Parton 1997), it normally involves a combination of home visits (including unannounced home visits), clinic-based care, community-based child and parenting services, and structured couple and family-focused work. Family support tends to work on a strengths-based approach rather than a deficit model, and aims to identify and build on competencies, achievements, resources, protective factors and resilience within families. By doing so, it attempts to minimize poor parenting practices and the risks and harms to children. Family support can also include specific interventions aimed at preventing the recurrence of child maltreatment and helping children recover from the effects of abuse or neglect.

Despite the push to intervene in the lives of families affected by problem drug use, the evidence on 'what works' is limited (Donohue, Romero and Hill 2006; Tunnard 2002). The strongest evidence in terms of reducing risks, increasing protective factors and reducing drug use and drug-related harm, is for cognitive and behavioural parent skills training, couple therapy, family therapy, social network interventions and children's skills training (Velleman and Templeton 2007b). Most well-evaluated interventions include a combination of these approaches and are intensive, highly structured and multi-component programmes.

Early intervention is crucial. Ideally, parenting support for the mother and father should begin during the antenatal period, well before the baby is born. Initiating a discussion about aspirations for motherhood, fatherhood and family life is a good starting point. This can usefully lead into a dialogue about the parent's preparations for the birth of the baby and how they plan to 'share the care' in the early postnatal period. Depending on their previous parenting experience and parenting confidence, parents can be encouraged to attend antenatal and parenthood education classes or to seek one-to-one support from the community midwife and health visitor. Early referral to a children's centre or parenting service is often helpful. Baby massage classes, 'dads' only services, mother and toddler groups and a range of other early years services for families (e.g. Sure Start) may be of interest. Many areas now have specialist family support services for drug-using parents and their young infants. These are often more flexible and offer outreach services.

Evaluations of parenting interventions with drug-using parents (see Catalano *et al.* 1999; Dawe *et al.* 2003; Johnson *et al.* 2006; Luthar and Suchman 2000; Velez *et al.* 2004), have reported a range of positive outcomes including: decreased parental drug use and risk behaviour, less time spent with drug-using peer group, improved psychological adjustment, increased involvement with children, improved parent–child relationships, parenting knowledge and skills, family functioning and decreased risk of child maltreatment.

Although there is no specific guidance on engaging and working with drug-using fathers, research on working with other disadvantaged fathers and those involved in the child protection system is potentially relevant (see Burgess 2008; Daniel and Taylor 2001; Ghate *et al.* 2000; Scourfield 2006). Research shows that fathers who are more involved in the pregnancy and 'share the care' with the mother during the child's first year of life are more likely to remain positively involved with their children as they grow up, even if they separate from the mother (Burgess 2008). Some studies have found that behavioural couples therapy, rather than individual-based parenting programmes for drug-using fathers result in greater improvement in the father's substance use, co-parental relationship with the mother and the child's psychological wellbeing (Fals-Stewart, O'Farrell and Birchler 2004).

Family-focused interventions have also been developed to prevent the children of drug users developing problems with substance use themselves (NICE 2007a; Velleman and Templeton 2007a). The Strengthening Families Programme (Kumpfer, Alvarado and Whiteside 2003), is one example of a well-evaluated community-based educational and therapeutic prevention programme which combines child, parent and family skills training.

The value of including and supporting non-drug-using partners and other family members has been clearly demonstrated (EIU 2002). They can benefit from advice about how to cope with the stresses of living with a drug user, how to manage the drug user's behaviour and their own responses towards them, and how to ensure their own health and wellbeing is maintained through extended social support networks. Copello *et al.*'s (2000) 'stress-coping-health' five-step brief intervention model, specifically designed for primary health care, is a good example of how family members can be helped in this way. The extended family (particularly the child's grandparents) may have a central role to play in the care and protection of children (Barnard 2003). Not only may they provide practical, emotional, material and financial assistance to the family, but when necessary, they may intervene to safeguard children and take over parenting responsibilities, either on a temporary or permanent basis.

Social behaviour and social network interventions, which aim to develop a protective informal and formal social support structure for the drug user and their family, have also been successfully employed (Copello *et al.* 2006). These approaches recognize the importance of wider contextual factors (e.g. drug-using peer groups and risky social environments) and work on developing positive social behaviours and support networks for all the network members. These ecological or community-based approaches involve a focus on the social ecology of drug-taking, parenting and child welfare. They understand the limitations of interventions which solely focus on individuals and risks within the home, and highlight instead, the role of social networks and the effects of various forms of 'capital' (social, cultural and economic). In practice, they focus on addressing the needs of the child by addressing risk and protective factors relating to the parents (Cabinet Office 2008a). 'Whole family' ecological approaches appear to be promising as they seek to work with resources within the community, as well as the family, to reduce drug-related harm and to prevent child maltreatment.

Conclusion

Intervening in the lives of families affected by problem drug use requires considerable skill and sensitivity as well as a thorough understanding of problem drug use and drug treatment, child development, child maltreatment, parenting and family functioning. More crucially, it involves an understanding of the socio-cultural environment of the family and the kind of stressors and hardships they face. Essentially, drug-using parents, both mothers and fathers, need to be encouraged to become part of the solution rather than just the crux of the problem.

Chapter Fifteen

The Limits, Challenges and Opportunities of Safeguarding Children in the Context of Primary Care

Markus Themessl-Huber, Anne Claveirole, Janette Pow,
Dona Milne and Lawrie Elliot

Introduction

The sexual health of young people is a concern for policy makers and practitioners alike in Scotland. Some young people are particularly vulnerable to the adverse consequences of early sexual behaviour and as such are widely recognized to be one of the most important groups for reproductive health interventions (Cowen 2002). In 2005, there were seven births for every 1000 women under 16 years (ISD Scotland Publications 2007) while in 2003, 25 per cent of young Scottish women aged under 20 years reported having had a pregnancy terminated (Scottish Executive 2006a). Moreover, abortion rates in all teenage age groups are rising, especially in the under 16s (ISD Scotland Publications 2007). Approximately one in seven attendances to Genito-urinary Medicine Clinics (GUM) are by young people aged under 20 years and between 2002 and 2003 there was a 40 per cent increase in Chlamydia diagnoses in females under 15 years (Scottish Executive 2006a). Over the last two decades, the sexual health of young people has seen virtually no improvements (ISD Scotland Publications 2007; Viner and Barker 2005), although the availability of information, education and services is improving throughout Scotland and there is no sign of further worsening of the situation (Scottish Executive 2006a).

Sexual health, however, cannot merely be defined as being free from infection or unplanned pregnancy. The lack of progress in safeguarding the sexual health of young people has occurred despite the sexual health of young people having long been a clinical and policy concern within primary care (Department of Health 2001a). The inability of society to be open and positive about sexuality and to accept adolescent sexuality, has produced a climate where it is difficult for adults, whether parents or professionals to be open and honest about sexual matters with children and young people (Crouch 2002; West 1999; Whitaker, Miller and Clarke 2000). Yet, young people themselves express the need to talk about sexuality and the need to be treated with respect and openness (West 1999). Young people usually make their first contact with the health service in a primary care context (Donaldson *et al.* 1994). This means that primary care professionals have regular contact with the majority of young people at some point. Indeed, three out of four young people visit their general practice at least once every year (Royal College of Paediatrics and Child Health 2003). Primary care professionals thus have a particular responsibility for safeguarding the sexual health of young people due to their skills, expertise as well as their role as gatekeepers or signposts to other health services (Intercollegiate Document 2006).

However, three fundamental issues regarding the sexual health care of young people in primary care have been identified. First, young people find it difficult to access primary care services to talk about sexual health matters (Jacobson *et al.* 2001; Royal College of General Practitioners and Brook 2000; Walker *et al.* 2002). Second, service providers are often uncomfortable about raising sexual health issues with young people due to lack of experience, embarrassment, or conflicting moral views (Evans 2004; Graham 2004; Gregg, Freeth and Blackie 1998). Third, young people in the most deprived areas are ten times more likely to deliver babies and have twice the rate of abortion than those in the least deprived areas (ISD Scotland Publications 2007). These three issues need urgent attention if the sexual health, and therefore the physical health and safety, of young people are to be improved. Young people need to be knowledgeable about sexual health matters, they need to be aware of available services and have the confidence and ability to use them. Service providers, likewise, need to have the knowledge, skills and confidence necessary to make sure their services are effective and acceptable to young people. This in turn, requires service providers to receive appropriate training and resources to enhance their capabilities and capacities (Viner and Barker 2005).

It is important to note here that general practitioners are only one of many professions in primary care (Polney 2001). The impact of primary care professionals and of community-based sexual health activities can be enhanced significantly by working in partnership with other public and private service providers (Fisher, Neve and Heritage 1999; Patouillard *et al.* 2007). Although few would deny the importance of collaborating, various personal and organizational hurdles need to be overcome to achieve effective and efficient partnership working in any such endeavour (Herbert *et al.* 2007; Horwath and Morrison 2007).

The availability and necessity of multiple professions engaging with the sexual health of young people, however, requires all professions involved to rethink the boundaries of their engagement (Milne and Chesson 2000). Primary care professionals have to accept that they play an important role in activities beyond the context of traditional health care, for instance in schools and community-based settings (Mellanby *et al.* 1995). They are key agents in raising awareness of and addressing myths and stigmas associated with young people's sexual health, the influence of which has implications far beyond health care matters (Evans 2004). In this context, primary care professionals include all those who contribute to the provision of sexual health education, information and services to young people, based on a definition of primary care (World Health Organization 1978), which goes beyond the traditional view of the health sector.

The wealth of different professions and organizations involved in safeguarding the sexual health of young people necessitates the co-ordination of activities and an efficient flow of information. To date, however, a lack of co-ordinated service provision (Milne and Chesson 2000) and the inverse care law, which states that the 'availability of good [health] care tends to vary inversely with the need for the population served' (Tudor Hart 1971, p.405), are still too often governing (sexual) health service provision for young people in the community (Webb 1998).

Close partnerships safeguard young people's sexual health

The effects of failed partnership working to safeguard young people are seen most drastically in children harmed or killed despite having been known by and referred to health and social care services (Laming 2003). However, to date the various sectors and service providers involved are struggling to close the gaps in the care and protection they provide to young people (Ferlie and McGivern 2003; Koeck 1998). Evidence still suggests that services for children are not well co-ordinated (HM Government 2006; Laming 2003). Indeed, working in partnership is a complex endeavour and its success depends on a variety of factors (Dowling, Powell and Glendinning 2004;

Flaherty *et al.* 2004; HM Government 2006; Hubbard and Themessl-Huber 2005; Scottish Executive 2006a; Sloper 2004; Taylor and Corlett 2007).

Yet, evidence suggests that collaborating and co-operating organizations are more effective at providing a complex array of community-based services than the same organizations would provide independently (Provan and Milward 1995). The benefits of inter-agency work are considered to be numerous and include rationalization of resources, a reduction in duplication of effort and more effective, integrated and supportive service provision for patients and professionals (Bloxham 1997). Collaborative approaches, offering a variety of services between them, are also more likely to meet the needs of young people (Health Development Agency 2001).

Effectively safeguarding the sexual health and wellbeing of children in primary care, therefore, arguably requires close collaboration between policy makers, professionals from different disciplines and organizations, parents and young people (HM Government 2006; Public Health Institute of Scotland 2003; Scottish Executive 2002, 2004b). In relation to sexual health services it is assumed that partnership working will provide the means to equip services providers with the capacity and capability to inform and empower people to have the knowledge and skills to make informed and responsible decisions about their sexual behaviour and improve access to supportive and high quality sexual health services (Scottish Executive 2006a).

A wealth of models, theories and research evidence promoting integration, partnership working, inter-agency collaborations and a focus on complexity and whole-systems approaches have emerged over the last decade to inform the development and co-ordination of services (Conner 2001; Dubbs *et al.* 2004; Foote and Plsek 2001; Iles and Sutherland 2001; Kirby 2001; Plsek and Wilson 2001; Swan *et al.* 2003; Williams and Imam 2007). However, before building services based on sound bites like partnership working, integrated care, or informed choice, the various aspects of the proposed collaborations have to be explicated in detail as their implications on the practical delivery of services is not always clear (Dieppe and Horne 2002).

A prerequisite for constructive partnership working and for selecting appropriate settings for collaborative service delivery is thus to build on explicit knowledge of services and their contexts. Effective partnership working in practice requires developing practical knowledge of services and service delivery (Eraut 1994; Schon 1987). Previous (published) experience provides some indication as to what factors are characteristic of successful partnerships (Asthana, Richardson and Halliday 2002; Dowling *et al.* 2004; Sloper 2004). Over and above the organizational intricacies of partnership working, the successful implementation, delivery and sustainability of sexual health interventions for young people further rely on them being delivered in a variety of contexts, i.e. schools, drop-in clinics and youth centres. Thus, no single service is likely to be able to address all relevant factors (Aggleton and Campbell 2000; Cheesbrough, Ingham and Massey 1999; Kane and Wellings 1998; Kirby, Laris and Rolleri 2006; McLeod 2001; West 1999).

In recent years, there have been local, regional and nationwide attempts to improve the sexual health and safety of young people in Scotland (Scottish Executive 2006a). Across the public and voluntary sectors a number of health and social care services have been adapted, augmented, or newly created to provide mainstream and special care (Department of Health 2001a; Scottish Executive 2006a). Many hospital- or community-based services have been newly implemented or re-structured and almost every region in Scotland attempted to increase the level of integration and collaboration of different services and agencies involved in addressing the sexual health and safety of young people.

Although services are often (re-)designed based on existing evidence and perceived local needs, their final shape is usually a result of numerous influences, including the planned structure, reactions to challenges posed by the local context and experiences managers and service providers gained in the course of implementing the planned services (Kushner 2000).

One challenge service providers, managers and funders alike face in working in partnership to safeguard the sexual health of young people is to assess the (cost-) effectiveness and efficiency of each service on its own as well as in comparison with others. Effective allocation of funds and development of health and social care services relies on information about the performance or potential of services to guide their decisions. Currently, a fair judgement of services is a challenging endeavour, especially when taking into account local contexts or the demands of the relevant clinical and administrative parties involved. This Gordian knot represents a hub in the complex system of care that needs to be untied or by-passed in order for services to have an impact on the sexual health and safety of young people.

The following portrayal of Healthy Respect and its effects on service providers aiming to improve young people's sexual health appraises one such attempt at untying this Gordian knot.

Healthy Respect: a demonstration project

In 2001, the Scottish Executive Health Department set up a national demonstration project, Healthy Respect (HR). HR was one of four national health demonstration projects announced in the *Towards a Healthier Scotland* White Paper (Scottish Executive 2003g). The demonstration projects were set up as test-beds for innovation to identify how to meet some of the health challenges in the 21st century and disseminate the learning across Scotland. The demonstration initiative was led by the then Health Minister and was therefore subject to much public scrutiny from professionals in the field, commissioners of programmes and services and the media. In order to assess the effectiveness of HR, the then Scottish Executive commissioned independent evaluations of impact on young people's health outcomes.

The project's aim was to help young people develop a positive attitude to their own sexuality and that of others and to improve their sexual health by taking a multi-faceted and co-ordinated approach (Scottish Executive 2003b). HR set out to integrate education, information and services for young people and parents, supported by an overarching communications strategy including the use of the HR brand and social marketing activities. Two tactics were used to pursue HR's aims. Activities, training and resources were aimed first at young people and parents and second at professionals. The latter tactic aimed at increasing service providers' capacity and capability to provide education, information and services as part of their work with young people and parents and to do so in a co-ordinated and consistent fashion.

Achieving improvements in young people's sexual health is challenging. There are strongly held views that increasing sex and relationships education and providing access to contraception will increase sexual activity among young people: this is not borne out in evidence (Fraser 2005) but has prevented many agencies from taking action in this area. What the evidence does suggest is that a multi-faceted approach combining education, information and services is most likely to deliver improvements in young people's sexual health outcomes (Kirby 2001). Evidence also suggests that collaborating organizations are more effective in the delivery of community-based services than those operating independently (Health Development Agency 2001).

As argued earlier, achieving such an approach cannot be delivered by a single agency: it requires partnership working which draws together statutory and voluntary sector partners to deliver combined education, information and services for young people. HR hoped to achieve this through establishing a sexual health and wellbeing partnership network.

A functioning partnership requires an understanding of the issues it faces and clearly articulated common goals that identify the part that all partners have to play (Mann, Pritchard and Rummery 2004). Partnership working is not just about the process of bringing agencies together to share resources, the benefits need to be apparent: two plus two really does need to make five, or in this case the benefits of linking education, information and services need to demonstrate clear benefits for young people, as recognized in the phase one evaluation of HR (Dugald Baird Centre for Research on Women's Health 2005).

Following the first phase of HR, the second phase (HR2) set out to create a partnership network that achieved more: leading to the school nurse working with the teacher to deliver sex and relationships education in school and the youth worker delivering the drop-in service as part of a local team with the school nurse. In creating this network, HR2 sought to identify key partners and agencies which had a role to play in improving young people's health and sexual health in particular. This involvement of staff within the wider primary care team led to a range of approaches being delivered which were able to take an evidence-based approach, work towards an agreed set of service standards while also responding to local need.

To support this local delivery, HR2 provided a number of programme co-ordination functions including advocacy and leadership, support to the partnership network, Lothian-wide integrated communications work, training, monitoring and evaluation (Healthy Respect 2003). The demonstration hypotheses being that increased confidence, capacity and capability of staff and agencies could lead to co-ordinated and consistent provision for young people (Healthy Respect 2003), something which was found to be lacking at an earlier stage in the work of the project.

The end product of partnership has to be improved service for young people (in this instance) and this needs to be the focus and yardstick against which partnership work is constantly measured. In the case of HR2, partnership working allowed innovative low threshold services to be developed, encouraged services to network and think of more imaginative ways of training and of framing youth issues. It also enabled access to more vulnerable and hard to reach groups and drew more professional groups into accepting responsibility for young people's sexual health and overall wellbeing.

Taking a population-based as well as a targeted approach, the HR2 network was created to support young people to access support through a range of professionals in recognition of young people's right to choose with whom they wanted to engage (Milne 2005) and the valued contributions that different professional groups had to make: whether that be a guidance teacher delivering sex and relationships education, a school nurse running a local drop-in service or a youth worker engaged in informal education.

The provider organizations involved in the HR2 initiative included primary and secondary schools; NHS services (school nurses, family planning, genito-urinary medicine, specialist teams, GP practices, child protection advisors, community paediatricians, some pharmacies); voluntary sector providers of sexual health services and community youth projects; and local authority (LA) teams of social workers, youth and community workers and special education units for young people unable to attend mainstream education. The primary schools delivered a teaching pack focused on respect and relationships while the secondary schools used the Sexual Health and Relationship Education (SHARE) teaching package, both of which were provided by HR2 together with training and ongoing support. The NHS, LA and the voluntary sector offered drop-in services within or close to high school communities.

A number of issues emerged throughout the establishment of the network, such as confidentiality, child protection, work with parents and the negotiation of local and national policy and protocols. The network co-ordination functions fulfilled by HR2 led to the establishment of formal partners' agreements, the provision of some resources to support local delivery and a greater level of expertise to support a functioning partnership.

Evaluation outcomes: the impact of Healthy Respect 2 on providers' ability to improve young people's sexual health

The external evaluation of HR2 aimed to assess the impact of the project on providers' ability to improve young people's sexual health in one defined Scottish area. Findings from a survey, which ran a year after the start of the project's second phase (Elliott *et al.* 2007), complemented by semi-structured interviews with some survey respondents (Claveirole *et al.* 2008) are reported here.

Service providers involved with Healthy Respect 2

The survey provided some insight into the type of providers involved with HR2 as partners as well as those who were less or not involved. The survey identified half of the participating service providers as being actively involved in the initiative. Four out of five involved service providers reported good partnership working with HR2. Partnership working lies at the heart of the project's approach to sexual provision for young people and thus these results were particularly encouraging. Furthermore, when asked if they would like to continue being involved with HR2, four out of five both confirmed and would also recommend HR2 to another organization.

With the exception of HR2 drop-ins and primary school, however, engagement levels varied across the involved service providers. Organizations with varying levels of involvement included HR2 secondary schools, NHS services and particularly local authority organizations (social work, youth community teams and special education units). Service providers also offered various reasons why HR2 had not been adopted uniformly across and within organizations.

The most important barrier identified by service providers was a lack of resources (time, funding and people) to undertake partnership work. Various service providers additionally had to deal with issues that were relevant to certain agencies.

Moreover, service providers not involved with HR2 either reported that they worked independently from HR2 and did not wish to engage with it; or in some cases a recent turnover of staff meant that those new in post knew very little about the project; some said the HR2 team had not invited them to take part; and for some, sexual health was not seen as a priority.

Education providers reported that the organizational structure of schools made it very difficult for them to become truly involved in partnership work with HR2. Many, although willing to undertake and be part of the continuing professional development sessions (offered by HR2), could not get out of school due to teaching commitments. Others felt that the initial SHARE training received was enough and there was no need for further contact with HR2 following this training (despite it being a recommendation from the phase one evaluation). The majority of those from the schools saw the partnership with HR2 as being very 'informal' and believed that the formal partnership was between the education department within the local authority and HR2. In secondary schools, particularly, an aging staff population meant a high turnover of teachers with the attendant risk of losing the HR2 culture that had been created.

In the NHS, some large services like family planning and genito-urinary medicine were generic, many of their staff working with adults more than with young people, sometimes part time. These providers would not have responded to the survey as partners but as informed commentators, giving the impression that the services were not fully engaged with HR2. In those teams, however, full-time senior workers were committed partners. Other important NHS providers of sexual health services surveyed, the general practitioners, were hardly involved with HR2 and did not feel the need to be.

In local authority organizations, the commitment to HR2 was patchy. Both the organizational structure and the necessary prioritization of managing acute situations (as in the case of child protection issues) left little time to undertake preventative work with young people. This acted both as a barrier to working with HR2 and meant that many could not or did not see the need to become involved or attend sexual health training.

Engagement with HR2 was lower among those working with vulnerable young people. Youth and street workers responded to HR2 unevenly and sometimes grudgingly. Many felt the joint working approach proposed by HR2 was not 'an equal partnership but rather commissioning on the cheap.' Still, youth workers were engaging in some sexual health work with their target groups but the influence of HR2 appeared to be limited. Social workers preferred to refer young people who needed sexual health and relationship input to other agencies.

Voluntary organizations in particular feared a 'loss of identity' and often felt marginalized by the bigger and more powerful organizations (namely health and local authority). This was particularly true when it came to the mainstreaming of initiatives; with one voluntary organization reporting that when services within a certain locality were being mainstreamed they were told that the 'voluntary sector would not be part of the mainstreaming'. These findings are consistent with what Mann *et al.* (2004) found when undertaking an evaluation of partnership working. They warned that partnership work instead of being a positive experience for organizations can in fact lead to losses for less powerful partners, particularly those from the voluntary sector.

Impact of HR2 on service providers' sexual health care capacity and capability

The main resources service providers received from HR2 were training, advice, support and information. Funding was also received by about one-third of service providers. Those receiving the most resources from HR2 were more likely to report a greater impact on their professional knowledge and skills. The amount of resources received was also the most important factor in helping them focus on the sexual health outcomes of young people including unintended teenage pregnancy. A high level of resource was related to good partnership working with HR2 and a small increase in organizational capacity. However, approximately half of HR2 partners also thought their general and administrative workload had increased following their involvement with HR2, perhaps due to the increase in quality standards and evaluation requirements of a demonstration programme.

About two-thirds of managers in partner organizations thought HR2 improved the quality and range of what they offered to young people for their sexual health and increased the level of staff training and staff time devoted to the sexual health of young people. A high level of managerial support for HR2 was further associated with a greater impact on professionals' knowledge and skills, improved support for parents and an increased focus on sexual health outcomes for young people. Managerial support also helped to establish good partnership working with HR2.

Almost all partners reported that HR2 helped them focus on enhancing young people's ability to make sexual health choices; increased the quality and consistency of sexual health and relationship education for young people; improved access to sexual health education and services; improved the quality of sexual health drop-ins. HR2 had also helped them to understand sexual health issues and young people's perspectives on sexual health and relationships; it had increased their confidence in approaching young people about sexual health and helped them share ideas about sexual health with other professionals.

Those service providers whose capacity and capability to do sexual health work with young people were most affected by HR2 resources were the schools and the providers of drop-ins. In the schools, the new teaching packages provided by HR2 and the impetus which sprang from their leadership had transformed sex and relationship education. In the drop-ins, partnership with HR2 at managerial level had meant high standards uniformly applied, good training and some financial support. However, service providers targeting vulnerable young people reported contrasting and uneven changes in their capacity and capability to do sexual health work with young people under the influence of HR2. Those working with identifiable groups, such as young people with learning disabilities or young people looked after by a local authority, or those providing alternative educational provision in an institutional setting reported improvements.

Those who claimed to be least able to use HR2 operated in the community and followed complex, multi-faceted agendas. They were social workers and youth workers. For them, young people's sexual health was only a small part of a very large remit. The majority of the providers also reported that HR2 did not reach some groups of vulnerable young people. The most common groups cited were young people not at school, those who were socially excluded and those with learning disabilities.

The impact of HR2 on forging new and existing partnerships between provider organizations

As mentioned earlier, partnership working is central to HR2. Service providers were asked about their partnerships with other organizations, to discover if partnership work was taking place prior to HR and whether HR had any impact on forging new or existing partnerships and networks. Social network analysis studies consider strong links or partnerships as those where each organization mentions the other as partners (Provan and Milward 1995). Many such 'confirmed ties' were reported between organizations working in this area. This suggests that partnership working and networking had been taking place between organizations. Nearly all (39 interviewees) confirmed that these 'ties' or partnerships with other organizations had been made prior to being engaged with HR2. Although many of the providers reported that these partnerships may be quite informal and are developed and maintained by the individual practitioners, fewer partnerships had been made at the organizational level. A few service providers mentioned that existing links with other organizations had been 'firmed up' through dialogue with HR2.

From a geographical perspective organizations tended to partner with other organizations in the same local area. There appeared to be a strong argument for the services available locally to be able to deliver 'a one stop shop', i.e. services that meet all of the clients' needs (advice, support, contraception, pregnancy testing and testing for sexually transmitted infections). Most service providers expressed fears over young people having to travel any distance to access services and felt it was more appropriate to have services available locally that they could direct young people to, therefore many of the partnerships were with local agencies. Service providers felt that if young people were then redirected to another service they might (a) never attend the other service and (b) lose faith in the first service as their needs were not being fully met.

The sustainability of Healthy Respect 2's impact on its partner organizations beyond the demonstration project

Service providers indicated that the impact of HR2 on professionals and their organization was affected by three factors: managerial support, resources received (which need not be solely financial, but could also include training, advice and information) and the type of organization in which people work. Changing any of these may affect the future impact of HR2. If the support which HR2 used to provide is not maintained by these organizations, the range and quality of sexual health support may be adversely affected. This view was shared by the majority of interviewees who expressed concern that aspects of the sexual health provision to young people, such as the resources, the leadership and the co-ordination role HR2 used to play, would be at risk. Half the informants, however, thought their organization would sustain the work previously supported by HR2 for a while. A small number of service providers thought the impact of HR2 on their organization had been too low to notice any difference. Some commented negatively on the mainstreaming process and the absence of consultation before activities were transferred from HR2 to their organization. Overall, the interviews confirmed and amplified the findings of the survey.

The limits, challenges and opportunities of partnership working

Addressing young people's sexual attitudes and behaviours is fraught with challenges for parents and service providers alike. Often, neither feel they have the skill, confidence or knowledge to raise this topic with young people. These insecurities, the sheer complexity of the task, but also the urgent need for improvement have encouraged parents, service providers and policy makers to join forces. Effective partnership working, however, is also difficult and requires committed partners and strategic co-ordination. Unfortunately, ineffective or dysfunctional partnership working can put young people at increased risk (Laming 2003).

Yet, a considerable evidence base of effective interventions has been accumulated. The Scottish Executive decided to build on this evidence and established the Healthy Respect Demonstration Project with the aims of supporting young people in developing positive attitudes towards sexuality and of improving their sexual health. HR2 comprised of various interventions, all of which relied heavily on working in partnership with relevant service providers in all public and private sectors.

The evaluation of HR2's activities showed that, for various reasons, it was difficult to actively involve all service providers in this initiative. Some service providers struggled with a lack of resources, others were at odds with HR2's approach to promoting sexual health and/or partnership working. Professionals working with vulnerable groups of young people were particularly difficult to engage and had considerable reservations about the benefits of HR2 for their work or their client group.

However, those providers who were actively involved were content with their role as partners. Service providers were not able to say whether the various HR2 initiatives had improved young people's sexual health. Yet, they thought that the training, advice, support and information they received from HR2 improved the quality and range of interventions they could offer young people and had a noticeable impact on their own sexual health care-related skills, knowledge and confidence. Service providers also reported that working with HR2 had resulted in strengthening already existing partnerships with other organizations and facilitated the forging of new collaborations.

Many service providers, irrespective of their level of engagement, expressed concern over the sustainability of HR2's achievements. They argued that the benefits of partnership working depended on continuing managerial support, the availability of resources and responsiveness of interventions to the needs and structures of different service providers. Without the co-ordinating and driving role of HR2 they were sceptical about whether HR2's achievements, including inter-organizational partnership working to promote young people's health, would prevail.

Chapter Sixteen

Safeguarding Children Where There May be Concerns about Ritualistic Abuse or Spirit Possession

Julie Taylor and Jane Cantrell

Introduction

The focus of this chapter is on those forms of abuse, usually sexual but also physical and neglectful and always emotional, that have a ritualistic element and may be linked to beliefs about witchcraft, the devil or spirit possession. However, it is important from the beginning to distinguish between individuals who may cynically use religion to inflict harm on children for their own gratification, and distressed parents who may genuinely believe that difficulties in their children's behaviour are due to possession by evil spirits. The terminology itself is difficult. Stobart's work (2006) suggested that no terms are entirely satisfactory, but that the most acceptable across faith-based organizations, non-governmental organizations and the public sector are 'possession by evil spirits' or 'witchcraft'.

It is also important to note that ritualistic behaviour may have nothing whatsoever to do with real or actual abuse. 'The offender may be involved in ritualistic activity with a child and may also be abusing a child, but one may have little or nothing to do with the other' (Lanning 2002). We have therefore structured this chapter to make a distinction between those who may use intimidating or occult props as part of the abuse of children and those who believe children can be possessed. We acknowledge, of course, that sometimes there may be overlap. Our priority is the support of practitioners in ensuring the safety of children. In many areas of abuse practitioners may never know the precise details of circumstances, events and interactions. We have to learn to live with uncertainty, while responding sympathetically and effectively to the suffering, harm and distress we encounter. Our attempts to safeguard and protect children need to recognize that a worst case scenario may be a possibility, without ruling out alternative explanations which may be compatible with limited evidence available.

We argue that forms of ritualistic or occult based abuses are very rare. While there are a few documented cases, high quality forensic evidence or objective video and audio recordings have not borne out the intense media attention that was paid to ritualistic sexual abuse in the 1980s and 1990s (Kirk Weir and Wheatcroft 1995). The intensive studies that have been undertaken (e.g. La Fontaine 1994; Lanning 1992) draw similar conclusions. However, we recognize that on occasion 'satanic' abuse may occur and also that allegations of ritual sexual abuse may arise from real sexual abuse that has little or nothing to do with demons or witchcraft. We suggest that dismissing everything is a danger and that there are some key triggers and stories that may yet point to abuse and harm, however sensational or unbelievable they apparently sound.

Following a discussion of satanic abuse and allegations of ritual sexual abuse, we turn to an area of increasing concern and evidence – belief in witchcraft and its associated practices. We use the 'muti' killings in southern Africa as an example. We then examine closely linked beliefs in spirit possession that many parents (and some religions) use to explain childhood behaviours or diseases. The practice of trying to cast out such demons is a worrying trend that seems to be associated with many current causes for concern and serious case reviews. While parents and carers may hold genuine beliefs about spirit possession, the effects of such beliefs on children are harmful. A small minority of churches, faiths or religious groups may be implicated as part of the problem, but there is much encouraging work that suggests they are also part of the solution.

Most of the kinds of abuse we describe in this chapter arise in homes and communities where primary health care practitioners are those most likely to encounter them first. Primary health care practitioners, therefore, need to be informed and vigilant.

Satanism

Through the 1990s there were many books and television documentaries examining claims and counter-claims about the existence of satanic ritual abuse. Just typing 'satanic ritual abuse' into a Google search box gets about three million hits. This is a subject that grabs the imagination. In a world where child abuse and neglect are already so abhorrent, the horror of witchcraft, ritual and mystery adds further to the 'otherness' of those who harm children, as well as reflecting increasing interest in sensationalist sex and violence.

According to FBI writer Lanning (2002), satanism and a variety of other terms, such as demonology, occultism and ritualism are used interchangeably, implying that all are part of a continuum of behaviour. Distinctions are often blurred and media representations are often used as 'evidence'. We do not yet have good enough knowledge about connections between belief systems and the crimes committed; nor do we have evidence about an organized conspiracy of satanic believers and interrelated serious abuse. Lanning suggests that as professionals we need to focus on facts. These facts are:

- Some individuals believe in and are involved in something commonly called satanism and the occult.

- Some of these individuals commit crimes.

- Some groups of individuals share these beliefs.

- Some members of these groups commit crime together.

In the early 1990s in the United States of America a wave of hysteria peaked: a shocking story of ritualistic satanic abuse, pornography, infanticide and torture had become a best-selling book. Lauren Stratford's story (1989), *Satan's Underground*, of her abusive childhood at the hands of a satanic cult was documented as factual and corroborated by a wealth of apparent evidence. Stratford's story became a validation of the 'repressed memory' frenzy, cited by many leading media and church authorities and broadcast widely as evidence of ritual sexual abuse. Stratford's story, however, appears to have been fabrication. According to Passantino, Passatino and Trott (1989), allegedly there was no evidence for her account and Stratford was a psychiatrically disturbed young woman, prone to self-harm and wild story invention. Stratford continually proclaimed the truth of her childhood (Stratford 1993). Despite the apparent fabrication, Stratford's story suggests a level of distress that needs to be taken seriously and responded to within the context of her reality.

Michelle Remembers was another best-selling book that triggered much of the furore on ritual abuse. In it psychiatrist Pazder documented the therapy of his long-term patient Michelle Smith (later his wife) who disclosed, under hypnosis, ritual abuse by her mother and others who 'belonged' to the Church of Satan when she was a young girl. During these rites Smith was allegedly tortured, locked in snake-filled cages, smeared with blood, forced to defecate on a crucifix, raped and sodomized with candles and made to witness murders (Pazder and Smith 1980). According to his account she repressed these memories until entering therapy with Pazder (Webster 1998). Although presented as a true story, Lanning (2002) claims that it has been shown by at least three independent investigations to have been a hoax. Nonetheless, there remain many people who believe such accounts and they are clearly indicative of agony of one kind or another.

Part of the problem in trying to ascertain what evidence base there is in this area is that some of the stories about ritualistic sexual abuse are so fantastic it is easy to dismiss them. Google provides a quite recent example from North Shields, UK (Van Fraser 2005). A woman writing in obvious personal anguish describes a huge conspiracy, but the 'facts' of such a story should be relatively easy to check. The author claims a Masonic plot at the highest levels of social services, police and justice systems that have orchestrated a cover-up of organized ritual sex-rings abusing children:

> I had thought that all the excrement, insects, perversions etc. were just sick...I also discovered that this kind of thing is prevalent in society. There is an organized court within authority which systematically damns mothers and children. I have met other mothers, all based in different parts of the country, with the same story. Some of the same judges, barristers and the Official Solicitor show up time and again. Psychiatrists are also prominent. All of us women have a gag order placed on us, with the threat of jail... The level of evil is very well planned and carried out ruthlessly... The authorities are not the solution, they are the problem. I would like to gather enough material to warrant a public enquiry.

The way such accounts are written, with similarities to accounts of alien abductions, means it is easy for us to dismiss them. In doing so, however, there is a danger that we put all such stories into the same box without rigorously investigating them. We have to remember too that practitioners may be influenced by the media. In Kitzinger's (2000) assessment of media templates in relation to sexual abuse she evidenced how the media influence people's perceptions and beliefs in regard to what had actually happened.

> The accumulation of 'social work scandals' around sexual abuse seems to have become a defining feature of the public debate encouraging suspicion of social services, justifying the demands for radical reform, informing parental fears and focusing concerns on false allegations. Just as phases such as 'another Vietnam, another Chernobyl or another Hitler' sum up a particular set of fears, so the phrase 'another Cleveland' provokes a set of powerful pre-packaged associations. (p.70)

We also need to be aware that these templates are so embedded that they might influence practitioners to be over-zealous, as was suggested in the Orkney case, or to be unwilling to admit to possibilities of organized abuse at all, because of their 'pre-packaged associations'. 'Professionals should cite reputable and scientific studies and note the sources of information. If they do not, when the exaggerations and distortions are discovered, their credibility and the credibility of the issue are lost' (Lanning 2002, p.1).

Although the zealousness in the early 1990s is now a distant memory, we need to be mindful that, on occasion, ritualistic sexual abuse may exist.

Rigorous, precise recording of what is said, observed or suspected, with clarity about facts and evidence and separation from opinion, is essential.

Allegations of ritual sexual abuse

We have already suggested that the evidence for satanic abuse is very limited. However, while it is argued that children rarely make false allegations of sexual abuse (less than 10%) (Jones and McGraw 1987), Kirk Weir and Wheatcroft (1995) suggest that they do sometimes make false accusations of *ritual* sexual abuse (RSA) and it is important to understand why. In an interesting UK study 20 case histories where allegations had been made of children being involved in RSA were examined. Each case was examined for:

- The nature of the allegation made by the child.

- Presence or absence of any sexualized behaviour.

- Presence or absence of circumstances known to increase the risk of child sexual abuse.

- Any non-specific signs or symptoms.

- Any forensic or medical evidence.

- The presence of any factors known to increase the risk of false allegations of child sexual abuse.

Of the 20 cases, systematic evaluation led to the conclusion that RSA had only been likely in five cases, although in another seven cases it was likely that sexual abuse had occurred. In the remaining eight cases it was likely that both allegations were fabricated. According to the researchers, the most worrying cases were those where the professionals involved believed the allegations based on consensus views and in spite of lack of evidence. In six cases they argue this led to a kind of 'professional crusade', seeking justice and using that as justification to abandon normal procedures.

> Children's general knowledge of ceremonies, witches and the occult may be much more than professionals appreciate and great care must be taken in evaluating the evidence gained from observations of young children's play. (Kirk Weir and Wheatcroft 1995, p.498)

In summary, the research offered the following explanations for why false allegations of ritualistic sexual abuse may be made:

- Children may have been sexually abused, but make false allegations of another kind when under pressure to please professionals interviewing them.

- Poor investigative practices combined with suggestible child leading to professional bias, leading questions.

- Maternal mental illness.

- Parental psychopathology, including coaching the child.

- Professional concerns regarding occult involvement of some family members.

Lanning (2002) has drawn similar conclusions, although his emphasis is always on a combination of answers as to why allegations may be false and each case is different. Lanning suggests the following:

- Pathological distortion: the allegations may be errors in processing reality influenced by underlying mental ill-health. They may be used to gain psychological benefits such as attention or sympathy.

- Traumatic memory: fear and severe trauma can cause distortions in recalling events. They may be part of an elaborate mental defence mechanism called 'splitting', where victims create a clear-cut manifestation of events that is psychologically more manageable,

- Normal childhood fears and fantasy: most young children fantasize and most are scared of monsters. While children very rarely invent stories about sexual activity, they may have been told about satanic activity (at church, at home, through the television) and may be 'dumping' all their fears together on an attentive listener.

We would also add that manipulative abusers may be very adept at using children's fears. There may be a further problem caused by access to or use of films and videos showing scenes of horror and the occult.

During the summer of 1983 in Manhattan Beach, California, Judy Johnson concluded that her two-year-old son had been abused anally by a male teacher at his daycare nursery. Johnson was said to be both devoutly religious and psychiatrically disturbed and to have no real evidence for her allegations (Webster 1998). Two hundred other parents began to pick up on her anxieties following letters they received from the police and the McMartin Preschool was portrayed as a cover for a sex ring. It was claimed that hundreds of children had been sexually abused, with disclosures from the children that they had seen witches flying or had been flushed down toilets to secret rooms where they were molested (Eberle 1993). An outside consultant was approached: Lawrence Padzer, who concluded that McMartin was the visible tip of a vast international satanic conspiracy. A full-scale national panic ensued. Eventually all charges against the accused in the McMartin case were rejected, but the rumours had reached the UK and similar satanic sexual abuse claims were reported here: Cheshire, Nottingham, Rochdale and Orkney. Eventually some 80 cases were reported in the UK alone (Webster 1998), but there are many other examples through the 1980s and 1990s: the Netherlands (Oude Pekele), Germany (Münsterland), Sweden (Södertälje and UmeD), Norway (Bjugn) and Denmark (Roum) (Henningsen 1996).

While it is extremely difficult to unpack exactly what happened at McMartin (and in some of the other places) and why no-one was ever prosecuted, it seems likely that widespread abuse did take place. That it was related to a conspiracy of satanic worship is, in this view, much more unlikely. There remains though a large group of people who are convinced that there is a vast and secretive world of intergenerational Satan worshippers abusing and murdering adults and children (Wenegrat 2001). On the basis of the limited evidence available it seems some incidents of abuse may be confounded by stories of the satanic element and after a media uproar, may be dismissed entirely, without always acknowledging the distress for parents and children and the possibility of actual abuse somewhere within the apparent fabrications.

Witchcraft

We now turn to witchcraft more specifically, which appears to be a strong belief system in many countries and cultures which has remained strong throughout history. An unexpected finding in a study comparing paranormal belief systems in 107 individuals with and without childhood physical abuse histories found a belief in witchcraft was the most strongly held belief in the abuse group (Perkins and Allen 2006). The researchers suggest such beliefs may offer a powerful emotional refuge to those who have endured the stress of abuse in childhood.

In Germany in the 16th century child witches were documented in some 400 accounts (Alexander 2007). Belief in witchcraft was common. Parents accused their children of intercourse with the devil, night travelling and eating of infants. Crop failures, sudden deaths and plagues were all blamed on witches. Children thus accused were beaten, starved, put in solitary confinement and forcibly woken from sleep. Alexander explores the witch-craze that spread through Europe between the 15th and mid-18th centuries, not all in the same place at the same time. Through times of peace and increased rational calculation, these beliefs and practices were eventually subdued.

It is essential that primary health care practitioners place child care and parenting debates within their historical and cultural context (Taylor, Spencer and Baldwin 2000). While in Europe beliefs and practices relating to witchcraft and the occult may have been largely suppressed, this is perhaps not the case in many African countries. High levels of immigration to the UK and other European countries may account for some of the current upsurge in beliefs about witchcraft. History tends to repeat itself and we need to pay attention to those phenomena that can return in new forms (Henningsen 1996).

Henningsen usefully differentiates between witchcraft and witch-craze. Witchcraft is based on long-term oral traditions; it can have an important social function (e.g. as part of a moral system) and is thought to be practised by only a few people in a community. Witch-craze, on the other hand, is a temporary phenomenon based on rumours and propaganda, characterized by unsystematic mythological belief structures, where a pact with the Devil is a fundamental tenet. Witch-craze outbreaks may lead to half the population falling under suspicion (as was demonstrated in the McMartin case). While witchcraft is a dying village tradition in European countries, witch-craze follows a repetitive pattern that appears in new and misleading disguises.

Witchcraft practices are not confined to story-telling, night travelling and crop failures. Muti is a Zulu word meaning 'medicine', usually implying traditional cures and is used commonly in southern African countries. In the years after apartheid the South African government set up a Commission of Inquiry into Witchcraft, Violence and Ritual Murders. A conservative estimate suggests that in the last decade at least 300 people have been murdered for their body-parts in South Africa. In the country's Northern provinces one child goes missing every three days and police suspect a link to muti-killings (Vallely 2007). Recent reports from other sub-Saharan countries are now beginning to unveil disturbing reports of children with albinism being murdered for their body-parts that are then used to make traditional medicines. At the time of writing this chapter there is intense media attention being paid to reports from Tanzania (a country that has an excellent record of the management of albinism), where there has been an alarming number of reports (28 already in the last year) where children with albinism have been killed for their body-parts to make muti (Gettleman 2008). What is clear is that in many countries in Africa, disability or 'differentness' is still often explained by witchcraft and sorcery.

Primary health care practitioners are working closely with local communities to promote education and reduce stigma. In Zambia teacher-targeted interventions aim to reduce stigma around epilepsy (Birbeck *et al.* 2006) and the plague (Ngulube *et al.* 2006), both diseases associated with witchcraft and possession; in Limpopo Province in South Africa designated 'witch villages' offer safe refuge for victims of witch-hunts; in the Democratic Republic of Congo (DRC) evangelical Christians give haven and education in 'witch-schools'.

Belief in spirit possession

The term 'belief in spirit possession' is defined as 'the belief that an evil force has entered a child and is controlling him or her' (HM Government 2007, p.5). This government report makes it very clear that abuse associated with such a belief is rare, but may be under-reported and under-recognized.

Most people are now familiar with the horrific events surrounding the death of Victoria Climbié in the UK in 2000. Lord Laming's review of the events and subsequent recommendations are rehearsed in most recent safeguarding literature and are well cited in other chapters in this book. One of the features of the case though concerns the beliefs Victoria's aunt and her boyfriend had regarding demonic possession of Victoria. Manning (the boyfriend) in particular had complained to church leaders that she was incontinent because of her demonic possessions. While advised that the pastor would pray and fast for her, Manning seems to have interpreted the advice as being an instruction to starve Victoria.

The casting out of demons is a fairly common tradition in many cults and churches and when belief systems are strong, it is easy to normalize behaviours that may be abusive in and of themselves, but importantly, lead to further abuse in the name of the faith. In 2006 a research report was commissioned in England to analyse the scope of the problem and any defining features regarding child abuse linked to accusations of possession and witchcraft since 2000 (Stobart 2006). From the beginning there were difficulties in identifying cases: police records were filed under various crime headings; public secure databases could not be searched by key terms; voluntary and non-governmental organizations often had very informal records; previous media coverage had made many very wary; there were concerns around confidential information; and some cases were still in the judicial system. A total of 93 cases was eventually reviewed, where a case was defined as: a household where a child or children were abused following an accusation of 'possession' or 'witchcraft'. The author did acknowledge some bias towards the Angolan and Congolese communities because much of the published research had concentrated on beliefs from Angola, Congo and the DRC. There was however, sufficient information for analysis from 38 cases involving 47 children. Some of the key findings from the analysis showed:

- More cases per year are now being found, likely due to better reporting and recognition.
- Gender of victim does not seem to play an important role.
- The majority of children are in the 8–14 age range.
- Schools appear to be the main source of referral.

- Children who were abused following accusations of possession or witchcraft showed behaviour consistent with distress.

- Although there is a perception that such abuse is more common among new immigrant communities, in fact about half of the children had been born in the UK.

- It was difficult to assess religion, but the majority described themselves as 'Christian'.

- Family structures were often very complex.

It was a common feature in the cases analysed that carers found it difficult to accept children with certain characteristics or behaviours, which were rationalized as being due to 'possession' or 'witchcraft'. Disability or illness, challenging behaviour, bed-wetting, nightmares and sleep-walking were all included as being traits of possession. Ridding a child of the 'evil spirit' included a number of measures, among them beatings, starvation, neglect, burning, cutting, bath-sleeping and threats of abandonment. Application of salt, ginger or chili peppers to the eyes and genitals was also reasonably common.

So where do practitioners go for guidance? Information for practitioners in this area of child protection is limited; however a recent document has been published by the UK government. *Safeguarding Children from Abuse Linked to a Belief in Spirit Possession* (HM Government 2007) gives non-statutory good practice guidance, which is multi-disciplinary and cross-sectoral in nature. It was produced to complement the statutory guidance in 'Safeguarding Children' (HM Government 2007) and builds on the principles outlined within this English document. The 2007 document is also being adopted by the Welsh Assembly.

The guidance is divided into various sections including:

- key considerations

- definitions and incidence

- why children are abused/neglected in this way

- how to identify child abuse or neglect linked to spirit possession

- what to do if you suspect such abuse or neglect

- concerns about a place of worship

- emerging best practice of agencies and institutions.

The document gives practitioners a useful list of actions to support their practice in this area of work and lists five additional areas of consideration, building on the statutory guidance. These include:

1. How do I understand this particular risk of harm to the child?
2. How do I best safeguard and promote the welfare of the child?
3. Which services are relevant in these cases of abuse?
4. Children being taken out of the UK?
5. Taking advice.

The document acknowledges that this type of abuse can be very difficult for professionals to understand and accept.

> It is necessary to emphasize the need for care in evaluating allegations for abuse because it has been noticeable that in cases where the possibility of ritual abuse occurs there can be such a level of professional anxiety that the normal procedures of investigation and protection of family rights are abandoned or curtailed. (Kirk Weir and Wheatcroft 1995, p.492)

Important aspects of this work are highlighted under the following as best practice of agencies and institutions.

1. An understanding of the wider context of abuse.
2. Early identification.
3. Developing partnerships with communities.
4. Working with place of worship and faith organizations.

Faiths, religion and the church

This chapter so far has discussed various types of ritual abuse and literature and evidence implicating various faiths and religious groups. Project Violet, established by the Metropolitan Police in London following the Kisanga case (see below) (Thompson 2005) continues to work to identify the scale of ritual and faith-based child abuse among ethnic minority groups. The team however, has so far only uncovered 31 cases since 2000, only five of which have gone to court (News24.com 2005). Although evidence is somewhat patchy, some recent events and issues for which there is substantial confirmation include:

- A child's headless torso was recovered from the Thames River in London in September 2001. In an attempt to humanize the boy, aged between four and seven, the police named him Adam. The contents of his stomach contained crushed bone and clay pellets impregnated with gold and quartz and detectives concluded this had been a ritualistic killing (News24.com 2005). Note however: there have been no other recorded instances of such grisly occurrences. During the subsequent enquiry, police confirmed that 300 African boys had gone missing from London schools during a three-month period in 2001 (Vallely 2007). Although there is no evidence that harm has occurred, there should be a concern at the unexplained loss of so many children. Perhaps they have returned to Africa, evaded immigration procedures, or been sent to live with other family members and a host of other plausible explanations.

• In London in late 2007, two women and a man were sentenced after 'beating the devil' out of an eight-year-old Angolan orphan know as 'Child B' and rubbing chili peppers in her eyes. Much was made of the church where the abuser-aunt, Kisanga, was a regular attendee and the pastor of the church was investigated (Or 2005). Kisanga had apparently discovered the girl's 'possession' through a prayer meeting. It should be however noted that the woman was thrown out of the church two years before the abuse took place and the church may not have been implicated in the abuse.

As Vallely points out, linking such abuse directly to churches can be misleading. Acts in the name of religion may not always take place in churches. Through interviews with a range of black community leaders Vallely demonstrates the underlying cultural ignorance in the media responses to such instances, where black churches have become linked to abuse without any direct evidence and heavy misrepresentation. What seems important here is that while the facts are confirmed, it is the interpretation of these facts that becomes challenging. There is a complex relationship between church and religion and while it would be wrong to overgeneralize, it should also be acknowledged that there are some churches whose practices could be questioned. Engaging with church and community leaders is therefore crucial and positive moves are being made in relation to the tighter regulation of minority churches and faith organizations. Africans Unite Against Child Abuse (Afruca) is a UK-based charity working in this area where they demonstrate the harm that even witnessing an exorcism can do to a child (Shuker 2006). Other locally based organizations across the world are doing likewise.

We know that changes can be made to faith-based practices. Female genital mutilation (FGM) is a good example of this. Previously (and erroneously) referred to as 'female circumcision', FGM is a traditional practice still performed on millions of young girls every year. While there is a firm commitment from many countries to abolish this practice, it remains common in many countries. However, there has been a strong shift in how it is viewed and there is a general political acceptance that FGM should be viewed as abuse and therefore eradicated. Working with particular groups is seen as helpful and there is strong commitment now in many of the countries where FGM is routinely practised to effect change through education and support. If we can work towards this aim in FGM, where there is a very firm founding in religious belief, we can do it in other areas.

Primary health care practitioners may often know of belief systems and the supportive structures that a strong faith can provide. They may be participants in these themselves. But sometimes it is useful to adjust the lenses to see things more clearly and prospectively. We need to be aware that sometimes, albeit rarely, children may be unwitting participants and victims in faith-based practices that are not helpful. This point was raised strongly in the Climbié Inquiry, when Lord Laming (2003) reflected on a number of assumptions that seem to have been held by a number of involved people about the cultural norms, practices and beliefs of Victoria and her family. He concluded that the misplacement of some of these ideas about Victoria's cultural circumstances may have shifted the focus away from her fundamental needs.

> The basic requirement that children are kept safe is universal and cuts across cultural boundaries... Cultural heritage is important to many people, but it cannot take precedence over standards of childcare embodied in law... There can be no excuse for failing to take adequate steps to protect a vulnerable child, simply because that child's cultural background would make the necessary action somehow inappropriate... A child is a child regardless of his or her colour and he or she must be kept safe. Cultural issues must be considered but the objective is the safety of the child...what cannot be ignored is that we live in a culturally diverse society and that safeguards must be in place to ensure that skin colour does not influence either the assessment of need or the quality of services delivered. (pp.345–347)

The NSPCC has produced an internal briefing paper on *Faith, Religion and Safeguarding Children* (Edwards 2007). It advises that there are 'inhibitors' to safeguarding children within the context that involves faith or religion and these 'inhibitors' come under the headings of (a) The Individual; (b) The Faith Organization; and (c) External Agency.

The section on the individual suggests that the practitioner should have an understanding of various faiths and religions and also their own values and beliefs. The section on the faith organizations considers the elements that influence safeguarding and also provides a useful list of why faith organizations and their leaders or representatives may not be challenged over various protection issues. The inhibitors that may effect external organizations are also considered.

It is important that practitioners and their managers are aware of these inhibiting factors and consider them as part of the overall assessment of the situation. Practitioners themselves working in the community are often a consistent and steady workforce that may be very much part of that community and indeed may live within the community that they serve. In the topic under discussion this can have a number of possible implications. It may be that practitioners are very well aware of what may be going on within a community and may wish to intervene and make allegations. Or it may be that the practitioner being part of the community perceives that this is the 'norm' or accepts and turns a 'blind eye', which may have the consequence of leaving children unprotected. Whether as professionals or as individuals, we all have responsibility for children's safety and wellbeing.

Conclusion

This chapter has attempted to demonstrate some of the links between various aspects of ritual abuse, the available evidence and possible responses and interventions by practitioners.

It seems clear within our analysis of this area of child protection that Satanism is over-represented in the media and culturally, without much evidence to support allegations of this type of abuse. However there seems to be an under-representation of abuse related to belief in spirit possession, which in reality may have just as serious implications for the families and individuals involved.

In an interview with the national media, Mary Marsh, chief executive of the NSPCC, pointed out that the law was extremely clear and psychological abuse of any sort was disallowed under the United Nations Convention on the Rights of the Child.

> Ritualistic treatment of a child in a context where they're being frightened or threatened, that has to be wrong. It's not protecting their rights... Children are entitled to protection. I'm not against people's beliefs, but I am against them harming children. We mustn't be seen as disrespectful, but be very clear what the boundaries are. (Carrell 2005)

Any assessment of what is happening in a child's life must be sufficiently probing to ensure that priority is given to the child's needs and that wellbeing and safety are protected.

The Contributors

Jane Cantrell is a Programme Director with NHS Education for Scotland (NES). She has a clinical background in community nursing and including health visiting and has been in nurse education for 20 years. During her educational career Jane has taught pre-registration, post registration and postgraduate students. In her current role she is leading an educational initiative on child protection to support staff with NHS Scotland.

Dr Anne Claveirole is Lecturer and Research Fellow at the Faculty of Health and Social Care of Napier University in Edinburgh, Scotland. Her work has focused on the needs of children and young people who are emotionally and mentally vulnerable. She is currently co-editing 'Understanding Children and Young People's Mental Health' for Wiley-Blackwell.

Professor Lawrie Elliott works in the Centre for Integrated Healthcare Research and Edinburgh Napier University. He has a substantial track record in conducting applied research in Public Health. He is a member of the MRC College of Experts and a member of the Editorial Board for the Journal of Mental Health and Psychiatric Nursing. He has also worked in an advisory capacity to government on a range of policy issues including public health nursing and addictions. In 2006 he co-authored a World Health Organisation report on health inequalities.

Dr Jacqueline Feather is a Clinical Psychologist and Lecturer in Psychology at Central Queensland University, Australia. She has practised as a clinician for many years in statutory child protection, specializing in assessment and treatment of abuse-related trauma. Her research focus is on the development and evaluation of treatment models based on an interweaving of local clinical practice with evidence-based approaches in order to ensure safe and effective outcomes for traumatized children and their families.

Lindsay Ferguson is Consultant Nurse for Child and Vulnerable Family Protection in NHS Tayside. following a long and varied career in health visiting across the UK. After moving to Scotland in 2002 she worked in health visiting and then as Child Protection Adviser for three years until 2005 when seconded to the Scottish Executive Health Department as Lead Consultant Nurse for Child Protection for Scotland.

Professor Ruth Freeman trained at Queen's University, Belfast and at the University of London. Prior to her appointment to the Chair of Dental Public Health Research, University of Dundee she worked at University College, London and was Professor of Dental Public Health at Queen's University, Belfast. She has researched and published extensively in the areas of behavioural sciences, oral health promotion and oral health inequalities. Her current research interests include theoretical and practical dimensions of health disparities in socially excluded groups.

Dr Martyn Jones is a Reader in School of Nursing and Midwifery, University of Dundee and Associate Director of the Social Dimensions of Health Institute in Universities of Dundee and St Andrews. Dr Jones has researched the effects of exercise promotion on people with severe/profound learning disabilities and challenging behaviour using rebound therapy and has explored service users' views on improving the accessibility of GP surgeries for people with learning disabilities.

Professor Barbara Juen is professor of Psychotraumatology, and Clinical Psychology at the Department of Psychology, University of Innsbruck, Austria. Her main research interests are psychotraumatology in children and adults. She is head of the Austrian Crisis Intervention in the Austrian Red Cross. She is author of several books on crisis intervention and psychotraumatology.

Dr Florian Juen is assistant professor of Developmental and Clinical Psychology at the Department of Psychology, University of Innsbruck, Austria. His main research interests are in socio-emotional development, attachment research and psychopathology in infancy and childhood. He has a special focus on early caregiver–child interaction processes.

Dr Toine Lagro-Janssen is a general practitioner and professor of gender in medicine at the Radboud University Nijmegen Medical Centre, the Netherlands. She is author of several publications on women's health, including sexual abuse and intimate partner violence.

Professor James Law is Director of the Centre for Integrated Healthcare Research (CIHR) and Professor of Language and Communication Science at Queen Margaret University Edinburgh. The main focus of his research activity relates to children with language learning difficulties, but he has also run a number of studies funded to examine specific aspects of user involvement.

Dr Anne Lazenbatt BSc (Hons) Psychology, DPhil, Queen's University Belfast. Dr Anne Lazenbatt is a health psychologist and NSPCC Reader in Childhood Studies, in the Institute of Child Care Research, School of Sociology, Social Policy and Social Work, Queen's University of Belfast, Northern Ireland. She has extensive research experience in multi-methods research methodologies, as well as theoretical and methodological models of evaluation of health and social care. She has published widely in areas such as child and domestic abuse, inequalities in health and social wellbeing; gender inequalities and evaluation and effectiveness. Anne is affiliated to the NSPCC and her research interests and publications are now in the area of 'vulnerability, violence and safeguarding children', with particular emphasis on domestic violence in pregnancy, health professionals' recognition and reporting of child physical abuse, the co-occurrence of domestic and child abuse, professionals' barriers to reporting child maltreatment concerns, and lessons learned from child death reviews.

Leila Mackie is a Psychology graduate and Speech and Language Therapist. She has over 10 years Speech and Language Therapy clinical experience working with children of all ages in health centre, mainstream and special school settings. She is currently carrying out a PhD at the Centre for Integrated Healthcare Research, investigating the link between Language Impairment and Emotional/ Behavioural Disorders.

Dona Milne is a Specialist in Public Health with NHS Lothian. She led and implemented the National Health Demonstration Programme, Healthy Respect. Dona has a background in youth work and young people's service provision working across local authorities, voluntary sector and public health, with a particular interest in confidentiality and child protection.

Dr Sarah Nelson has carried out research and has published papers on a wide range of issues related to childhood sexual abuse and its effects in adult life most recently on the support needs of male survivors. Her other research has included neighbourhood prevention programmes to keep children safe from sexual crime; the mental and physical health effects of CSA; organized sadistic abuse; and the future of child protection. In 2008 *See Us Hear Us*, for school staff working with sexually abused children, was published. She is also joint lead professional to the Scottish Government on their national strategy for survivors of childhood sexual abuse.

Dr Michelle O'Neill has a background in working with children and young people with Additional Support Needs. She is passionate about the wellbeing and care of children and young people. Having recently completed a PhD at the University of Dundee on the use of imitation with children with Autistic Spectrum Disorder and their parents/carers, she now works in the field of Research and Development.

Janette Pow (RGN, BN, BSc, MPH) is currently a PhD Research Student with Napier University, Edinburgh, Scotland. She is a member of the research team evaluating the Healthy Respect 2 Project. Janette has a background in nursing and has a significant interest in research associated with the promotion and protection of young people's health and wellbeing.

Dr Catherine Powell is a Consultant Nurse Safeguarding Children at Portsmouth City Teaching Primary Care Trust and holds the designated nurse responsibility across the City. She has a background as a general nurse, children's nurse and health visitor and has specialized in safeguarding children since 1994 as both a practitioner and an academic. Catherine is the nurse representative on the Hampshire, Isle of Wight, Portsmouth and Southampton Local Safeguarding Children Boards Child Death Overview Panel.'

Professor Kevin Ronan is currently in the position of Professor of Clinical Psychology in the Department of Behavioural and Social Sciences at Central Queensland University. He is an advisor to Queensland's Department of Child Safety and sits on a number of national panels having to do with children's welfare.

Caroline Selkirk is the Director of Change of Innovation for NHS Tayside (Scotland) and the Boards Commissioner for Child Health. She is currently: a member of the Children and Young People's Advisory Group which advises the Cabinet Secretary for Health on matters related to the health and wellbeing of children and young people in Scotland, Chair of the National Child and Adolescent Mental Health Steering Group, Chair of the LAAC 'Being Emotionally, Mentally and Physically Healthy Working Group', a member of the LAAC Implementation Board and Chair of the National Delivery Plan Specialist Children and Young People's Services Implementation Group.

Ruth Skelton is Consultant Paediatrician and Designated Doctor Child Protection Bradford Hospitals Foundation Trust / Bradford and Airedale PCT. Ruth trained in Paediatrics in Nottingham, Blackburn, Sydney and Leeds and worked as a consultant Neonatologist in Hull before further developing interest in child protection and returning to Leeds as a paediatrician and Designated/Named Doctor for child protection. Ruth moved to Bradford in 2007 and is developing the service further, including establishing a sexual abuse service. Ruth has a particular interest in neglect and factitious and fabricated illness/medical abuse and is also developing the Leeds MMEDSCI child protection module.

Professor Julie Taylor is Research Dean and Professor of Family Health in the School of Nursing and Midwifery at the University of Dundee, Scotland. With Brigid Daniel she is co-author of *Engaging with Fathers: Practice Issues for Health and Social Care* and co-editor of *Neglect: Issues for Health and Social Care*. Julie has a significant background in research projects that seek to explore better ways of recognizing and responding to child care and protection issues. She is associate editor of the journal *Child Abuse Review*, co-founding member of the Scottish Child Care and Protection Network; and co-founder of the international Gender and Child Welfare network.

Dr Markus Themessl-Huber is Senior Lecturer in Clinical Psychology in the Behavioural and Social Sciences Department at Central Queensland University, Australia. Markus has been involved in numerous research projects, including an assessment of the mental wellbeing of children and young people in a Scottish region.

Dr Floris van de Laar works as a general practitioner and as physician in an Infant Welfare Centre in Lent, the Netherlands. Furthermore he works as teacher and researcher at the department of general practice of Radboud University Nijmegen Medical Centre. He is author of publications about several topics such as eating psychology, type 2 diabetes and nutrition.

Dr Anne Whittaker is Primary Care Facilitator in NHS Lothian, Scotland, where she is involved in policy and practice development, teaching and research. After qualifying as a nurse in 1983, Anne worked in a wide range of health and social care settings, specializing in learning disabilities, mental health, drug and alcohol problems, and blood borne viruses. She has a special interest in gender, parenthood and problem substance use within a harm reduction and family welfare framework. Following post-graduate training in drug and alcohol studies and a degree in psychology, Anne completed her doctoral study on problem drug use and fatherhood in 2008.

Dr Suzanne Zeedyk is a Senior Lecturer in Developmental Psychology at the University of Dundee, with expertise in parent–infant communication. She now brings the insights that have been gained about these early years to understanding how social interactions can be nurtured when one of the partners is defined as having a 'communicative impairment'. She is the author of a number of academic publications and several books exploring this challenging puzzle.

References

Ackerman, P. T., Newton, J. E. O., McPherson, W. B., Jones, J. G. and Dykman, R. A. (1998) 'Prevalence of post traumatic stress disorder and other psychiatric diagnoses in three groups of abused children (sexual, physical and both).' *Child Abuse and Neglect 22,* 759–774.

ACMD (2003) *Hidden Harm: Responding to the Needs of Children of Problem Drug Users. The Report of an Inquiry by the Advisory Council on the Misuse of Drugs.* London: Home Office.

Act 28 168 (2006) *Regeling van de aanspraak op, de toegang tot en de bekostiging van jeugdzorg (Wet op de jeugdzorg) [Regulation on claims, access and finance of the care for minors (Act on youth care)].* Amsterdam. Justice Volksgexondheid, Welzijn en Sport.

Aggleton, P. and Campbell, C. (2000) 'Working with young people – towards an agenda for sexual health.' *Sexual and Relationship Therapy 15*(3), 283–297.

Ainsworth, M. D. S. (1985) 'Patterns of infant–mother attachments: antecendents and effects on development.' *Bulletin of the New York Academy of Medicine 61*(9), 771–791.

Alderson, A. (2005) 'Dozens of African children beaten, abused and accused of withcraft.' http://moderntribalist.blogspot.com/2005/06/dozens-of-african-children-beaten.html (accessed 5/1/08).

Aldgate, J. and McIntosh, M. (2006) *Looking After the Family: A Study of Children Looked After in Kinship Care in Scotland* Edinburgh: Social Work Inspection Agency.

Alexander, S. (2007) 'The witch and the child: women's historical writing and the unconscious.' *Women: A Cultural Review 18*(3), 327–344.

Allan, W. D., Kashani, J. H. and Reid, J. C. (1998) 'Parental hostility: impact on the family.' *Child Psychiatry and Human Development 28,* 169–178.

Allen, R. E. and Oliver, J. M. (1982) 'The effects of child mistreatment on language development.' *Child Abuse and Neglect 6*(3), 299–305.

Amaro, H., Fried, L. E., Cabral, H. and Zuckerman, B. (1990) 'Violence during pregnancy and substance use.' *American Journal of Public Health 80*(5), 575–579.

American Academy of Pediatrics and American Academy of Pediatric Dentistry (1999) 'Oral and dental aspects of child abuse and neglect. Joint statement of the American Academy of Pediatrics and the American Academy of Pediatric Dentistry.' *Pediatrics 104,* 348–350.

American Academy of Pediatrics Committee on Child Abuse and Neglect (2007) policy statement. Available at www.aappolicy.aappublications.org/cgi/search, accessed on 9 May 2009.

American Psychiatric Association (1987) *Diagnostic and Statistical Manual of Mental Disorders, 3rd edn (DSM-III).* Washington, DC: APA.

American Psychiatric Association (1994) *Diagnostic and Statistical Manual of Mental Disorders, 4th edn (DSM-IV).* Washington, DC: American Psychiatric Association.

American Psychiatric Association (2000) *Diagnostic and Statistical Manual of Mental Disorders (Text rev., 4th edn).* Washington, DC: APS.

Angus, W. (1996) 'A patient who changed my life.' *British Medical Journal 313,* 210.

Appel, A. E. and Holden, G. W. (1998) 'The co-occurrence of spouse and physical child abuse: a review and appraisal.' *Journal of Family Psychology 12,* 578–599.

Appleton, J. V. (1996) 'Working with vulnerable families: a health visiting perspective.' *Journal of Advanced Nursing 23*(5), 912–918.

Arias, I. (2004) 'The legacy of child maltreatment: long-term health consequences for women.' *Journal of Women's Health and Gender-Based Medicine 13*(5), 468–473.

Asher, S. R. and Gazelle, H. (1999) 'Loneliness, peer relations and language disorder in childhood.' *Topics in Language Disorder 19*(2), 16–33.

Ashton, M. (2008) 'The new abstentionists.' *Druglink* (Dec/Jan), 1–16.

Asthana, S., Richardson, S. and Halliday, J. (2002) 'Partnership working in public policy provision: a framework for evaluation.' *Social Policy and Administration 36,* 780–795.

Bacchus, L., Mezey, G. and Bewley, S. (2002) 'Women's perceptions and experiences of routine enquiry for domestic violence in a maternity service.' *British Journal of Obstetrics and Gynaecology 109,* 9–16.

Bacchus, L., Mezey, G. and Bewley, S. (2005) 'Prevalence of domestic violence when midwives routinely enquire in pregnancy.' *Obstetrical and Gynaecological Survey 60*(1), 11–13.

Baird, G., Simonoff, E., Pickles, A., Chandler, S. *et al.* (2006) 'Prevalence of disorders of the autism spectrum in a population cohort of children in South Thames: the Special Needs and Autism Project (SNAP).' *Lancet 368*, 210–215.

Baker, A.W. and Duncan, S.P. (1985) 'Child sex abuse: a study of prevalence in Great Britain.' *Child Abuse and Neglect 9*, 453–467.

Bancroft, A., Wilson, S., Cunningham-Burley, S., Backett-Milburn, K. and Masters, H. (2004) *Resilience and Transition: Young People's Experience of Drug and Alcohol Misusing Parents.* Edinburgh: Scottish Executive and University of Edinburgh.

Bannon, M. J. and Carter, Y. H. (2003) 'Paediatricians and child protection: the need for effective education and training.' *Archives of Disease in Childhood 88*(7), 560–562.

Banwell, C. and Bammer, G. (2006) 'Maternal habits: narratives of mothering, social position and drug use.' *International Journal of Drug Policy 17*, 504–513.

Barlow, J. (2006) 'Home visiting for parents of pre-school children in the UK.' In C. McCauley, P. J. Pecora and W. Rose (eds) *Enhancing the Wellbeing of Children and Families Through Effective Interventions.* London: Jessica Kingsley Publishers.

Barlow, J. and Parsons, J. (2002) 'Group-based parent-training programmes for improving emotional and behavioural adjustment in 0–3 year old children.' *Cochrane Database of Systematic Reviews.*

Barnard, M. (2003) 'Between a rock and a hard place: the role of relatives in protecting children from the effects of parental drug problems.' *Child and Family Social Work 8*, 291–299.

Barnard, M. and Barlow, J. (2003) 'Discovering parental drug dependence: silence and disclosure.' *Children and Society 17*(1), 45–46.

Barnish, M. (2004) *Domestic Violence: A Literature Review.* London: Home Office.

Baron-Cohen, S., Leslie, A. M. and Frith, U. (1985) 'Does the autistic child have a "theory of mind?"' *Cognition 21*, 37–46.

Barrett, P. M., Duffy, A. L., Dadds, M. R. and Rapee, R. M. (2001) 'Cognitive-behavioral treatment of anxiety disorders in children: long-term (6-year) follow-up.' *Journal of Consulting and Clinical Psychology 69*, 135–141.

Barrett, P.M., Dadda, M. and Ryan, S. (1996) 'Family enhancement of cognitive style in anxious and aggressive children.' *Journal of Abnormal Child Psychology 24*, 187–203.

Bayatpour, M., Wells, R. D. and Holford, S. (1992) 'Physical and sexual abuse as predictors of substance use and suicide among pregnant teenagers.' *Journal of Adolescent Health 13*(2), 128–132.

Beers, S. R. and De Bellis, M. D. (2002) 'Neuropsychological function in children with maltreated-related posttraumatic stress disorder.' *American Journal of Psychiatry 159*, 438–486.

Beitchman, J. H., Wilson, B., Johnson, C. J., Atkinson, L., Young, A., Adlaf, E., Escobar, M. and Douglas, L. (2001) 'Fourteen-year follow-up of speech/language-impaired and control children: psychiatric outcome.' *Journal of the American Academy of Child and Adolescent Psychiatry 40*(1), 75–82.

Beitchman, J. H., Zucker, K. J., Hood, J. E., daCosta, G. A., Akman, D. and Cassavia, E. (1992) 'A review of the long-term effects of child sexual abuse.' *Child Abuse and Neglect 16*(1), 101–118.

Benner, G. J., Nelson, J. R. and Epstein, M. H. (2002) 'Language skills of children with EBD.' *Journal of Emotional and Behavioral Disorders 10*, 43–59.

Best, D. and Abdulrahim, D. (2005) *Women in Drug Treatment Services.* London: National Treatment Agency for Substance Misuse (NTA).

Bewley, S. (1997) 'Pregnancy and violence.' In S. Bewley, J. Friend and G. Mezey (eds) *Violence Against Women.* London: RCOG Press.

Bewley, S., Friend, J. R. and Mezey, G. C. (1997) *Violence Against Women.* London: Royal College of Obstetricians and Gynaecologists Press.

Bhatia, M. S. and Sapra, S. (2005) 'Pseudo-seizures in children: a profile of 50 cases.' *Clinical Paediatrics 44*(7), 617–621.

Birbeck, G. L., Chomba, E., Atadzhanov, M., Mbewe, E. and Haworth, A. (2006) 'Zambian teachers: what do they know about epilepsy and how can we work with them to decrease stigma?' *Epilepsy and Behavior 9*, 275–280.

Birchall, E. and Hallett, C. (1995) *Working Together in Child Protection.* London: HMSO.

Bisset, A. F. and Hunter, D. (1992) 'Child sexual abuse in general practice in north east Scotland.' *Health Bulletin (Edinburgh) 50*(3), 237–247.

Black, B. and Logan, A. (1995) 'Links between communication patterns in mother–child, father–child and child–peer interactions and children's social status.' *Child Development 66*, 255–271.

Bleeker, G., Vet, N. J., Haumann, T. J., Van Wijk, L. and Gemke, R. J. (2005) 'Increase in the number of reported cases of child abuse following adoption of a structured approach in the VU Medical Centre, Amsterdam, in the period 2001–2004 [Toename van het aantal gemelde gevallen van kindermishandeling na een gestructureerde aanpak in het VU Medisch Centrum, Amsterdam, 2001/'04].' *Nederlands Tijdschrift voor Geneeskdunde 149*, 1620–1624.

Bloomfield, L., Kendall, S., Applin, L., Attarzadeh, V., *et al.* (2005) 'A qualitative study exploring the experiences and views of mothers, health visitors and family support centre workers on the challenges and difficulties of parenting.' *Health and Social Care in the Community 13*, 46–55.

Bloxham, S. (1997) 'The contribution of interagency collaboration to the promotion of young people's sexual health.' *Health Education Research 12*(1), 91–101.

BMA (1998) *Domestic Violence: A Health Care Issue?* London: British Medical Association.

BMA (2004) *Doctors' Responsibilities in Child Protection Cases; Guidance from the Ethics Department*
www.bma.org.uk/ap.nsf/AttachmentsByTitle/PDFchild04/$FILE/child04.pdf (accessed 6/12/08).

BMA (2007a) *Domestic Abuse: A Report from the BMA Board of Science.* London: British Medical Association.

BMA (2007b) *Fetal Alcohol Spectrum Disorders: A Guide for Healthcare Professionals.* London: British Medical Association.

Bosely, S. (2008) 'Paediatrician reluctant to court backlash.' *Guardian:*
www.guardian.co.uk/society/2008/mar/19/children.health (accessed 6/12/08).

Bowlby, J. (1969) *Attachment and Loss, Vol.1: Attachment.* New York: Basic Books.

Bowlby, J. (1973) *Attachment and Loss, Vol.2: Separation, Anxiety and Anger.* London: Hogarth Press.

Bowlby, J. (1997) *Attachment and Loss, Vol. 1: Attachment, 2nd edn.* London: Pimlico.

Boyd, S. (1999) *Mothers and Illicit Drugs: Transcending the Myths.* Toronto: University of Toronto Press.

Bradley, F., Smith, M., Long, J. and O'Dowd, T. (2002) 'Reported frequency of domestic violence: cross sectional survey of women attending general practice.' *British Medical Journal 324,* 271.

Brandon, M., Belderson, P., Warren, C., Howe, D., Gardner, R., Dodsworth, J. and Black, J. (2008) *Analysing Child Deaths and Serious Injury through Abuse and Neglect: What can we Learn? A Biennial Analysis of Serious Case Reviews 2003–2005.* London: Department for Children, Schools and Families.

Brandon, M., Dodsworth, J. and Rumball, D. (2005) 'Serious case reviews: learning to use expertise.' *Child Abuse Review 14,* 160–176.

Brandon, M., Thoburn, J., Lewis, A. and Way, A. (1999) *Safeguarding Children with the Children Act 1989.* London: The Stationery Office.

Bremberg, S. (2006) 'Reduction of social inequalities in child accidental injuries through environmental preventive measures.' *An Evidence-Based Approach to Public Health and Tackling Inequalities: Opportunities and Challenges* www.health-inequalities.eu/object.php?id=summaryandidx=84 (accessed 16/1/08).

Brennan, K. and Keen, A. (2007) *Joint Statement by DCSF and DH on the Duties of Doctors and Other Health Professionals in Investigations of Child Abuse.* London: HMSO.

Bretherton, I., Ridgeway, D. and Cassidy, J. (1990) 'Assessing internal working models of the attachment relationship: an attachment story completion task.' In M. T. Greenberg, D. Ciccetti and E. M. Cummings (eds) *Attachment in the Preschool Years.* Chicago: University Press.

Briere, J. and Elliott, D. (1994) 'Immediate and long term impacts of child sexual abuse.' *The Future of Children 4*(2), 54–69.

Briere, J. and Scott, C. (2006) *Principles of Trauma Therapy: A Guide to Symptoms, Evaluation and Treatment.* Thousand Oaks, CA: Sage Publications.

Brinton, B., Fujiki, M. and Highbee, L. M. (1998) 'Participation in cooperative learning activities by children with specific language impairment.' *Journal of Speech, Language and Hearing Research 41*(5), 1193–1206.

Brinton, B., Fujiki, M. and McKee, L. (1998) 'Negotiation skills of children with specific language impairment.' *Journal of Speech, Language and Hearing Research 41*(4), 927–940.

Brinton, B., Fujiki, M., Spencer, J. C. and Robinson, L. A. (1997) 'The ability of children with specific language impairment to access and participate in an ongoing interaction.' *Journal of Speech, Language and Hearing Research 40*(5), 1011–1025.

British Society of Paediatric Dentistry and Royal College of Physicians (2005) *Procedures to be Adopted by the Dental Professional who Suspects Child Abuse.* London. www.cpdt.org.uk/f_info/dload/BSPDRCPCHNov05.pdf (accessed 7/2/08).

Browne, A. and Finkelhor, D. (1986) 'The impact of child sexual abuse: a review of the research.' *Psychological Bulletin 99,* 66–77.

Bruni, M. (2003) 'Anal findings in sexual abuse of children (a descriptive study).' *Journal of Forensic Sciences 48*(6), 1343–6.

Buck, L. (2007) 'Why don't midwives ask about domestic violence?' *British Journal of Midwifery 15*(12), 753–758.

Buckner, J. C., Beardslee, W. R. and Bassuk, E. L. (2004) 'Exposure to violence and low-income children's mental health: direct, moderated and mediated relations.' *American Journal of Orthopsychiatry 74,* 413–423.

Bunting, L. and Reid, C. (2005) 'Reviewing child deaths – learning from the American Experience.' *Child Abuse Review 14,* 82–96.

Burgess, A. (2008) *The Costs and Benefits of Active Fatherhood: Evidence and Insights to Inform the Development of Policy and Practice.* www.fathersdirect.com accessed on 16 May 2009

Burke, F. and Freeman, R. (2004) *Preparing for Dental Practice.* Oxford: Oxford University Press.

Burns, B. J., Phillips, S. D., Wagner, R. W., Barth, R. P. *et al.* (2004) 'Mental health need and access to mental health services by youths involved with child welfare: a national survey.' *Journal of the American Academy of Child and Adolescent Psychiatry 43,* 960–970.

Burns, C., O'Driscoll, M. and Wason, G. (1996) 'The health and development of children whose mothers are on methadone maintenance.' *Child Abuse Review 5,* 113–122.

Butchart, A. and Villaveces, A. (2003) *Violence against Women and the Risk of Infant and Child Mortality.* Geneva: WHO.

Butler, S. (1996) 'Child protection or professional self preservation by the baby nurses? Public health nurses and child protection in Ireland.' *Social Science and Medicine 43*(3), 303–314.

Butler-Sloss, E. (1987) *Report of the Inquiry into Child Abuse in Cleveland.* London: HMSO.

Cabinet Office (2007) *Families at Risk: Background on Families with Multiple Disadvantages.* London: Social Exclusion Task Force, Cabinet Office.

Cabinet Office (2008a) *Think Family: A Literature Review of Whole Family Approaches* London: Social Exclusion Task Force, Cabinet Office.

Cabinet Office (2008b) *Think Family: Improving the Life Chances of Families at Risk* London: Social Exclusion Task Force, Cabinet Office.

Cairns, A. M., Mok, J. Y. and Welbury, R. R. (2005) 'The dental practitioner and child protection in Scotland.' *British Journal of Dentistry 199*(8), 517–520.

Cairns, A., Murphy, M. and Welbury, R. (2004) 'An overview and pilot study of the dental practitioner's role in child protection.' *Child Abuse Review 13*, 65–72.

Caldwell, P. (2004) *Crossing the Minefield: Establishing Safe Passage through the Sensory Chaos of Autistic Spectrum Disorder.* Brighton: Pavilion Publishing.

Caldwell, P. (2006) *Finding You, Finding Me: Using Intensive Interaction to get in Touch with People whose Severe Learning Disabilities are Combined with Autistic Spectrum Disorder.* London: Jessica Kingsley Publishers.

Caldwell, P. (2007) *From Isolation to Intimacy: Making Friends Without Words.* London: Jessica Kingsley Publishers.

Caldwell, P. (2008) *Using Intensive Interaction and Sensory Integration: A Handbook for those who Support People with Severe Autistic Spectrum Disorder.* London: Jessica Kingsley Publishers.

Campbell, J., García-Moreno, C. and Sharps, P. (2003) 'Abuse during pregnancy in industrialized and developing countries.' *Violence Against Women 10*(7), 770–789.

Campbell, J. L. and Lewandowski, L. (1997) 'Mental and physical health effects of intimate partner violence on women and children.' *The Psychiatric Clinics of North America 20*, 353–374.

Cantwell, D. B. and Baker, L. (1987) 'Prevalence and types of psychiatric disorders in three speech and language groups.' *Journal of Communication Disorders 20*, 151–160.

Cardol, M., Van Dijk, L., De Jong, J. D., De Bakker, D. H. and Westert, G. P. (2004) *Second National Study about Diseases and Actions in General Practice: What is the Gatekeeper Doing? [Tweede Nationale Studie naar Ziekten en Verrichtingen in de Huisartspraktijk: Huisartsenzorg: wat Doet de Poortwachter?].* Utrecht: Bilthoven, NIVEL, Rijksinstituut voor Volksgezondheid en Milieu.

Care Co-ordination Network (2004) *Care Co-ordination Key Worker Standards.* www.ccnuk.org.uk (accessed 11/12/07).

Carlson, B. E. (2000) 'Children exposed to intimate partner violence: research findings and implications for intervention.' *Trauma, Violence and Abuse 1*(4), 321–340.

Carrell, S. (2005) 'London 2005. A child is "tried" for witchcraft. How many more?' news.independent.co.uk/uk/legal/article224494.ece (accessed 11/11/07).

Carson, P. (1998) *Paediatric Sedation and Dental General Anaesthesia: Choices for the Future.* (Unpublished PhD Thesis). Belfast: Queen's University of Belfast

Carter, J. and Schechter, S. (1997) *Child Abuse and Domestic Violence: Creating Community Partnerships for Safe Families–Suggested Components of an Effective Child Welfare Response to Domestic Violence.* San Francisco, CA: Family Violence Prevention Fund.

Carter, Y. H. and Bannon, M. J. (2002) *The Role of Primary Care in the Protection of Children from Abuse and Neglect. A Position Paper for the Royal College of General Practitioners* www.rcgp.org.uk/pdf/ childprotection.pdf (accessed 17/1/08).

Casanueva, C. E. and Martin, S. L. (2007) 'Intimate partner violence during pregnancy and mothers child abuse potential.' *Journal of Interpersonal Violence 22*(5), 603–622.

Catalano, R. F., Gainey, R. R., Fleming, C. B., Haggerty, K. P. and Johnson, N. O. (1999) 'An experimental intervention with families of substance abusers: one-year follow-up of the focus on families project.' *Addiction 94*(2), 241–254.

Cattanach, A. (1992) *Play Therapy with Abused Children.* London: Jessica Kingsley Publishers.

Catto, G. (2008) 'GMC's reply.' *British Medical Journal 336*, 231.

Catts, H. W. and Kamhi, A. G. T. (2005) *The Connections between Language and Reading Disabilities* Mahwah, New Jersey, New York: Lawrence Elrbaum Associates.

Cawson, P. (2003) *Child Maltreatment in the United Kingdom: A Study of the Prevalence of Child Abuse* London: NSPCC.

Cawson, P., Wattam, C., Brooker, S. and Kelly, G. (1995) *Child Maltreatment in the United Kingdom: A Study of the Prevalence of Child Abuse and Neglect* London: NSPCC.

Cawson, P., Wattam, C., Brooker, S. and Kelly, G. (2000) *Child Maltreatment in the United Kingdom: A Study of the Prevalence of Child Abuse and Neglect* London: NSPCC.

CEMACH (2008) *Confidential Enquiry into Maternal and Child Health, Why Children Die: A Pilot Study, 2006.* London: CEMACH.

Chadwick, D. L., Krous, H. F. and Runyan, D. K. (2006) 'Meadow, Southall and the General Medical Council of the United Kingdom.' *Pediatrics 117*(6), 2247–2251.

Chakrabati, S. and Fombonne, E. (2001) 'Pervasive developmental disorders in preschool children.' *Journal of the American Medical Association 285*, 3093–3099.

Charles, M. and Stevenson, O. (1991) *Multidisciplinary is Different. Child Protection: Working Together, Part II: Sharing Perspectives.* Nottingham: Nottingham University.

Cheesbrough, S., Ingham, R. and Massey, D. (1999) *Reducing the Rate of Teenage Conceptions. A Review of the International Evidence: The United States, Canada, Australia and New Zealand* London: Health Education Authority.

Child Health Commissioners (2004) *Unpublished paper on role of the Child Health Commissioner.* Dundee City Council.

Child Health Support Group (2001) *A Template for Child Health Services Within Unified NHS Board Areas.* Edinburgh: Scottish Executive.

Children 1st (2007) *Getting the Balance Right: Report by Children 1st and Childline Scotland of Key Concerns Around the Child Protection System in Scotland.* Edinburgh: Children 1st.

Children (Scotland) Act (1995) *Chapter 36. Office of Public Sector Information.* www.opsi.gov.uk/ACTS/acts1995/ukpga_19950036 (accessed 6/12/08).

Chorpita, B., Albano, A. and Barlow, D. (1996) 'Cognitive processing in children: relation to anxiety and family influences.' *Journal of Clinical Child Psychology 25,* 170–176.

Cicchetti, D. and Rogosch, F. A. (2002) 'A developmental psychopathology perspective on adolescence.' *Journal of Consulting and Clinical Psychology 70,* 6–20.

Claveirole, A., Elliott, L., Pow, J. and Themessl-Huber, M. (2008) *Qualitative Interviews with Providers of Sexual Health and Education for Young People.* Edinburgh: Napier University.

Cleaver, H., Unell, I. and Aldgate, J. (1999) *Children's Needs – Parenting Capacity: The Impact of Parental Mental Illness, Problem Alcohol and Drug Use and Domestic Violence on Children's Development.* London: HMSO.

Cohen, J. A. and Mannarino, A. P. (1996) 'A treatment study for sexually abused preschool children: initial findings.' *Journal of the American Academy of Child and Adolescent Psychiatry 35,* 42–50.

Cohen, J. A. and Mannarino, A. P. (1997) 'A treatment study of sexually abused preschool children: outcome during 1-year follow-up.' *Journal of American Academy of Child and Adolescent Psychiatry 36,* 1228–1235.

Cohen, J. A., Berliner, L. and Mannarino, A. P. (2003) 'Psychological and pharmacological interventions for child crime victims.' *Journal of Traumatic Stress 16,* 175–186.

Cohen, J. A., Deblinger, E., Mannarino, A. P. and Steer, R. A. (2004) 'A multisite, randomised controlled trial for children with sexual abuse-related PTSD symptoms.' *Journal of American Academy of Child and Adolescent Psychiatry 43,* 393–402.

Cohen, J. A., Mannarino, A. P. and Deblinger, E. (2006) *Treating Trauma and Traumatic Grief in Children and Adolescents.* New York: The Guilford Press.

Cohen, N. and Lipsett, L. (1991) 'Recognized and unrecognized language impairment in psychologically disturbed children: child symptomatology, maternal depression and family dysfunction: preliminary report.' *Canadian Journal of Behavioral Science 23*(3), 376–389.

Cohen, N., Barwick, M. A., Horodezky, N. B., Vallance, D. D. and Im, N. (1998a). 'Language, achievement and cognitive processing in psychiatrically disturbed children with previously identified and unsuspected language impairments.' *Journal of Child Psychology and Psychiatry 39*(6), 865–877.

Cohen, N., Menna, R., Vallance, D. D., Barwick, M. A., Im, N. and Horodezky, N. B. (1998b) 'Language, social cognitive processing and behavioral characteristics of psychiatrically disturbed children with previously identified and unsuspected language impairments.' *Journal of Child Psychology and Psychiatry 39*(6), 853–864.

Coia, P. and Jardine Handley, A. (2008) 'Developing relationships with people with profound learning disabilities through intensive interactions.' In M. S. Zeedyk (ed.) *Promoting Social Interaction for Individuals with Communicative Impairments: Making Contact.* London: Jessica Kingsley Publishers.

Coker, A. L., Sanderson, M. and Dong, B. (2004) 'Partner violence during pregnancy and risk of adverse pregnancy outcomes.' *Paediatric and Perinatal Epidemiology 18,* 260–269.

Commission for Health Improvement (2004) *Protecting Children and Young People: Results of an Audit of NHS Organisations in England.* www.chi.nhs.uk/eng/about/publications/childprotection/index.shtml (accessed 4/5/08).

Community Practitioners' and Health Visitors' Association (1998) *Domestic Violence: The Role of the Community Nurse.* London: CPHV.

Conner, M. (2001) 'Developing network-based services in the NHS.' *International Journal of Health Care Quality Assurance 14*(6), 237–244.

Connolly, A., Katz, V. I. and Bash, K. L. (1997) 'Trauma and pregnancy.' *American Journal of Perinatology 14*(6), 331–336.

Conti-Ramsden, G. and Botting, N. (2000) 'Social and behavioural difficulties in children with language impairment.' *Child Language Teaching and Therapy 16*(2), 105–120.

Conti-Ramsden, G. and Botting, N. (2004) 'Social difficulties and victimization in children with SLI at 11 years of age.' *Journal of Speech Language and Hearing Research 47*(1), 145–161.

Copello, A., Orford, J., Vellerman, R., Templeton, L. and Krishnan, M. (2000) 'Methods for reducing alcohol and drug related harm in non-specialist settings.' *Journal of Mental Health 9*(3), 329–343.

Copello, A., Williamson, E., Orford, J. and Day, E. (2006) 'Implementing and evaluating social behaviour and network therapy in drug treatment practice in the UK: a feasibility study.' *Addictive Behaviors 31*(5), 802–810.

Coren, E. and Barlow, J. (2001) Individual and group-based parenting programmes for improving psychosocial outcomes for teenage parents and their children: Cochrane Database of Systematic Reviews.

Corkey, B. and Freeman, R. (1994) 'Predictors of dental anxiety in six-year-old children: findings from a pilot study.' *ASCD Journal of Dentistry for Children 61,* 267–271.

Coster, W. and Cicchetti, D. (1993) 'Research on the communicative development of maltreated children: clinical implications.' *Topics in Language Disorders 13*(4), 25–38.

Covington, T., Foster, V. and Rich, S. (2005) *A Program Manual for Child Death Review.* Okemos, MI: The National Center for Child Death Review.

Cowen, F. M. (2002) 'Adolescent reproductive health interventions.' *Sexually Transmitted Infections 78,* 315–318.

Craft, A. (2007) 'Working together to protect children: who should be working with whom?' *Archives of Disease in Childhood 92*, 571–573.

Craig, C. (2003) *Domestic Violence and Health Professionals.* Belfast: Northern Ireland Women's Aid Federation.

Creighton, S. (2004) *Prevalence and Incidence of Child Abuse: International Comparisons.* London: NSPCC.

Crime and Victims Act (2004) *Domestic Violence, Crime and Victims Act 2004.* London: Office of Public Sector Information.

Crisp, B. and Lister, P. (2004) 'Child protection and public health: nurses' responsibilities.' *Journal of Advanced Nursing 47*(6), 656–663.

Crisp, B. and Lister Green, P. (2006) 'Nurses' perceived training needs for child protection issues.' *Health Education 106*(5), 381–399.

Cross, M. (2005) *Children with Emotional and Behavioural Difficulties and Communication Problems: There is Always a Reason.* London: Jessica Kingsley Publishers.

Crouch, V. (2002) 'Teenage pregnancy and sexual health.' *Community Practitioner 75*(3), 82–84.

Cuffe, S. P., Addy, C. L., Garrison, C. Z., Waller, J. L., Jackson, K. L. and McKeown, R. E. (1998) 'Prevalence of PTSD in a community sample of older adolescents.' *Journal of the American Academy of Child and Adolescent Psychiatry 37*, 147–154.

Culp, R., Watkins, R., Lawrence, H., Letts, D., Kelly, H. and Rice, M. (1991) 'Maltreated children's language and speech and development: abused, neglected and abused.' *First Language 11*, 377–389.

Dale, P. (1999) *Adults Abused as Children.* London: Sage.

Dale, P., Green, R. and Fellows, R. (2002) *What Really Happened? Child Protection Case Management of Young Children with Serious Injuries and Discrepant Parental Explanations.* London: NSPCC Publications Unit.

Daniel, B. and Taylor, J. (2001) *Engaging with Fathers. Practice Issues for Health and Social Care.* London: Jessica Kingsley Publishers.

Daniel, B. M. and Taylor, J. (2006) 'Gender and child neglect: theory, research and policy.' *Critical Social Policy 26*(2), 426–439.

Davies, L. (2004) 'The difference between child abuse and child protection could be you: creating a community network of protective adults.' *Child Abuse Review 13*(6), 426–432(427).

Davis, L. and Siegel, L. J. (2000) 'Posttraumatic stress disorder in children and adolescents: a review and analysis.' *Clinical Child and Family Psychology Review 3*, 135–154.

Dawe, S., Harnett, P. H., Rendalls, V. and Staiger, P. (2003) 'Improving family functioning and child outcomes in methadone maintained families: the "Parents Under Pressure" programme.' *Drug and Alcohol Review 22*, 299–307.

Dawson, G. and Adams, A. (1984) 'Imitation and social responsiveness in autistic children.' *Journal of Abnormal Child Psychology 12*, 209–226.

Dawson, G. and Galpert, L. (1990) 'Mothers' uses of imitative play for facilitating social responsiveness and toy play in young autistic children.' *Development and Psychopathology 2*, 151–162.

Deblinger, E. and Heflin, A. H. (1996) *Treating Sexually Abused Children and Their Nonoffending Parents: A Cognitive Behavioral Approach.* Thousand Oaks, CA: Sage Publications.

Deblinger, E., McLeer, S. V., Atkins, M. S., Ralphe, D. and Foa, E. (1989) 'Post-traumatic stress in sexually abused, physically abused and nonabused children.' *Child Abuse and Neglect 13*, 403–404.

Deblinger, E., Steer, R. and Lippmann, J. (1999) 'Two-year follow-up study of cognitive-behavioural therapy for sexually abused children suffering posttraumatic stress symptoms.' *Child Abuse and Neglect 23*, 1371–1378.

Delago, C., Deblinger, E., Schroeder, C. and Finkel, M. (2008) 'Girls who disclose sexual abuse: urogenital symptoms and signs after genital contact.' *Pediatrics 122*(2), 281–286.

Delta Dental (2008) 'The PANDA program [on-line].' Kansas City. www.deltadentalks.com/DDKS/ DentistsPANDA.aspx?DView=DentistsPANDAProgram (accessed 21/10/08).

Denham, S., Caverly, S., Schmidt, M., Blair, K., *et al.* (2002) 'Preschool understanding of emotions: contributions to classroom anger and aggression.' *Journal of Child Psychology and Psychiatry 43*(7), 901–916.

Department for Children, Schools and Families (2008a) 'Patterns and causes of child death: information sheet [online].' www.everychildmatters.gov.uk/socialcare/safeguarding/childdeathreview/trainingmaterials (accessed 1/10/08).

Department for Children, Schools and Families (2008b) *Responding to an Unexpected Child Death.* London: HMSO.

Department for Education and Skills (2004a) *Every Child Matters, Change for Children.* London: HMSO.

Department for Education and Skills (2004b) *National Service Framework for Children, Young People and Maternity Services: Core Standards.* London: Department of Health.

Department for Education and Skills (2006) *Working Together to Safeguard Children: A Guide to Inter-Agency Working to Safeguard and Promote the Welfare of Children.* London: Department of Health.

Department of Health (2000) *Domestic Violence: A Resource Manual for Health Care Professionals.* London: Department of Health.

Department of Health (2001a) *Better Prevention, Better Services, Better Sexual Health – The National Strategy for Sexual Health and HIV.* London: Department of Health.

Department of Health (2001b) *Children in Northern Ireland: Domestic Violence and Professional Awareness.* Belfast: Department of Health.

Department of Health (2002) *The Children's Act Report.* London: HMSO.

Department of Health (2003a) *Green Paper Consultation Document: Every Child Matters.* London: HMSO.

Department of Health (2003b) *What to do if You're Worried a Child is Being Abused.* London: HMSO.

Department of Health (2004a) *Framework for the Assessment of Children in Need and their Families.* London: Department of Health.

Department of Health (2004b) *National Service Framework for Children, Young People and Maternity Services: Care Standards.* London: Department of Health. www.dh.gov.uk/PolicyAndGuidance/HealthAndSocialCareTopics/ChildrenServices/ ChildrenServicesInformation/fs/en (accessed 23/5/05).

Department of Health (2005) *Child Protection and the Dental Team.* www.cpdt.org.uk/tab01/ 1_1_1_3_0.htm (accessed 6/12/08).

Department of Health (2006) *Tackling the Health and Mental Health Effects of Domestic and Sexual Violence and Abuse.* London: Department of Health.

Department of Health (2007a) *Child Protection and the Dental Team.* www.dh.gov.uk/en/Publicationsandstatistics/Publications/PublicationsStatistics/DH_081280/ (accessed 30/01/08).

Department of Health (2007b) *Drug Misuse and Dependence: UK Guidelines on Clinical Management.* London: Department of Health (England), the Scottish Government, Welsh Assembly Government and Northern Ireland Executive.

Department of Health (2007c) *Healthy Inequality Target Monitoring – Infant Mortality.* www.dh.gov.uk/en/Publicationsandstatistics/Publications/PublicationsStatistics/DH_081280 (accessed 18/1/08).

Dieppe, P. and Horne, R. (2002) 'Soundbites and patient centred care.' *British Medical Journal 325*(7364), 605.

Dietz, P. M., Gazmararian, J. A., Goodwin, M., Bruce, F. C., Johnson, C. H. and Rochat, R. (1997) 'Delayed entry into prenatal care: the effects of physical violence.' *Obstetrics and Gynaecology 90*(2), 221–224.

Dixon, L., Browne, K. and Hamilton-Giachritsis, C. (2005) 'Risk factors of parents abused as children: a mediational analysis of the intergenerational continuity of child maltreatment (Part I).' *Journal of Child Psychology and Psychiatry 46*, 47–57.

Dodsworth, J., Belderson, P., Black, J., Brandon, M. *et al.* (2008) *Biennial Analysis of English Serious Case Reviews 2003–2005.* London: NSPCC.

Donaldson, L. J. and O'Brien, S. (1995) 'Press coverage of the Cleveland child sexual abuse enquiry: a source of public enlightenment?' *Journal of Public Health 17*(1), 70–76.

Donaldson, M., Yordy, K. and Vanselow, N. (1994) *Defining Primary Care: An Interim Report.* www.nap.edu/catalog.php?record_id=9153 (accessed 16/1/08).

Donohue, B., Romero, V. and Hill, H. H. (2006) 'Treatment of co-occurring child maltreatment and substance abuse.' *Aggression and Violent Behaviour 11*, 626–640.

Dowling, B., Powell, M. and Glendinning, C. (2004) 'Conceptualising successful partnerships.' *Health and Social Care in the Community 12*(4), 309–317.

Dozier, M., Stovall, K. C. and Albus, K. E. (1999) 'Attachment and psychopathology in adulthood.' In J. Cassidy and P. Shaver (eds) *Handbook of Attachment.* New York: Guilford Press.

Drossman, D. A., Talley, N. J., Leserman, J., Olden, K. W. and Barreiro, M. A. (1995) 'Sexual and physical abuse and gastrointestinal illness. Review and recommendations.' *Annals of Internal Medicine 123* (10), 782–794.

DrugScope (2005) *Substance Misuse in Pregnancy: A Resource Book for Professionals.* London: DrugScope.

Dubbs, N. L., Bazzoli, G. J., Shortell, S. M. and Kralovec, P. D. (2004) 'Re-examining organizational configurations: an update, validation and expansion of the taxonomy of health networks and systems.' *Health Services Research 39*(1), 207–220.

Dube, S. R., Aanda, R. F., Felitti, V. J., Edwards, V. J. and Croft, J. B. (2002) 'Adverse childhood experiences and personal alcohol abuse as an adult.' *Addictive Behaviors 27*(5), 713–725.

Dube, S. R., Felitti, V. J., Dong, M., Chapman, D. P., Giles, W. H. and Anda, R. F. (2003) 'Childhood abuse, neglect and household dysfunction and the risk of illicit drug use: the adverse childhood experiences study.' *Paediatrics and Child Health 111*, 564–572.

Dubner, A. E. and Motta, R. W. (1999) 'Sexually and physically abused foster care children and posttraumatic stress disorder.' *Journal of Consulting and Clinical Psychology 67*(3), 367–373.

Dugald Baird Centre for Research on Women's Health (2005) *Healthy Respect: Executive summary.* www.healthyrespect.org.uk/downloads-and-campaigns/evidence-and-reports-phase-1.htm?pageindex=1 (accessed 3/7/08).

Durfee, M., Tilton Durfee, D. and West, P. M. (2002) 'Child fatality review: an international movement.' *Child Abuse and Neglect 26*, 619–636.

Durkin, K. and Conti-Ramsden, G. (2007) 'Language, social behaviour and the quality of friendships in adolescents with and without a history of specific language impairment.' *Child Development 78*(5), 1441–1457.

Dyer, C. (2004) 'Inexpert witness.' *The Guardian:* www.guardian.co.uk/world/2004/apr/06/law.children (accessed 6/12/08).

Eberle, P. (1993) *The Abuse of Innocence: The McMartin Preschool Trial.* New York: Prometheus Books.

Edelson, J. L. (2001) 'Studying the co-occurrence of child maltreatment and woman battering in families.' In S. A. Graham-Bermann and J. L. Edelson (eds) *Domestic Violence in the Lives of Children: The Future of Research, Intervention and Social Policy.* Washington, D.C: American Psychological Association.

Edwards, H. (2007) *Faith, Religion and Safeguarding Children – NSPCC Internal Briefing Paper.* London: NSPCC Training and Consultancy.

Edwards, P., Green, J., Roberts, I. and Lutchmun, S. (2006) 'Deaths from injury in children and employment status in family: analysis of trends in class specific death rates.' British Medical Journal (doi:10.1136/bmj.38875,757488.4F [published 7 July 2006]).

Ehlers, A. and Clark, D. M. (2000) 'A cognitive model of posttraumatic stress disorder.' Behaviour Research and Therapy 38, 319–345.

Eiden, R. D., Edwards, E. P. and Leonard, K. E. (2002) 'Mother–infant and father–infant attachment among alcoholic families.' Development and Psychopathology 14(2), 253–278.

EIU (2002) Supporting Families and Carers of Drug Users: A Review. Edinburgh: Effective Interventions Unit, Scottish Executive.

Elliott, L., Claveirole, A., Pow, J. and Themessl-Huber, M. (2007) Survey of Professionals Working in Sexual Health and Education for Young People: First Sweep. Edinburgh: Napier University.

EMCDDA (2006) The State of the Drugs Problem in Europe. Lisbon: European Monitoring Centre for Drugs and Drug Addiction.

Ephraim, G. (1986) A Brief Introduction to Augmented Mothering, Playtrack Pamphlet. Radlet: Herts: Harpebury Hospital School.

Eraut, M. (1994) Developing Professional Knowledge and Competence. London: Falmer Press.

Erickson, M. F. and Egeland, B. (1987) 'A developmental view of the psychological consequences of mistreatment.' School Psychology Review 16(2), 156–168.

Escalona, A., Field, T., Nadel, J. and Lundy, B. (2002) 'Brief Report: imitation effects on children with autism.' Journal of Autism and Developmental Disorders 32, 141–144.

Espinosa, L. and Osborne, K. (2002) 'Domestic violence during pregnancy: implications for practice.' Journal of Midwifery and Women's Health 47, 305–317.

Evans, D. T. (2004) 'Continuing professional development: behind the headlines: sexual health implications for nursing ethics and practice.' Primary Health Care 14(8), 40–50.

Evans, R. G. and Stoddart, G. L. (1994) 'Producing health, consuming health care.' In R. G. Evans, M. L., Barer and T. R. Marmor (eds) Why are Some People Healthy and Others Not? The Determinants of Health of Populations. Berlin, New York: Walter de Gruyter.

Ezard, N. (2001) 'Public health, human rights and the harm reduction paradigm: from risk reduction to vulnerability reduction.' International Journal of Drug Policy 12, 207–219.

Fairholm, J. and Juen, B. (2008) Children and Child Protection, Module 6; IFRC Reference Centre for Psychosocial Support: Community based Psychosocial Support: Revised Version of The Trainer's Manual, 2008. Unpublished manuscript.

Fals-Stewart, W., Fincham, F. D. and Kelley, M. L. (2004) 'Substance-abusing parents' attitudes toward allowing their custodial children to participate in treatment: a comparison of mothers versus fathers.' Journal of Family Psychology 18(4), 666–671.

Fals-Stewart, W., O'Farrell, T. J. and Birchler, G. R. (2004) 'Behavioral couples therapy for substance abuse: rationale, methods and findings.' Science and Practice Perspective 30–43.

Famularo, R., Fenton, T., Kinscherff, R., Ayoub, C. and Barnum, R. (1994) 'Maternal and child posttraumatic stress disorder in cases of child maltreatment.' Child Abuse and Neglect 18, 27–36.

Farmer, E. and Moyers, S. (2005) Children Placed with Family and Friends: Placement Patterns and Outcomes. Bristol: School for Policy Studies, University of Bristol.

Farrell, P., Critchley, C. and Mills, C. (1999) 'Attainment of pupils with emotional and behavioural difficulties.' British Journal of Special Educational and Child Psychology 26(1), 50–53.

Farrell, S. P., Haines, A. A. and Davies, W. H. (1998) 'Cognitive behavioural interventions for sexually abused children exhibiting PTSD symptomatology.' Behavior Therapy 29, 241–255.

Feather, J. S. and Ronan, K. R. (2004) Te Ara Whetu: Trauma-focused Cognitive Behavioural Therapy for Abused Children: A Treatment Manual. Unpublished manuscript.

Feather, J. S. and Ronan, K. R. (2006) 'Trauma-focused cognitive-behavioural therapy for abused children with posttraumatic stress disorder.' New Zealand Journal of Psychology 35, 132–145.

Feather, J. S., Ronan, K. R., Murupaenga, P., Berking, T. and Crellin, K. (2007) 'Trauma-focused cognitive-behavioural therapy for Maori and Samoan children with multiple-abuse and PTSD in a New Zealand child protection setting: a single-case multiple-baseline study.' Manuscript in preparation.

Featherstone, B. (2006) 'Rethinking family support in the current policy context.' British Journal of Social Work 36, 5–19.

Fergusson, D. M. and Lynskey, M. T. (1997) 'Physical punishment/maltreatment during childhood and adjustment in young adulthood.' Child Abuse and Neglect 21(7), 617–630.

Fergusson, D. M., Horwood, L. J. and Lynskey, M. T. (1996) 'Childhood sexual abuse and psychiatric disorder in young adulthood I: prevalence of sexual abuse and factors associated with sexual abuse.' Journal of the American Academy of Child and Adolescent Psychiatry 35, 1355–1364.

Ferlie, E. and McGivern, G. (2003) Relationship between Health Care Organisations. London: National Co-ordinating Centre for NHS Service Delivery and Organisation R&D.

Festinger, L. (1962) 'Cognitive dissonance.' Science America 207, 93–102.

Field, T., Sanders, C. and Nadel, J. (2001) 'Children with autism display more social behaviours after repeated imitation sessions.' Autism 5, 317–323.

Filipas, H. H. and Ullman, S. E. (2006) 'Child sexual abuse, coping responses, self-blame, posttraumatic stress disorder and adult sexual revictimization.' Journal of Interpersonal Violence 21, 652–672.

Finkelhor, D. (1994) 'The international epidemiology of child sexual abuse.' *Child Abuse and Neglect 18*(5), 409–417.

Finkelhor, D. and Dziuba-Leatherman, J. (1994) 'Children as victims of violence: a national survey.' *Pediatrics 94*, 413–420.

Finkelhor, D., Ormond, R., Turner, H. and Hamby, S. L. (2005) 'The victimisation of children and youth: a comprehensive, national survey.' *Child Maltreatment 10*, 5–25.

Fisher, B., Neve, H. and Heritage, Z. (1999) 'Community development, user involvement and primary health care.' *British Medical Journal 318*(7186), 749–750.

Flaherty, E. G., Jones, R. and Sege, R. (2004) 'Telling their stories: primary care practitioners' experience evaluating and reporting injuries caused by child abuse.' *Child Abuse and Neglect 28*, 939–945.

Flaherty, E. G., Sege, R., Binns, H. J., Mattson, C. L. and Christoffel, K. K. (2000) 'Health care providers' experience of reporting child abuse in the primary care setting.' *Archive Pediatric Adolescent Medicine 154*, 489–493.

Flaherty, E.G., Sege, R., Mattson, C.L. and Binns, H.J. (2002) 'Assessment of suspicion of abuse primary care setting.' *Ambulatory Pediatrics 2*, 120–126.

Fleck-Henderson, A. F. (2002) 'Domestic violence in the child protection system: seeing double.' *Children and Youth Services Review 22*, 333–354.

Fleming, P., Blair, P., Sidebotham, P. and Hayler, T. (2004) 'Investigating sudden unexpected deaths in infancy and childhood and caring for bereaved families: an integrated multiagency approach.' *British Medical Journal 328*, 331–334.

Fonagy, P. (2001) *Attachment Theory and Psychoanalysis.* New York: Other Press.

Fonagy, P. (1994) 'Mental representations from an intergenerational cognitive science perspective.' *Infant Mental Health Journal 15*(1), 57–68.

Fonagy, P. (1999) *Attachment and Psychoanalysis.* New York: Other Press.

Fonagy, P., Gergely, G., Jurist, E. L. and Target, M. (2002) *Affect Regulation, Mentalization and the Development of the Self* Stuttgart: Klett-Cotta.

Foote, C. and Plsek, P. (2001) 'Thinking out of the box.' *Health Service Journal 12 April*, 32–33.

Fowler, J. and Chevannes, M. (1998) 'Evaluating the efficacy of reflective practice in the context of clinical supervision.' *Journal of Advanced Nursing 27*, 379–382.

Fox, J. (2008) *A Contribution to the Evaluation of Recent Developments in the Investigation of Sudden Unexpected Death in Infancy.* University of Surrey/National Policing Improvement Agency www.baspcan.org.uk/sudibriefingpaperjohnfox.pdf (accessed 16/6/08).

Fox, L., Long, S. H. and Langlois, A. (1988) 'Patterns of language comprehension deficit in abused and neglected children.' *Journal of Speech and Hearing Disorders 53*, 239–244.

Frankel, A., Graydon-Baker, E., Neppl, C., Simmonds, T., Gustafson, M. and Ganhi, T. (2003) 'Patient safety leadership walkrounds.' *Joint Commission Journal on Quality Improvement 29*(1), 16–26.

Fraser, S. (2005) *Promoting a Healthy Respect: What does the Evidence Support?* Edinburgh: Health Scotland.

Frederick, J. and Goddard, C. (2007) 'Exploring the relationship between poverty, childhood adversity and child abuse from the perspective of adulthood.' *Child Abuse Review 16*, 323–341.

Freel, R. and Robinson, E. (2005) *Experience of Domestic Violence in Northern Ireland: Findings from the 2003/04 Northern Ireland Crime Survey.* Belfast: Northern Ireland Office.

Freeman, R. (1999) 'A psychodynamic understanding of the dentist–patient interaction.' *British Dental Journal 186*, 503–506.

Freeman, R. (2000) *The Psychology of Dental Patient Care.* London: BDJ Books.

Freeman, R. (2007) 'An anxious child attends: a psychoanalytic explanation of children's responses to dental treatment.' *International Journal of Paediatric Dentistry 17*, 407–418.

Freeman, R. and Kells, B. (1996) 'A dysmorphophobic reaction to cosmetic dentistry: observations and responses to psychotherapeutic intervention.' *Psychoanalytic Psychotherapy 10*, 21–31.

Freeman, R., Russell, M., Lazenbatt, A. and Marcenes, W. (2003) *Victoria Climbié – Can We Get the Lessons Right?* www.bmj.com/egi/eletters/326/7384/293 (accessed 25/01/08).

Freemantle, J. and Read, A. (2008) 'Preventing child deaths.' *British Medical Journal 336*, 1083–1084.

French, E., Pituch, M., Brandt, J. and Pohorecki, S. (1998) 'Improving interactions between substance-abusing mothers and their substance-exposed newborns.' *Journal of Obstetric Gynecologic and Neonatal Nursing 27*(3), 262–269.

Freud, A. (1952) 'The role of bodily illness in the mental life of children.' *Psychoanalytic Study of the Child 7*, 69–81.

Freud, S. (1914) *Remembering, Repeating and Working-Through.* SE XII. London: Hogarth Press.

Friedrich, W. N. (2002) *Psychological Assessment of Sexually Abused Children and their Families.* Thousand Oaks, California: Sage.

Frith, U. (1989) *Autism: Explaining the Enigma.* Oxford: Blackwell Publishing.

Frith, U. (2003) *Autism: Explaining the Enigma.* Oxford: Blackwell Publishing.

Fujiki, M., Brinton, B., Hart, C. H. and Fitzgerald, A. H. (1999) 'Peer acceptance and friendship in children with specific language impairment.' *Topics in Language Disorder 19*(2), 34–48.

Gallagher, T. M. (1999) 'Interrelationships among children's language, behavior and emotional problems.' *Topics in Language Disorders 19*(2), 1–15.

Gauthier, Y. (2003) 'Infant mental health as we enter the third millennium: can we prevent aggression?' *Infant Mental Health Journal 24*(3), 296–308.

Gazmararian, J. A., Lazorick, S., Spitz, A. M., Goodwin, M., Saltzman, L. E. and Marks, J. S. (1996) 'Prevalence of violence against pregnant women: a review of the literature.' *Journal of the American Medical Association 275*, 1915–1920.

Geddes, J. F. and Plunkett, J. (2004) 'Editorial: the evidence base for shaken baby syndrome.' *British Medical Journal 328*, 719–720.

Geddes, J. F., Vowles, G. H., Hackshaw, A. K., Nickols, C. D., Scott, I. S. and Whitwell, H. L. (2001) 'Neuropathology of inflicted head injury in children II Microscopic brain injury in infants.' *Brain 124*, 1299–1306.

General Dental Council (2005) *Standards for Dental Professionals*. London: General Dental Council.

George, C. and Solomon, J. (1996) 'Representational models of relationships: links between caregiving and attachment.' *Infant Mental Health Journal 17*(3), 198–216.

Gerhart, S. (2004) *Why Love Matters: How Affection Shapes a Baby's Brain*. Hove: Brunner-Routledge.

Gettleman, J. (2008) 'Victims of a witch-hunt.' http://scotlandonsunday.scotsman.com/spectrum/Victims-of-a-witch-hunt.4305870.jp (accessed 20/7/08).

GGD Rotterdam (2008) 'Statute for the reporting of child abuse [Rotterdamse meldcode voor kindermishandeling][on-line].' www.huiselijkgeweld.rotterdam.nl/ (accessed 15/7/08).

Ghate, D., Shaw, C. and Hazel, N. (2000) *Fathers and Family Centres: Engaging Fathers in Preventive Services*. York: Joseph Rowntree Foundation.

Giacona, R. M., Reiknherz, H. Z., Silverman, A. B., Pakiz, B., Frost, A. K. and Cohen, E. (1995) 'Traumas and PTSD in a community sample of older adolescents.' *Journal of the American Academy of Child and Adolescent Psychiatry 34*, 1369–1380.

Gielen, A. C., O'Campo, P. J., Faden, R. R., Kass, N. E. and Xue, X. (1994) 'Interpersonal conflict and physical violence during the childbearing year.' *Social Science and Medicine 39*, 781–787.

Gil, E. (2006) *Helping Abused and Traumatized Children: Integrating Directive and Nondirective Approaches* New York: The Guilford Press.

Gilmour, J., Hill, B., Place, M. and Skuse, D. H. (2005) 'Social communication deficits in conduct disorder: a clinical and community survey.' *Journal of Child Psychology and Psychiatry 45*(5), 967–978.

Gipson, M. and Connolly, F. (1975) 'The incidence of schizophrenia and severe psychological disorders in patients 10 years after cosmetic rhinoplasty.' *British Journal of Plastic Surgery 28*, 155–159.

Glaser, D. (2000) 'Child abuse and the brain – a review.' *Journal of Child Psychology and Psychiatry 41*, 97–116.

GMC (2007) *0–18 Years: Guidance for all Doctors*. London: www.gmc-uk.org/guidance/ethical_guidance/children_guidance/77_prescribing_medicines.asp (accessed 6/12/08).

GMC (2008) *Acting as an Expert Witness*. www.gmc uk.org/guidance/ethical_guidance/children_guidance/77_prescribing_medicines.asp (accessed 6/12/08).

Goldman, L. (2000) *Life and Loss: A Guide to Help Grieving Children*. Philadelphia: Taylor and Francis.

Goodall, E. and Lumley, T. (2007) *Not Seen and Not Heard – Child Abuse: A Guide for Donors and Funders* London. New Philanthropy Capital

Goodwin, M., Gazmararian, J. A., Johnson, C. H., Gilbert, B. C., Saltzman, L. E. and Group, P. W. (2000) 'Pregnancy intendedness and physical abuse around the time of pregnancy: findings from the Pregnancy Risk Assessment Monitoring System, 1996–1997.' *Maternal and Child Health Journal 4*(2), 85–92.

Gorin, S. (2004) *Understanding what Children Say: Children's Experiences of Domestic Violence, Parental Substance Misuse and Parental Health Problems*. London: National Children's Bureau.

Gornall, J. (2008) 'Three doctors and a GMC prosecution.' *British Medical Journal 337*, a907.

Graham, A. (2004) 'Sexual health.' *British Journal of General Practice 54*, 382–387.

Greco, V., Sloper, P. and Barton, K. (2004) *Coordination and Key Worker Services for Disabled Children in the UK*. York: Social Policy Research Unit, The University of York.

Greene, P. and Chiswick, M. (1995) 'Child abuse/neglect and the oral health of children's primary dentition.' *Military Medicine 160*, 290–293.

Greene, P., Chiswick, M. and Aaron, G. (1994) 'A comparison of oral health status and need for dental care between abused/neglected children and nonabused/non-neglected children.' *Pediatric Dentistry 16*, 41–45.

Gregg, R., Freeth, D. and Blackie, C. (1998) 'Teenage health and the practice nurse: choice and opportunity for both?' *British Journal of General Practice 48*(426), 909–910.

Gross, J. J. (1998) 'The emerging field of emotion regulation: an integrative review.' *Review of General Psychology 2*, 271–299.

Grubbs, G. A. (1994) 'An abused child's use of sandplay in the healing process.' *Clinical Social Work Journal 22*(2), 193–209.

Gruenert, S., Ratnam, S. and Tsantefski, M. (2004) *The Nobody's Clients Project: Identifying and Addressing the Needs of Children with Substance Dependent Parents*. Victoria: Odyssey Institute of Studies.

Guterman, N. B. and Lee, Y. (2005) 'The role of fathers in risk for physical child abuse and neglect: possible pathways and unanswered questions.' *Child Maltreatment 10*(2), 136–149.

Haines, L. and Turton, J. (2008) 'Complaints in child protection.' *Archives of Disease in Childhood 93*, 4–6.

Hall, D. (2003) 'Child protection-lessons from Victoria Climbié.' *British Medical Journal 326*, 293–294.

Hall, D. and Elliman, D. (2003) *Health for All Children: 4th Report*. Oxford: Oxford University.

Happé, F. G. E. (1999a) 'Autism: cognitive deficit or cognitive style?' *Trends in Cognitive Sciences 3*, 216–222.

Happé, F. G. E. (1999b) 'Understanding assets and deficits in autism – why success is more interesting than failure.' *The Psychologist 12*, 540–547.

Harbin, F. and Murphy, M. (eds) (2000) *Substance Misuse and Childcare: How to Understand, Assist and Intervene when Drugs Affect Parenting.* Lyme Regis: Russell House.

Harris, S. L., Handleman, J. S. and Fong, P. L. (1987) 'Imitation of self-stimulation: impact on the autistic child's behavior and affect.' *Child and Family Behavior Therapy 9*, 1–21.

Hartley, C. C. (2002) 'The co-occurrence of child maltreatment and domestic violence: examining both neglect and child physical abuse.' *Child Maltreatment 7*(4), 349–358.

Hartley, C. C. (2004) 'Severe domestic violence and child maltreatment: considering child physical abuse, neglect and failure to protect.' *Children and Youth Services Review 23*, 373–392.

Hartup, W. W. (1995) 'The company they keep: friendships and their developmental significance.' *Child Development 67*(1), 1–13.

Health Development Agency (2001) *Teenage Pregnancy: An Update on Key Characteristics of Effective Interventions.* London: Health Development Agency.

Healthy Respect (2003) *A Review of Specialist Sexual Health Services for Young People: A Short Report (All I Want).* Edinburgh: Healthy Respect.

Heger, A., Ticson, L., Velasquez, O. and Bernier, R. (2002) 'Children referred for possible sexual abuse: medical findings in 2384 children.' *Child Abuse and Neglect 26*(6–7), 645–659.

Heimann, M., Laberg, K. E. and Nordren, B. (2006) 'Imitative interaction increases social interest and elicited imitation in non-verbal children with autism.' *Infant and Child Development 15*, 297–309.

Hendricks, S., Freeman, R. and Sheiham, A. (1990) 'Why inner city mothers take their pre-school children for medical and dental check-ups.' *Community Dental Health 7*, 33–42.

Henningsen, G. (1996) 'The child witch syndrome: satanic child abuse of today and child witch trials of yesterday.' *Journal of Forensic Psychiatry and Psychology 7*(3), 581–593.

Hepburn, M. (2004) 'Caring for the pregnant drug user.' In B. Beaumont (ed.) *Care of Drug Users in General Practice: A Harm Reduction Approach.* Oxford: Radcliffe.

Herbert, C. P., Bainbridge, L., Bickford, J., Baptiste, S., *et al.* (2007). 'Factors that influence engagement in collaborative practice: how 8 health professionals became advocates.' *Canadian Family Physician 53*(8), 1318–1325.

Herman, D. B., Slusser, E. S., Sturening, E. L. and Link, B. L. (1997) 'Adverse childhood experiences: are they risk factors for adult homelessness?' *American Journal Public Health 87*(2), 249–255.

Herman, J. L., Perry, J. C. and van der Kolk, B. A. (1989) 'Childhood trauma in borderline personality disorder.' *American Journal Psychiatry 146*(10), 1358–1359.

Herrenkohl, E. C., Herrenkohl, R. C. and Egolf, B. P. (2003) 'The psychosocial consequences of living environment instability on maltreated children.' *American Journal of Orthopsychiatry 73*(4), 367–380.

Hester, M. and Radford, L. (1996) *Domestic Violence and Child Contact Arrangements in England and Denmark.* Bristol: Policy Press.

Hester, M., Pearson, C. and Harwin, N. (1998) *Making an Impact: Children and Domestic Violence.* Bristol: University of Bristol.

Hester, M., Pearson, C. and Harwin, N. (2000) *Making an Impact: Children and Domestic Violence.* London: Jessica Kingsley Publishers.

Hewitt, S. K. (1999) *Assessing Allegations of Abuse in Preschool Children.* Thousand Oaks, California: Sage.

Higgins, D. J. and McCabe, M. P. (2003) 'Maltreatment and family dysfunction in childhood and the subsequent adjustment of children and adults.' *Journal of Family Violence 18*(2), 107–120.

Hill, E. (2004a) 'Executive dysfunction in autism.' *Trends in Cognitive Sciences 8*, 26–32.

Hill, E. (2004b) 'Evaluating the theory of executive dysfunction in autism.' *Developmental Review 24*, 189–233.

HM Government (2004) *Every Child Matters: Change for Children.* London: The Stationery Office.

HM Government (2006) *Working Together to Safeguard Children: A Guide to Inter-Agency Working to Safeguard and Promote the Welfare of Children.* London: Department for Education and Skills.

HM Government (2007) *Safeguarding Children from Abuse Linked to a Belief in Spirit Possession.* London: Department for Education and Skills.

HM Government (2008) *Drugs: Protecting Families and Communities. The 2008 Drug Strategy.* London: Home Office.

HMIE Her Majesty's Inspectorate for Education (2007) www.hmie.gov.uk/Publications.aspx (accessed 6/12/08).

Hobbs, C., Hanks, H. and Wynne, J. (1999) *Child Abuse and Neglect: A Clinician's Handbook.* London: Churchill Livingstone.

Hoffman, L. and Hatch, M. (2000) 'Depressive symptomatology during pregnancy: evidence for an association with deceased fetal growth in pregnancies of lower social class women.' *Health Psychology 19*(6), 535–543.

Hogan, D. M. (1998) 'Annotation: the psychological development and welfare of children of opiate and cocaine users: review and research needs.' *Journal of Child Psychology and Psychiatry 39*(5), 609–620.

Hogan, D. M. and Higgins, L. (2001) *When Parents use Drugs: Key Findings from a Study of Children in the Care of Drug-Using Parents.* Dublin: Trinity College.

Home Office (1999) *The Home Office Agenda on Violence Against Women.* www.homeoffice.gov.uk/domesticviolence/hoagen.htm (accessed 21/7/08).

Home Office (2003) *British Crime Survey.* London: Home Office.

Home Office (2006) *A Coordinated Prostitution Strategy and a Summary of Responses to Paying the Price* London: Home Office.

Home Office and Cabinet Office (1999) *Domestic Violence: Findings from a New British Crime Survey Self-completion Questionnaire.* London: Home Office Research Study 191.

Home Office Circular (2000) Domestic Violence, London: Home Office.

Horton, R. (2008a) 'Margaret Chan puts primary health care centre stage at WHO [editorial].' *Lancet 371*, 1811.

Horton, R. (2008b) 'A renaissance in primary health care [editorial].' *Lancet 372*, 863.

Horwath, J. and Morrison, T. (2007) 'Collaboration, integration and change in children's services: critical issues and key ingredients.' *Child Abuse and Neglect 31*(1), 55–69.

Hosking, G. and Walsh, I. (2005) *The Wave Report 2005. Violence and What to Do about It* London: Wave Trust.

Howarth, J. and Morrison, T. (1999) *Effective Staff Training in Social Care, From Theory to Practice* London: Routledge.

Hubbard, G. and Themessl-Huber, M. (2005) 'Professional perceptions of joint working in primary care and social care services for older people in Scotland.' *Journal of Interprofessional Care 19*(4), 371–385.

Hummel, R. and Gross, A. (2001) 'Socially anxious children: an observational study of parent–child interaction.' *Child and Family Behavior Therapy 23*, 19–41.

Humphreys, C., Thiara, R. K. and Regan, L. (2005) 'Domestic violence and substance misuse: tackling complexity.' *British Journal of Social Work 35*(8), 1303–1320.

Hunt, S. and Martin, A. (2001) *Pregnant Women, Violent Men: What Midwives Need to Know.* Hale: Books for Midwives Press.

Hunter, B. (2004) 'Conflicting ideologies as a source of emotion work in midwifery.' *Midwifery 20*, 261–272.

Huygen, F. J. A. (1978) *Family Medicine: The Medical Life History of Families* Nimegen, The Netherlands: Dekker and Van de Vegt.

Hwang, B. and Hughes, C. (2000) 'Increasing early social-communicative skills of preverbal preschool children with autism through social interactive training.' *Journal of the Association for Persons with Severe Handicaps 25*, 18–28.

IFRC (2003) *Community Based Psychosocial Support, A Trainer's Manual.* Unpublished manuscript, Copenhagen.

IJzendoorn, M. H., Prinzie, P., Euder, E. M., Groeneveld, M. G., *et al.* (2007) *Child Abuse: Leiden Attachment Research Program.* Leiden: Cashmir Publishers, Universiteit Leiden, Fac. Sociale wetenschappen, Algemene en Gezinspedagogiek – Datatheorie, WODC.

Iles, V. and Sutherland, K. (2001) *Organisational Change: A Review for Health Care Managers, Professionals and Researchers* London: NCCSDO.

Ingersoll, B. and Schreibman, L. (2006) 'Teaching reciprocal imitation skills to young children with autism using a naturalistic behavioral approach: effects on language, pretend play and joint attention.' *Journal of Autism and Developmental Disorders 36*, 487–505.

Institute for Healthcare Improvement (2005) *Going Lean in Healthcare* Cambridge, Mass: IHI.

Intercollegiate Document (2006) *Safeguarding Children and Young People: Roles and Competences for Health Care Staff.* London: Royal College of Paediatrics and Child Health.

ISD Scotland Publications (2007) *Sexually Transmitted Infections and Other Sexual Health Information for Scotland* www.isdscotland.org/isd/991.html (accessed 13/2/08).

Itard, J. M. G. (1932) *The Wild Boy of Aveyron (Rapports et memories sur le Sauvage de l'Aveyron)* Translated by George and Muriel Humphrey. New York: Century Co.

Iwaniec, D., Larkin, E. and Higgins, S. (2006) 'Research review: risk and resilience in cases of emotional abuse.' *Child and Family Social Work 11*, 73–82.

Jackson, K. (2005) 'The roles and responsibilities of newly qualified children's nurses.' *Paediatric Nursing 17*(6), 26–30.

Jacobson, L., Richardson, G., Parry-Langdon, N. and Donovan, C. (2001) 'How do teenagers and primary healthcare providers view each other? An overview of key themes.' *British Journal of General Practice 51*, 811–816.

Janoff-Bulman, R. (1989) 'Assumptive worlds and the stress of traumatic events: applications of the schema construct.' *Social Cognition 7*(2), 113–136.

Järbrink, K. and Knapp, M. (2001) 'The economic impact of autism in Britain.' *Autism 5*, 7–22.

Järbrink, K., Fombonne, E. and Knapp, M. (2003) 'Measuring the parental, service and cost impacts of children with autistic spectrum disorder: a pilot study.' *Journal of Autism and Developmental Disorders 33*, 395–402.

Jasinski, J. L. (2004) 'Pregnancy and domestic violence: a review of the literature.' *Trauma Violence Abuse 5*(1), 47–64.

Jenny, C. (2007) 'The intimidation of British paediatricians.' *Paediatrics 119*(4), 797–799.

Jenny, C. and Isaac, R. (2006) 'The relationship between child death and child maltreatment.' *Archives of Disease in Childhood 91*, 265–269.

Jewkes, R. I., Levin, J. and Loveday, P. (2002) 'Risk factors for domestic violence: findings from a South African cross-sectional study.' *Social Science and Medicine 55*, 1603–1617.

Johnson, M. A., Stone, S., Lou, C., Ling, J., Claassen, J. and Austin, M. J. (2006) *Assessing Parent Education Programs for Families Involved with Child Welfare Services: Evidence and Implications* Berkeley: Centre for Social Services Research, University of California.

Johnstone, F. D. (1998) 'Pregnant drug users.' In J. R. Robertson (ed.) *Management of Drug Users in the Community: A Practical Handbook.* London: Arnold.

Jones, D. P. H. and McGraw, J. M. (1987) 'Reliable and fictitious accounts of sexual abuse to children.' *Journal of Interpersonal Violence 2*, 27–45.

Jones, L. P., Gross, E. and Becker, I. (2002) 'The characteristics of domestic violence victims in a child protective service caseload.' *Families in Society 83*, 405–415.

Juen, F., Peham, D., Juen, B. and Benecke, C. (2007) 'Emotion, aggression and the meaning of prevention in early childhood.' In G. Steffgen and M. Gollwitzer (eds) *Emotions and Aggressive Behaviour.* Göttingen: Hofgrefe.

Kaduson, H. G. (2006) 'Release play therapy for children with posttraumatic stress disorder.' In H. G. Kaduson and C. E. Schaefer (eds) *Short-term Play Therapy for Children.* New York: Guilford Press.

Kaduson, H. G. and Schaefer, C. E. (eds) (2004) *101 Favorite Play Therapy Techniques.* Lanham, Maryland: Rowman and Littlefield.

Kane, M. T. and Kendall, P. C. (1989) 'Anxiety disorders in children: a multiple baseline evaluation of a cognitive-behavioral treatment.' *Behavior Therapy 20,* 499–508.

Kane, R. and Wellings, K. (1998) Reducing the rate of teenage conceptions. An international review of the evidence (data from Europe) – Part 1. www.nice.org.uk/niceMedia/documents/ pregnancyinternationalpt1.pdf (accessed 13/2/08).

Kavle, G., Berg, E., Nilsen, C., Raadal, M., Nielsen, G. and Johnsen, T. (1997) 'Validation of the dental fear scale and dental belief survey in a Norwegian sample.' *Community Dentistry and Oral Epidemiology 25,* 160–164.

Kazdin, A. E. (2000) *Psychotherapy for Children and Adolescents: Directions for Research and Practice.* New York: Oxford University Press.

Kellogg, N. (2005a) 'Oral and dental aspects of child abuse and neglect.' *Pediatrics 116(6),* 1565–1568.

Kellogg, N. and committee on child abuse and neglect (2005b) 'The evaluation of sexual abuse in children'. *Pediatrics 116(2)* 506–542.

Kendall, P. C. (1994) 'Treating anxiety disorders in children: results of a randomised clinical trial.' *Journal of Consulting and Clinical Psychology 62,* 100–110.

Kendall, P. C., Chansky, T. E., Kane, M. T., Kim, R. S. (1992) *Anxiety Disorders in Youth: Cognitive-behavioral Interventions.* Needham Heights, MA: Allyn and Bacon.

Kendall, P. C., Kane, M., Howard, B. and Siqueland, L. (1990) *Cognitive-behavioral Treatment of Anxious Children: Treatment Manual.* Available from Phillip C. Kendall, Department of Psychology, Temple University, Philadephia, PA 19122.

Kendall-Tackett, K. (2001) 'Chronic pain: the next frontier in child maltreatment research.' *Child Abuse and Neglect 25(8),* 997–1000.

Kendall-Tackett, K. (2002) 'The health effects of childhood abuse: four pathways by which abuse can influence health.' *Child Abuse and Neglect,26* (6–7), 715–729.

Kenney, J. and Laming, L. (2006) *Domestic Violence.* London: Forensic Science International.

Keys, M. (2007) *The Role of Nurses and Midwives in Child Protection.* A report for the Scottish Executive (unpublished).

Kilpatrick, N. M., Scott, J. and Robinson, S. (1999) 'Child protection: a survey of experience and knowledge within the dental profession of New South Wales.' *International Journal of Paediatric Dentistry 9(3),* 153–159.

King, M. C. and Ryan, J. (1996) 'Woman abuse: the role of nurse-midwives in assessment.' *Journal of Nurse-Midwifery 41(6),* 436–441.

Kirby, D. (2001) *Emerging Answers: Research Findings on Programs to Reduce Unwanted Teenage Pregnancy.* Washington, DC: National Campaign to Prevent Teen Pregnancy.

Kirby, D., Laris, B. and Rolleri, L. (2006) *Sex and HIV Education Programs for Youth: Their Impact and Important Characteristics.* Washington, DC: Family Health International.

Kirk Weir, I. and Wheatcroft, M. S. (1995) 'Allegations of children's involvement in ritual sexual abuse: clinical experience in 20 cases.' *Child Abuse and Neglect 19(4),* 491–505.

Kitzinger, J. (2000) 'Media templates: patterns of association and the (re)construction of meaning over time.' *Media, Culture and Society 22,* 61–84.

Kitzmann, K. M., Gaylord, N. K., Holt, A. R. and Kenny, E. D. (2003) 'Child witnesses to domestic violence: a meta-analytic review.' *Journal of Consulting and Clinical Psychology 71(2),* 339–352.

Klee, H. (1998) 'Drug-using parents: analysing the stereotypes.' *International Journal of Drug Policy 9,* 437–448.

Klee, H., Jackson, M. and Lewis, S. (2002) *Drug Misuse and Motherhood.* London: Routledge.

KNMG (2008) 'Reporting statute concerning child abuse [IX.01 Meldcode inzake kindermishandeling][on-line].' http://knmg.artsennet.nl/vademecum/ (accessed 15/7/08).

Knox, E. and Conti-Ramsden, G. (2007) 'Bullying in young people with a history of specific language impairment (SLI).' *Educational and Child Psychology 24(4),* 130–141.

Koeck, C. (1998) 'Time for organisational development in healthcare organisations.' *British Medical Journal 317,* 1267-1268.

Kolbo, J. R., Blakely, E. H. and Engleman, D. (1996) 'Children who witness domestic violence: a review of empirical literature.' *Journal of Interpersonal Violence 11(2),* 281–293.

Kotch, J. (1999) 'Predicting child maltreatment in the first four years of life from characteristics assessed in the neonatal period.' *Child Abuse and Neglect 23(4),* 305–319.

Kroll, B. and Taylor, A. (2003) *Parental Substance Misuse and Child Welfare.* London: Jessica Kingsley.

Kumpfer, K., Alvarado, R. and Whiteside, H. (2003) 'Family-based interventions for substance use and misuse prevention.' *Substance Use and Misuse 38(11–13),* 1759–1787.

Kumpfer, K. L. and Bluth, B. (2004) 'Parent/child transactional processes predictive of resilience or vulnerability to "Substance abuse disorders".' *Substance Use and Misuse 39(5),* 671–698.

Kuritane, I. S. (2005) 'Childhood trauma in the aetiology of borderline personality disorder.' *Psychiatrica Hungarica 20(4),* 256–270.

Kushner, S. (2000) *Personalizing Evaluation.* London: Sage.

Kuyvenhoven, M. M., Hekkink, C. F. and Voorn, T. B. (1998) 'Deaths due to abuse for the age group 0–18 years; an estimate of 40 cases in 1996 based on a survey of family practitioners and pediatricians [Overlijdensgevallen onder 0–18-jarigen door vermoede mishandeling: naar schatting 40 gevallen in 1996 gebaseerd op een enquLte onder huisartsen en kinderartsen]. 'Nederlands Tijdschrift voor Geneeskunde 142, 2515–2518.

La Fontaine, J. (1994) *The Extent and Nature of Organised and Ritual Abuse: Research Findings.* London: HMSO.

Lalanda, M. and Haslam, J. (2008) *Child complaints. MPS Casebook.* www.medicalprotection.org/uk/casebook/child-complaints (accessed 6/12/08).

Laming, Lord (2003) *The Victoria Climbié Inquiry: Report of an Inquiry by Lord Laming.* London: The Stationery Office.

Laming, Lord (2008) *Deadly Care* – Radio 4 programme. http://news.bbc.co.uk/1/hi/programmes/file_on_4/3708232.stm (accessed 22/7/08).

Laming, Lord (2009) *The Protection of Children in England: A Progress Report.* London: Department of Health.

Landenburger, K., Campbell, D. W. and Rodriguez, R. (2004) 'Nursing care of families using violence.' In J. C. Campbell and J. Humphreys (eds) *Family Violence and Nursing Practice.* Philadelphia: Lippincott Williams and Wilkins.

Langley, G. J., Nolan, K. N., Nolan, T. W. and Provost, L. P. (1996) *The Improvement Guide: A Practical Approach to Enhancing Organizational Performance.* San Francisco: Jossey-Bass Business and Management Services.

Lanning, K. V. (1992) *Investigator's Guide to Allegations of 'Ritual' Child Abuse.* New York: Quantico.

Lanning, K. V. (2002) 'Guide to allegations of childhood sexual abuse.' www.religioustolerance.org/ fbi_02.htm (accessed 5/3/08).

Law, J. (2002) 'Feral, autistic or neglected.' *Bulletin of the Royal College of Speech and Language Therapists* December 8-9.

Law, J. and Conway, J. (1992) 'Effect of abuse and neglect on the development of children's speech and language.' *Developmental Medicine and Child Neurology 34,* 943–948.

Law, J. and Garrett, Z. (2004) 'Speech and language therapy: its potential role in CAMHS.' *Child and Adolescent Mental Health 9*(2), 50–55.

Law, J. and Plunkett, C. *The Interaction Between Behaviour and Speech and Language Difficulties: Does Intervention for One Affect Outcome on the Other?* London: Institute of Education (in press).

Law, J., Lindsay, G., Peacey, N., Gascoigne, M. *et al.* (2000) *Provision for Children with Speech and Language Needs in England and Wales: Facilitating Communication Between Education and Health Services* Nottingham.

Lawn, J. E., Rohde, J., Rifkin, S., Were, M., Paul, V. K. and Chopra, M. (2008) 'Alma-Ata 30 Years on: revolutionary, relevant and time to revitalise'. *Lancet 372,* 917–927.

Lawson, W. (2001) *Understanding and Working with the Spectrum of Autism.* London: Jessica Kingsley Publishers.

Lazenbatt, A. and Freeman, R. (2006) 'Recognizing and reporting child physical abuse: a cross sectional survey of primary health care professionals.' *Journal of Advanced Nursing 56*(3), 227–237.

Lazenbatt, A., Cree, L. F. and McMurray. (2005) 'The use of exploratory factor analysis in evaluating midwives' attitudes and stereotypical myths related to the identification and management of DV in practice.' *Midwifery: An International Journal 21,* 322–334.

Lazenbatt, A., Taylor, J. and Cree, L. (2008) 'A healthy settings framework: an evaluation and comparison of midwives' responses to addressing domestic violence in pregnancy.' *Midwifery* (in press).

Lea-Cox, C. and Hall, A. (1991) 'Attendance of general practitioners at child protection case conferences.' *British Medical Journal 302*(8), 1378–1379.

Lemon, S. C., Verhoek-Oftedahl, W. and Donnelly, E. F. (2002) 'Preventive healthcare use, smoking and alcohol use among Rhode Island women experiencing intimate partner violence.' *Journal of Women's Health and Gender-Based Medicine 11*(6), 555–562.

Lentsch, K. A. and Johnson, C. F. (2000) 'Do physicians have adequate knowledge of child sexual abuse? The results of two surveys of practicing physicians, 1986 and 1996.' *Child Maltreatment 5,* 72–78.

Leonard, L. B. (1998) *Children with Specific Language Impairment.* Massachusetts: MIT Press.

Leserman, J., Li, Z., Drossman, D., Toomey, T., Nachman, G. and Glogau, L. (1997) 'Impact of sexual and physical abuse dimensions on health status: development of an abuse severity measure.' *Psychosomatic Medicine 59,* 152–160.

Leventhal, J. M. (1999) 'The challenges of recognising child abuse: seeing is believing.' *Journal of the American Medical Association 281,* 657–659.

Lewis, G. and Drife, J. (2001) *Why Mothers Die: Report from the Confidential Enquiries into Maternal Deaths in the UK 1997–9, Commissioned by Department of Health from RCOG and NICE.* London: Department of Health, RCOG Press.

Lewis, G. and Drife, J. (2005) *Why Mothers Die 2000–2002: Report on Confidential Enquiries into Maternal Deaths in the United Kingdom.* London: CEMACH.

Lewy, A. L. and Dawson, G. (1992) 'Social stimulation and joint attention in young autistic children.' *Journal of Abnormal Child Psychology 20,* 555–566.

Liiva, C. A. and Cleave, P. L. (2005) 'Roles of initiation and responsiveness in access and participation for children with specific language impairment.' *Journal of Speech, Language and Hearing Research 48*(3), 868–883.

Lindsay, G. and Dockrell, J. (2000) 'The behaviour and self-esteem of children with specific speech and language difficulties.' *British Journal of Educational Psychology 70,* 503–681.

Linning, L. M. and Kearney, C. A. (2004) 'Post-traumatic stress disorder in maltreated youth: a study of diagnostic comorbidity and child factors.' *Journal of Interpersonal Violence 19,* 1087–1101.

Lloyd, D. and Myserscough, E. J. (2006) *Neonatal Abstinence Syndrome. A New Intervention: A Community Based, Structured Health Visitor Assessment.* Edinburgh: Scottish Executive.

Lloyd, N., O'Brien, M. and Lewis, C. (2003) *Fathers in Sure Start.* London: Institute for the Study of Children, Families and Social Issues, Birkbeck, University of London.

Lo Fo Wong, S. H. and Lagro-Janssen, A. L. (2005) 'Intimate partner abuse of women: identification of victims in medical practice [Mishandeling van vrouwen binnen de partnerrelatie: signalering in de medische praktijk].' *Nederlands Tijdschrift voor Geneeskunde 149,* 6–9.

Lo Fo Wong, S. H., Wester, F., Mol, S. S. and Lagro-Janssen, T. L. (2006) 'Increased awareness of intimate partner abuse after training: a randomised controlled trial.' *British Journal of General Practice 56,* 249–257.

Locke, T. F. and Newcomb, M. D. (2003) 'Childhood maltreatment, parental alcohol/drug-related problems and global parental dysfunction.' *Professional Psychology: Research and Practice 34*(1), 73–79.

Lord Goldsmith (2006) The review of infant death cases; addendum to report Shaken Baby Syndrome. www.attorneygeneral.gov.uk/attachments/shaken_baby_syndrome_review_report.doc (accessed 12/4/08).

Lucas, D. R., Wezner, K., Milner, J. S., McCanne, T. *et al.* (2002) 'Victim, perpetrator, family and incident characteristics of infant and child homicide in the United States Air Force.' *Child Abuse and Neglect 26,* 167–186.

Luig-Arlt, H. L. (2004) Modellprojekt Schutzengel e.V.: Abschlussbericht – Evaluation. www.schutzengel-flensburg.de/dateien/Modellprojekt-Schutzengel.pdf (accessed 16/1/08).

Lundy, M. and Grossman, S. F. (2005) 'The mental health and service needs of young children exposed to domestic violence.' *Families and Sociology 86*(1), 17–29.

Lupton, N., North, I. and Khan, N. (2001) *Working Together or Pulling Apart? The National Health Service and Child Protection Networks.* Bristol: The Policy Press.

Luthar, S. S. and Suchman, N. E. (2000) 'Relational psychotherapy mother's group: a developmentally informed intervention for at-risk mothers.' *Development and Psychopathology 12*(2), 235–253.

Lynch, M. and Roberts, J. (1982) *Consequences of Child Abuse.* London: Academic Press.

Lyons-Ruth, K., Connell, D. B., Grunebaum, H. U. and Botein, S. (1990) 'Infants at social risk: maternal depression and family support services as mediators of infant development and security of attachment.' *Child Development 61*(1), 85–98.

Maat-Van Manen, J., Mol, S., Kuyvenhoven, M. and Schellevis, F. (2005) 'Child abuse, a changeling? [Kindermishandeling, een ondergeschoven kind?].' *Huisarts Wet 48,* 265.

Macdonald, K., Lambie, I. and Simmonds, L. (1995) *Counselling for Sexual Abuse: A Therapist's Guide to Working with Adults, Children and Families.* Auckland, NZ: Oxford University Press.

Maguire, S., Sibert, J., Kemp, A., Hunter, B., Hunter, L. and Mann, M. (2007) 'Diagnosing abuse: a systematic review of torn frenum and other oral injuries.' *Archives of Disease of Childhood 92,* 1113–1117.

Main, M. (1995) 'Desorganisation im Bindungsverhalter (Disorganisation in attachment behaviour).' In G. Spangler and P. Zimmermann (eds) *Die Bindungstheorie.* Stuttgart: Klett-Cotta.

Mankell, H. (2004) *Die, But the Memory Lives on. The World Aids Crises and the Memory Book Project.* London: The Harvill Press.

Mann, P., Pritchard, S. and Rummery, K. (2004) 'Supporting interorganizational partnerships in the public sector.' *Public Management Review 6*(3), 417–439.

Marcellus, L. (2005) 'The ethics of relation: public health nurses and child protection clients.' *Journal of Advanced Nursing 51*(4), 414–420.

Marmot, M. (2008) *Closing the Gap in a Generation: Health Equity Through Action on the Social Determinants of Health. Final Report of the Commission on Social Determinants of Health.* Geneva: World Health Organization.

Marsh, J. and Cao, D. (2005) 'Parents in substance abuse treatment: implications for child welfare practice.' *Children and Youth Services Review 27,* 1259–1278.

Masten, A. S. (2001) 'Ordinary magic: resilience processes in development.' *American Psychologist 56,* 227–238.

Masten, A. S. (2004) 'Regulatory process, risk and resilience in adolescent development.' *Annals of the New York Academy of Sciences 1021,* 310–319.

Masten, A. S. and Gewirtz, A. H. (2006) 'Vulnerability and resilience in early child development.' In K. McCartney and D. D. Phillips (eds) *Handbook of Early Childhood Development.* Malden: Blackwell.

Masten, C., Guyer, A., Hodgdon, H., McClure, E., *et al.* (2008) 'Recognition of facial emotions among maltreated children with high rates of post-traumatic stress disorder.' *Child Abuse Neglect 32,* 139–153.

McCartan, B. and McCreary, C. (2006) 'History taking and examination.' In P. A. Mossey, G. J. Holsgrove, D. R. Stirrups and E. S. Davenport (eds) *Essential Skills for Dentists.* Oxford: Oxford University Press.

McCloskey, L. A. and Walker, M. (1999) 'Posttraumatic stress in children exposed to family violence and single incident trauma.' *Journal of the American Academy of Child and Adolescent Psychiatry 39*(1), 108–115.

McFarlane, A. C. and Yehuda, R. (2000) 'Clinical treatment of posttraumatic stress disorder: conceptual challenges raised by recent research.' *Australian and New Zealand Journal of Psychiatry 34,* 940–953.

McFarlane, J., Campbell, J. C., Sharps, P. and Watson, K. (2002) 'Abuse during pregnancy and femicide.' *Obstetrics and Gynecology 100,* 27–36.

McFarlane, J., Parker, B. and Soeken, K. (1996a) 'Abuse during pregnancy: Associations with maternal health and infant birth.' *Nursing Research 45,* 37–42.

McFarlane, J., Parker, B. and Soeken, K. (1996b) 'Physical abuse, smoking and substance use during pregnancy: prevalence, interrelationships and effects on birth weight.' *Journal of Obstetric, Gynecologic and Neonatal Nursing 25*(4), 313–320.

McFarlane, J., Parker, B., Soeken, K. A. and Bulloack, L. (1992) 'Assessing for abuse during pregnancy: frequency and extent of injuries and entry into prenatal care.' *Journal of American Medical Association 267*(23), 3176–3178.

McGee, C. (2000) 'Childhood experiences of domestic violence.' *Adoption and Fostering 20*, 8–15.

McGee, H. (2003) *The SAVI Report: Sexual Abuse and Violence in Ireland.* Dublin Rape Crisis Centre, Liffey Press.

McGuigan, W. M. and Pratt, C. C. (2001) 'The predictive impact of domestic violence on three types of child maltreatment.' *Child Abuse Neglect 25*(7), 869–883.

Mckeown, K., Haase, T. and Pratschke, J. (2001) *Springboard: Promoting Family Well-being Through Family Support Services.* www.dohc.ie/publications/pdf/springb.pdf?direct=1 (accessed 16/1/08).

McLeer, S., Dixon, J. and Henry, D. 'Psychopathology in non-clinically referred sexually abused children.' *Journal of the American Academy of Child and Adolescent Psychiatry 37*, 1326–1333.

McLeod, A. (2001) 'Changing patterns of teenage pregnancy: population-based study of small areas.' *British Medical Journal 323*, 199–203.

McMahon, T. J., Winkel, J. D. and Rounsaville, B. J. (2008) 'Drug abuse and responsible fathering: a comparative study of men enrolled in methadone maintenance treatment.' *Addiction 103*(2), 269–283.

McMahon, T. J., Winkel, J. D., Suchman, N. E. and Rounsaville, B. J. (2007) 'Drug-abusing fathers: patterns of pair bonding, reproduction and paternal involvement.' *Journal of Substance Abuse Treatment 33*(3), 295–302.

McMillan, C., Zuravin, S. and Rideout, G. (1995) 'Perceived benefits from childhood sexual abuse.' *Journal of Consulting and Clinical Psychology 63*, 1037–1043.

McVeigh, C., Hughes, K., Bellis, M. A., Reed, E., Ashton, J. R. and Syed, Q. (Cartographer). (2005) *Violent Britain: People, Prevention and Public Health.* Liverpool: Centre for Public Health, John Moores University.

McWilliams, M. and McKiernan, J. (1993) *Bringing it Out Into the Open.* Belfast: HMSO.

Meier, P. S., Donmall, M. C. and McElduff, P. (2004) 'Characteristics of drug users who do or do not have care of their children.' *Addiction 99*(8), 955–961.

Mellanby, A., Phelps, F., Crichton, N. J. and Tripp, J. (1995) 'School sex education: an experimental programme with educational and medical benefit.' *British Medical Journal 311*, 414–417.

Messer, D. (1994) *The Development of Communication: From Social Interaction to Language.* Chichester: Wiley.

Mezey, G. C. and Bewley, S. (1997) 'Domestic violence and pregnancy.' *British Medical Journal 314*, 1295.

Mezey, G. C., Bacchus, L., Bewley, S. and White, S. (2005) 'Domestic violence, lifetime trauma and psychological health of childbearing women.' *British Journal of Obstetrics and Gynaecology: An International Journal of Obstetrics and Gynaecology 112*(2), 197–204.

Mezey, G. C., Bacchus, L., Haworth, A. and Bewley, S. (2003) 'Midwives' perceptions and experiences of routine enquiry for domestic violence.' *British Journal of Obstetrics and Gynaecology 110*(8), 744–752.

Mezzich, A. C., Bretz, W. A., Corby, P. M., Kirisci, L., *et al.* (2007) 'Child neglect and oral health problems in offspring of substance-abusing fathers' *American Journal of Addictions 16*, 397–402.

Millichamp, J., Martin, J. and Langley, J. (2006) *On the Receiving End: Young Adults Describe their Parents' use of Physical Punishment and other Disciplinary Measures During Childhood.* www.nzma.org.nz//journal/119-1228/1818/ (accessed 8/3/07).

Milne, A. C. and Chesson, R. (2000) 'Health services can be cool: partnership with adolescents in primary care.' *Family Practitioner 17*(4), 305–308.

Milne, D. (2005) *Healthy Respect Phase Two: A Proposal to the Scottish Executive Health Improvement Strategy Division for Phase Two of the National Health Demonstration Project on Young People's Sexual Health.* Edinburgh: NHS Lothian.

Mirrlees-Black, C. (1999) *Domestic Violence: Findings from the British Crime Survey Self Completion Questionnaire.* London: Home Office.

Moran, T. E. and O'Hara, M. W. (2006) 'Maternal psychosocial predictors of pediatric health care use: use of the common sense model of health and illness behaviours to extend beyond the ususal suspects.' *Clinics in Effective Nursing 9*, e171–e180.

Muldoon, L. K., Hogg, W. E. and Levitt, M. (2008) 'Primary Care (PC) and Primary Health Care (PHC).' *Canadian Journal of Public Health 97*(5), 409–411.

Mullender, A. (2004) *Tackling Domestic Violence: Providing Support for Children who Have Witnessed Domestic Violence.* London: Home Office, Crown.

Mullender, A. (2005) 'What children tell us: "He said he was going to kill our mum".' In C. Humphreys and N. Stanley (eds) *Domestic Violence and Child Protection.* London: Jessica Kingsley Publishers.

Mullender, A., Burton, S., Hague, G., Imam, U. *et al.* (2003a) *'Stop Hitting Mum!' Children Talk about Domestic Violence.* East Molesey, Surrey: Young Voice.

Mullender, A., Hague, G., Imam, U., Kelly, L., Malos, E. and Regan, L. (2003b) *Children's Perspectives on Domestic Violence.* London.

Mullender, A., Hague, G., Imam, U., Kelly, L., Malos, E. and Regan, L. (2003b) *'Could Have Helped but they Didn't': The Formal and Informal Support Systems Experienced by Children Living with Domestic Violence.* London: Routledge, Falmer.

Murphy, C. C., Schei, B., Myhr, T. L. and Du Mont, J. (2001) 'Abuse: a risk factor for low birth weight? A systematic review and meta-analysis.' *Canadian Medical Association Journal 164*, 1567–1515.

Murphy, J. and Welbury, R. (1998) 'The dental practitioner's role in protecting children from abuse. The child protection system.' *British Dental Journal 184*, 7–10.

Murphy, M. (2004) *Developing Collaborative Relationships in Interagency Child Protection Work.* Lyme Regis: Russell House Publishing.

Murupaenga, P., Feather, J. S. and Berking, T. (2004) *CBT with children of indigenous and migrant families: Interweaving of cultural context and psychological/therapeutic models with Maori and Pacific Island children and families traumatised by abuse.* Paper presented at the 15th International Congress on Child Abuse and Neglect (ISPCAN), Brisbane, Australia.

Naar-King, S., Silvern, L., Ryan, V. and Sebring, D. (2002) 'Type and severity of abuse as predictors of psychiatric symptoms in adolescence.' *Journal of Family Violence 17*(2), 133–149.

Nadel, J., Croué, S., Mattlinger, M.-J., Canet, P. *et al.* (2000) 'Do children with autism have expectancies about the social behaviour of unfamiliar people?' *Autism 4*, 133–145.

Naidoo, S. (2000) 'A profile of the oro-facial injuries in child physical abuse at a children's hospital.' *Child Abuse Neglect 24*, 521–534.

Nasir, K. and Hyder, A. A. (2003) 'Violence against pregnant women in developing countries.' *The European Journal of Public Health 13*(2), 105–107.

Nayda, R. (2004) 'Registered nurses' communication about abused children: rules, responsibilities and resistance.' *Child Abuse Review 13*(3), 188–199.

Nelson, J. R., Benner, G. J. and Cheney, D. (2005). 'An investigation of the language skills of students with emotional disturbance served in public school settings.' *Journal of Special Education 39*(2), 97–105.

Nelson, S. (2001) *Beyond Trauma: Mental Health Care Needs of Women who Survived Childhood Sexual Abuse* Edinburgh: Health in Mind.

Nelson, S. (2002) 'Physical symptoms in sexually abused women: somatisation or undetected injury?' *Child Abuse Review 11*(1), 51–64.

Nelson, S. and Baldwin, N. (2004) 'The Craigmillar Project: neighbourhood mapping to improve children's safety from sexual abuse.' *Child Abuse Review 13*, 415–525.

Nelson, S. and Hampson, S. (2008) *Yes You Can! Working with Survivors of Childhood Sexual Abuse*, 2nd edn. Edinburgh: The Scottish Government.

Nemeroff, C. B. (2004) 'Neurobiological consequences of childhood trauma.' *Journal of Clinical Psychiatry 65*, 18–28.

News24.com (2005) 'Black magic fear grips Britain.' www.news24.com/News24/World/News/ 0,,2-10-1462_1716531,00.html (accessed 20/7/08).

Newton, M. (2002) *Savage Girls and Wild Boys: A History of Feral Children* London: Faber and Faber.

Ngulube, T. J., Muula, C., Mwanza, A. S. and Njobvu, K. (2006) 'Knowledge, attitudes and public health response towards plague in Petauke, Zambia.' *Tropical Doctor 36*(4), 223–225.

NHS Modernization Agency (2005) *The Clinician's Guide to Applying the 10 High Impact Changes.* www.modern.nhs.uk/highimpactchanges (accessed 6/12/08).

NHS Tayside Board (2007) *Collaborative Commissioning.* Dundee: NHS Tayside Board.

NICE (2006) *Depression in Children and Young People.* www.nice.org.uk/pdf/CG028 (accessed 6/12/08).

NICE (2007a) *Community-based Interventions to Reduce Substance Misuse Among Vulnerable and Disadvantaged Children and Young People.* London: National Institute for Health and Clinical Excellence.

NICE (2007b) *Drug Misuse: Opioid Detoxification.* London: National Institute for Clinical Excellence.

NICE (2007c) *Drug Misuse: Psychosocial Interventions.* London: National Institute for Clinical Excellence.

NICE (2007d) *Methadone and Buprenorphine for the Management of Opioid Dependence.* London: National Institute for Clinical Excellence.

NICE (2008) *Antenatal Care: Routine Care for the Healthy Pregnant Woman.* London: National Institute for Clinical Excellence.

Nicolau, B., Marcenes, W. and Sheiham, A. (2003) 'The relationship between traumatic dental injuries and adolescents' development along the life course.' *Community Dentistry and Oral Epidemiology 31*, 306–313.

Nind, M. (1999) 'Intensive interaction and autism: a useful approach?' *British Journal of Special Educational and Child Psychology 26*, 96–102.

Nind, M. (2000) 'Intensive interaction and children with autism.' In S. Powell (ed.) *Helping Children with Autism to Learn.* London: David Fulton.

Nind, M. and Hewitt, D. (2001) *A Practical Guide to Intensive Interaction* Plymouth: BILD.

Nind, M. and Kellet, M. (2002) 'Responding to individuals with severe learning difficulties and stereotyped behaviour: challenges for an inclusive era.' *European Journal of Special Needs Educations 3*, 265–282.

Norton, L. B., Peipert, J. F., Zierler, L. B. and Hume, L. (1995) 'Battering in pregnancy: an assessment of two screening methods.' *Obstetrics and Gynecology 85*, 321–325.

NSPCC (2007) NSPCC publications, posters, leaflets and training packs can be ordered via their website at www.nspcc.org.uk/inform/publications/publications_-wda48207.html (accessed 6/12/08).

NTA (2004) *Engaging and Retaining Clients in Drug Treatment* London: National Treatment Agency for Substance Misuse.

Nursing and Midwifery Council (2004) *Rules and Standard.* London: Nursing and Midwifery Council.

NVMW (1999) *Professional Profile of the Social Worker [Beroepsprofiel van de maatschappelijkwerker].* Utrecht: Nederlandse Vereniging van Maatschappelikj Werkers.

O'Neill, M. B. (2007) *Imitation as an intervention for children with Autistic Spectrum Disorder and their parents/carers* Unpublished doctoral thesis. University of Dundee, Dundee.

Oates, R. K. (2004) 'Sexual abuse and suicidal behaviour.' *Child Abuse and Neglect 28*(5), 487–489.

Office of Chief Researcher (2006) *What do we Measure and Why? An Evaluation of the CitiStat model of Performance Management and its Applicability to the Scottish Public Sector.* Edinburgh: Scottish Executive Social Research.

Ohno, T. (1988) *The Toyota Production System: Beyond Large-Scale Production* Portland, OR: Productivity Press.

Olivan, G. (2003) 'Untreated dental caries is common among 6 to 12-year-old physically abused/neglected children.' *European Journal of Public Health 13*, 91–92.

Or, E. K. Y. (2005) 'Child abuse exorcism unveiled among evangelical African churches in UK.' www.christiantoday.com/article/child.abuse.exorcism.unveiled.among.evangelical.african.churches.in.uk/3078. htm (accessed 20/7/08).

Ornoy, A., Michailevskaya, V. and Lukashov, L. (1996) 'The developmental outcome of children born to heroin-dependent mothers, raised at home or adopted.' *Child Abuse and Neglect 20*(5), 385–396.

Orr, S. T., James, S. A. and Blackmore Prince, C. (2002) 'Maternal prenatal depressive symptoms and spontaneous preterm births among African-American women in Baltimore, Maryland.' *American Journal of Epidemiology 156*, 797–802.

Osofsky, J. D. (1995) 'The effects of violence exposure on young children.' *American Psychologist 50*, 782–788.

Osofsky, J. D. (2003) 'Prevalence of children's exposure to domestic violence and child maltreatment: implications for practice and intervention.' *Clinical Child and Family Psychology Review 6*(3), 161–170.

Paluzzi, P. A. and Houde-Quimbly, C. H. (1996) 'Domestic violence implications for the American College of Nurse-Midwives and Its Members.' *Journal of Nurse-Midwifery 41*(6), 430–435.

Pandit, S. and Shah, L. (2000) 'Post-traumatic stress disorder: causes and aetiological factors.' In K. N. Dwivedi (ed.) *Post-traumatic Stress Disorder in Children and Adolescents.* London: Whurr Publishers.

Papousek, M., Schieche, M. and Wurmser, H. (2004) *Regulationsstörungen der frühen Kindheit* (Regulatory disorders in early childhood). Bern, Toronto, Seattle: Hans Huber.

Parson, E. R. (1997) 'Posttraumatic child therapy (P-TCT): assessment and treatment factors in clinical work with inner-city children exposed to catastrophic community violence.' *Journal of Interpersonal Violence 12*, 172–194.

Parsons, L. H., Zaccaro, D., Wells, B. and Stovall, T. G. (1995) 'Methods of and attitudes towards screening obstetrics and gynecology clients for domestic violence.' *American Journal of Obstetrics and Gynecology 173*(2), 381–388.

Parton, N. (ed.) (1997) *Child Protection and Family Support: Tensions, Contradictions and Possibilities.* London: Routledge.

Passantino, B., Passantino, G. and Trott, J. (1989) 'Satan's sideshow.' *Cornerstone 18*(90), 23–28.

Patouillard, E., Goodman, C. A., Hanson, K. G. and Mills, A. J. (2007) 'Can working with the private for-profit sector improve utilization of quality health services by the poor? A systematic review of the literature.' *International Journal for Equity in Health 6*, 17–26.

Patrick, M., Hobson, R., Castle, D., Howard, R. and Maughan, B. (1994) 'Personality disorder and the mental representation of early social experience.' *Developmental Psychopathology 6*, 375–388.

Pauly, B. (2008) 'Harm reduction through a social justice lens.' *International Journal of Drug Policy 19*, 4–10.

Pazder, L. and Smith, M. (1980) *Michelle Remembers.* New York: Pocket Books.

Pearce, J. W. and Pezzot-Pearce, T. D. (1994) 'Attachment theory and its implications for psychotherapy with maltreated children.' *Child Abuse and Neglect 18*, 425–438.

Peckover, S. (2003) 'Health visitors' understanding of domestic violence.' *Journal of Advanced Nursing 44*(2), 200–208.

Pecora, P. J., Wittaker, J. K. and Maluccio, T. (2006) 'Child welfare in the US.' In C. McCauley, P. J. Pecora and W. Rose (eds) *Enhancing the Wellbeing of Children and Families Through Effective Interventions.* London: Jessica Kingsley Publishers.

Perez, T. and Rushing, R. (2007) *How Data-Driven Government Can Increase Efficiency and Effectiveness.* www.americanprogress.org (accessed 6/12/08).

Perkins, D. F. and Jones, D. F. (2004) 'Risk behaviours and resiliency within physically abused adolescents.' *Child Abuse and Neglect 28*, 547–568.

Perkins, S. F. L. and Allen, R. (2006) 'Childhood physical abuse and differential development of paranormal belief systems.' *Journal of Nervous and Mental Disease 194*(5), 349–355.

Perry, B. D., Pollard, R. A., Blakely, T. L., Baker, W. L. and Vigilante, D. (1995) 'Childhood trauma, the neurobiology of adaptation and "use dependent" development of the brain: How "states" become "traits".' *Infant Mental Health Journal 16*(4), 271–290.

Petersilia, J. (2000) 'Invisible victims: violence against persons with developmental disabilities.' *Human Rights 27*(1), 9–13.

Pfefferbaum, B., Nixon, S., Tucker, P., Tivis, R., *et al.* (1999) 'Posttraumatic stress response in bereaved children after Oklahoma City bombing.' *Journal of the American Academy of Child and Adolescent Psychiatry 38*, 1372–1379.

Pfefferbaum, B., Searle, T., McDonald, N., Brandt, E., *et al.* (2000). 'Posttraumatic stress two years after the Oklahoma City bombing in youths geographically distant from the explosion.' *Psychiatry 63*, 358–370.

Pilkington, B. and Kremer, J. (1995) 'A review of the epidemiological research on child sexual abuse: community and college student samples.' *Child Abuse Review 4*(2), 84–98.

Plsek, P. and Wilson, T. (2001) 'Complexity, leadership and management in healthcare organisations.' *British Medical Journal 322*, 746–749.

Poland, B., Green, L. and Rootman, I. (2000) *Settings for Health Promotion: Linking Theory and Practice.* London. Sage, Thousand Oaks.

Polney, J. (2001) 'Why child protection management is different from other medical problems.' In J. Polney (ed.) *Child Protection in Primary Care.* Abingdon: Radcliffe Medical Press.

Pound, A. and Mills, M. (1985) 'A pilot evaluation of NEWPIN, a home visiting and befriending scheme in South London.' *Association of Child Psychology and Psychiatry Newsletter 7*, 13–15.

Powell, C. (2007) *Safeguarding Children and Young People: A Guide for Nurses and Midwives.* Maidenhead: Open University Press.

Powis, B., Gossop, M., Bury, C., Payne, K. and Griffiths, P. (2000) 'Drug-using mothers: social, psychological and substance use problems of women opiate users with children.' *Drug and Alcohol Review 19*, 171–180.

Price, S., Baird, K. and Salmon, D. (2005) 'Asking the question: antenatal domestic violence.' *The Practising Midwife 8*(3), 21–25.

Protheroe, L., Green, J. and Spiby, H. (2001). 'An interview study of the impact of domestic violence training on midwives.' *Midwifery 20*(1), 94–103.

Provan, K. G. and Milward, H. B. (1995) 'A preliminary theory of interorganisational network effectiveness: a comparative study of four community mental health systems.' *Administrative Science Quarterly 40*(1), 1–33.

Public Health Institute of Scotland (2001) *Needs Assessment Report: Autistic Spectrum Disorders.* Glasgow: Public Health Institute of Scotland, NHS.

Public Health Institute of Scotland (2003) *Needs Assessment Report on Child and Adolescent Mental Health Final Report – May 2003.* Glasgow: Public Health Institute of Scotland.

Putnam, F. W. (2003) 'Ten-year research update review: child sexual abuse.' *Journal of the American Academy of Child and Adolescent Psychiatry 42*(3), 269–278.

Pynoos, R. S. (1994) 'Traumatic stress and developmental psychopathology in children and adolescents.' In R. S. Pynoos (ed.) *Posttraumatic Stress Disorder: A Clinical Review.* Lutherville, MD: The Sidran Press.

Pynoos, R. S., Fredrick, C., Nader, K., Arroyo, W., Steinberg, A. and Eth, S. (1987) 'Life threat and posttraumatic stress in school-age children.' *Archives of General Psychiatry 44*, 1057–1063.

Radford, L., Blacklock, N. and Iwi, K. (2006) 'Domestic violence risk assessment and safety planning in child protection – assessing perpetrators.' In C. Humphreys and N. Stanley (eds) *Domestic Violence and Child Protection: Directions for Good Practice.* London: Jessica Kingsley Publishers.

Ramos-Gomez, F., Rothman, D. and Blain, S. (1998) 'Knowledge and attitudes among Californian dental care providers regarding child abuse and neglect.' *JADA 129*, 340–348.

Ramsay, J., Richardson, J., Carter, Y. H., Davidson, L. and Feder, G. (2002) 'Should health professionals screen women for domestic violence? Systematic review.' *British Medical Journal 325*, 1–13.

Ramsay, J., Rivas, C. and Feder, G. (2005) *Interventions to reduce violence and promote the physical and psychosocial well being of women who experience partner violence: a systematic review of controlled evaluations* London: Department of Health.

RCGP (2005) *Keep me Safe. Strategy for Child Protection.* London: Royal College of General Practitioners.

RCGP (2007) *An Introduction to Child Protection.* London: Royal College of General Practitioners. www.rcgp.org.uk/default.aspx?page=2587 (accessed 6/12/08).

RCGP (2008) *Safeguarding Children – A Toolkit.* (With NSPCC.) London: Royal College of General Practitioners.

RCM (1997) *Domestic Abuse in Pregnancy (Position Paper No 19).* London: Royal College of Midwives.

RCN (2000) *Domestic Abuse: Guidance for Nurses.* London: Royal College of Nursing.

RCN (2005) *Child Protection – Everyone's Responsibility. Guidance for Nursing Staff.* London: Royal College of Nursing.

RCPCH (2004a) *Child Protection Complaints Survey.* London: RCPCH. www.rcpch.ac.uk/Health (accessed 6/12/08).

RCPCH (2004b) *Responsibilities of Doctors in Child Protection with Regard to Confidentiality.* www.rcpch.ac.uk/Health-Services/Child-Protection/Child-Protection-Publications (accessed 6/12/08).

RCPCH (2005a) *Model Job Description for Named and Designated Doctor for Child Protection.* www.rcpch.ac.uk/Health-Services/Child-Protection/Named-and-Designated-Doctors (accessed 6/12/08).

RCPCH (2005b) *Safeguarding Children and Young People: Roles and Competencies for Health Care Staff.* Intercollegic Document London: Royal College of Paediatrics and Child Health.

RCPCH (2006) *Child Protection Companion.* London: Royal College of Paediatrics and Child Health.

RCPCH (2008a) *The Physical Signs of Child Sexual Abuse. An Evidence-based Review and Guidance for Best Practice* London: Royal College of Paediatrics and Child Health.

RCPCH (2008b) *Standards for Radiological Investigation of Suspected Non Accidental Injury. Intercollegic report of Royal College of Radiologists and Royal College of Paediatrics and Child Health.* London: Royal College of Paediatrics and Child Health.

RCPCH, NSPCC and ALSG (2007) *Recognition and Response in Child Protection. Developed by the RCPCH and the Advanced Life Support Programme (ALSG).* Paper presented at the http://ww.rcpch.ac.uk/Education/Education-Courses-and-Programmes/Safeguarding-Children/Safeguarding-Children-One-Day-Course (accessed 6/12/08).

RCPCH and The Association of Forensic Physicians (2007) *Guidance on Paediatric Forensic Examination in Relation to Possible Child Sexual Abuse.* www.rcpch.ac.uk/Health-Services/ Child-Protection-Publications (accessed 6/12/08).

Redmond, S. M. and Rice, M. L. (1998) 'The socioemotional behaviors of children with SLI: social adaptation or social deviance?' *Journal of Speech Language and Hearing Research 41*, 688–700.

Reijnders, U. J., van Baasbank, M. C. and van der Wal, G. (2005) 'Diagnosis and interpretation of injuries: a study of Dutch general practitioners.' *Journal of Clinical Forensic Medicine 12*, 291–295.

Reuter, P. and Stevens, A. (2007) *An Analysis of UK Drug Policy: A Monograph Prepared for the UK Drug Policy Commission* London: UK Drug Policy Commission.

Rew, L., Taylor-Seehafer, M. and Fitzgerald, M. L. (2001) 'Sexual abuse, alcohol and other drug use and suicidal behaviours in homeless adolescents.' *Issues in Comprehensive Pediatric Nursing 24*(4), 225–240.

Rhodes, T. (2002) 'The "risk environment": a framework for understanding and reducing drug-related harm.' *International Journal of Drug Policy 13*, 85–94.

Richardson, J., Coid, J., Petruckevitch, A., Chung, W. S., Moorey, S. and Feder, G. (2002) 'Identifying domestic violence: cross sectional study in primary care.' *British Medical Journal 324*, 1–6.

Richter, K. P. and Bammer, G. (2000) 'A hierarchy of strategies heroin-using mothers employ to reduce harm to their children.' *Journal of Substance Abuse Treatment 19*(4), 403–413.

Rimza, M. E., Schackner, R. A., Bowen, K. A. and Marshall, W. (2002) *Can child deaths be prevented? The Arizona Child Fatality Review Programme Experience.* www.pediatrics.org/cgi/content/full/110/1/ell (accessed 12/6/08).

Ripley, K. and Yuill, N. (2005) 'Patterns of language impairment in boys excluded from school'. *British Journal of Educational Psychology 75*, 37–50.

Robertson, R. (ed.) (1998) *Management of Drug Users in the Community: A Practical Handbook.* London: Arnold.

Rogosch, F. A., Cicchetti, D. and Aber, J. L. (1995) 'The role of child maltreatment in early deviations in cognitive and affective processing abilities and later peer relationship problems.' *Development and Psychopathology 7*, 591–609.

Ronan, K. R. and Johnson, D. M. (2005) *Promoting Community Resilience in Disasters: The Role for Schools, Youth and Families.* New York: Springer.

Rosenbaum, M. and Irwin, K. (2000) 'Pregnancy, drugs and harm reduction.' In J. A. Inciardi and L. D. Harrison (eds) *Harm Reduction. National and International Perspectives.* Thousand Oaks: Sage.

Royal College of General Practitioners and Brook (2000) *Confidentiality and Young People. Improving Teenagers' Uptake of Sexual and Other Health Advice.* London: Royal College of General Practitioners and Brook.

Royal College of Paediatrics and Child Health (2003) *Bridging the gaps: healthcare for adolescent.* www.rcpsych.ac.uk/files/pdfversion/cr114.pdf (accessed 31/1/08).

Royal College of Paediatrics and Child Health (2004) *Responsibilities of Doctors in Child Protection Cases with Regard to Confidentiality.* London: RCPCH.

Royal College of Paediatrics and Child Health (2008) *Guidance on Child Death Review Processes.* London: RCPCH.

Runyon, M. K. and Kenny, M. C. (2002) 'Relationship of attributional style, depression and posttrauma distress among children who suffered physical or sexual abuse.' *Child Maltreatment 7*(3), 254–264.

Rymer, R. (1993) *Genie: Escape from a Silent Childhood.* London: Michael Joseph.

Saigh, P. A. (1987) 'In vitro flooding of an adolescent's posttraumatic stress disorder.' *Journal of Child Clinical Psychology 16*, 147–150.

Salt, J., Sellars, V., Shemilt, J., Boyd, S., Coulson, T. and McCool, S. (2001) 'The Scottish Centre for Autism preschool treatment programme. I: a developmental approach to early intervention.' *Autism 5*, 362–373.

Saltman, R. B., Rico, A. and Boerma, W. (eds) (2005) *Primary Care in the Driver's Seat.* Maidenhead: McGrawHill.

Sandman, C. A., Wadhwa, P. D., Chicz-DeMet, A., Dunkel-Schetter, C. and Porto, M. (2007) 'Maternal stress, HPA activity and fetal/infant outcome.' *Annals of New York Academy Science 814*, 266–275.

Saunders, B. E. (2003) 'Understanding children exposed to violence: toward an integration in overlapping fields.' *Journal of Interpersonal Violence 18*(4), 356–376.

Saunders, B. E., Berliner, L. and Hanson, R. F. (2004) *Child Physical and Sexual Abuse: Guidelines for Treatment.* http://tfcbt.musc.edu (accessed 21/6/06).

Scaife, V. H. (2008) 'Maternal and paternal drug misuse and outcomes for children: identifying risk and protective factors.' *Children and Society 22*(1), 53–62.

Schon, D. (1987) *Educating the Reflective Practitioner: Towards a New Design for Teaching and Learning in the Professions.* San Francisco: Jossey-Bass.

Schweitzer, R. D., Buckley, L., Harnett, P. and Loxton, N. J. (2006) 'Predictors of failure by medical practitioners to report suspected child abuse in Queensland, Australia.' *Australian Health Review 30*, 298–304.

Scobie, R. and McGuire, M. (1999). 'The silent enemy: domestic violence in pregnancy.' *British Journal of Midwifery 7*, 259–262.

Scottish Executive (2002) *'It's Everyone's Job to Make Sure I'm Alright': Report of the Child Protection Audit and Review.* Edinburgh: The Stationery Office Bookshop.

Scottish Executive (2003a) *Responding to Domestic Abuse: Guidelines for Health Care Workers in NHS Scotland.* Edinburgh: Scottish Executive.

Scottish Executive (2003b) *Getting Our Priorities Right, Policy and Practice Guidelines for Working with Children and Families Affected by Problem Drug Use.* Edinburgh: Scottish Executive.

Scottish Executive (2003c) *Making it Work for Scotland's Children: Child Health support Group Overview Report:* Scottish Executive.

Scottish Executive (2003d) *Growing Support, A Review of Services for Vulnerable Families with Young Children.* Edinburgh: Scottish Executive.

Scottish Executive (2003e) *Getting Our Priorities Right: Good Practice Guidance for Working with Children and Families Affected by Substance Misuse.* Edinburgh: Scottish Executive.

Scottish Executive (2003f) *Health For All Children: Guidance on Implementation in Scotland.* Edinburgh: Scottish Executive.

Scottish Executive (2003g) *Towards a Healthier Scotland.* Edinburgh: Scottish Executive.

Scottish Executive (2004a) *Children's Charter, Framework for Standards and Guidance for Child Protection Committees.* www.scotland.gov.uk/Publications/2004 (accessed 6/12/08).

Scottish Executive (2004b) *Integrated Children's Services Planning 2005–2008: Guidance.* Edinburgh: Scottish Executive.

Scottish Executive (2004c) *Sharing Information about Children at Risk of Abuse or Neglect. A Guide to Good Practice.* Edinburgh: Scottish Executive.

Scottish Executive (2005a) *Getting it Right for Every Child: Proposals for Action.* Edinburgh: Scottish Executive.

Scottish Executive (2005b) *Health for all Children 4: Guidance on Implementation in Scotland.* Edinburgh: Scottish Executive.

Scottish Executive (2006a) *Respect and Responsibility: Sexual Health Strategy Annual Report.* Edinburgh: Scottish Executive.

Scottish Executive (2006b) *Hidden Harm Next Steps, Supporting Children Working with Parents.* Edinburgh: Scottish Executive.

Scottish Executive (2006c) *Career Framework for Health.* Edinburgh: Scottish Executive.

Scottish Executive (2006d) *Quality Improvement Framework for Children and Young People and Their Families.* Edinburgh: Scottish Executive.

Scottish Executive (2007a) *Delivering Health: An Action Framework for Children and Young People's Health in Scotland.* Edinburgh: Scottish Executive.

Scottish Executive (2007b) *Strengthening the Role of Managed Clinical Networks NHS. HDL.* Edinburgh: Scottish Executive Health Department.

Scottish Government (2007a) *2008/2009 HEAT Targets.* Edinburgh: Scottish Government.

Scottish Government (2007b) *Better Health Better Care: An Action Plan.* Edinburgh: Scottish Executive.

Scottish Nationalist Party (2007) *Manifesto: It's Time to Move Forward.* www.snp.org (accessed 17/12/08).

Scottish Office (1998) *Acute Services Review Report.* Edinburgh: Scottish Executive.

Scourfield, J. (2006) 'The challenge of engaging fathers in the child protection process.' *Critical Social Policy 26*(2), 440–449.

Scourfield, J. and Coffey, A. (2002) 'Understanding gendered practice in child protection.' *Qualitative Social Work 1*(3), 319–340.

SCRA (2007) *Scottish Children's Reporter Service Annual Report 2006–2007.* Edinburgh: Scottish Children's Reporter Service.

Sege, R. and Flaherty, E. (2008) 'Inconsistencies in reporting child abuse.' *Archives of Disease in Childhood 93,* 822–824.

Selkirk, S. (2007) *NHS Tayside Board paper on Collaborative Commissioning.* Dundee NHS Tayside Board.

Seung, H. K., Ashwell, S., Elder, J. H. and Valcante, G. (2006) 'Verbal communication outcomes in children with autism after in-home father training.' *Journal of Intellectual Disability Research 50,* 139–150.

Shadigian, E. M. and Bauer, S. T. (2004) 'Screening for partner violence during pregnancy.' *International Journal of Gynecology and Obstetrics 84*(3), 273–280.

Shardlow, S., Davis, C., Johnson, M., Long, M., *et al.* (2004) *Education and Training for Inter Agency Working: New Standards.* Salford Centre for Social Research, Salford Centre for Nursing Midwifery and Collaborative Research.

Shaw, A., Egan, J. and Gillespie, M. (2007) *Drugs and Poverty: A Literature Review.* Glasgow: Scottish Drugs Forum (SDF).

Shengold, L. (2006) *Haunted by Parents.* New Haven: Yale University Press.

Shipman, K. L., Rossman, B. B. R. and West, J. C. (1999) 'Co-occurrence of spousal violence and child abuse: conceptual implications.' *Child Maltreatment 4,* 93–102.

Shuker, S. (2006) 'African children "at risk of ritual abuse".' http://news.bbc.co.uk/1/hi/england/london/6177001.stm (accessed 9/11/07).

Shumway, J., O'Campo, P. and Gielen, A. (1999) 'Preterm labour, placental abruption and premature rupture of membranes in relation to maternal violence or verbal abuse.' *Journal of Maternal-Fetal Medicine 8*(3), 76–80.

Sidebotham, P. (2001) 'An ecological approach to child abuse: a creative use of scientific models in research and practice.' *Child Abuse Review 10,* 97–112.

Sidebotham, P. (2003) 'Red skies, risk factors and early indicators.' *Child Abuse Review 12,* 41–45.

Sidebotham, P., Fox, J., Horwath, J., Powell, C. and Perwez, S. (2008) *Preventing Childhood Deaths: A Study of 'Early Starter' Child Death Overview Panels in England.* London: Department for Children, Schools and Families,.

Silverman, M. R., Decker, E., Reed, A. and Raj, A. (2006) 'Intimate partner violence victimization prior to and during pregnancy among women residing in 26 US states: associations with maternal and neonatal health.' *American Journal of Obstetrics and Gynecology 195,* 140–148.

Simkin, Z. and Conti-Ramsden, G. (2006) 'Evidence of reading difficulty in subgroups of children with specific language impairment.' *Child, Language Teaching and Therapy 22*(3), 315–331.

Sinclair, R. and Bullock, R. (2002) *Learning from Past Experiences – A Review of Significant Case Reviews.* London: The Stationery Office.

Skuse, D. (1984) 'Extreme deprivation in childhood: II Theoretical issues and a comparative view.' *Journal of Child Psychology and Psychiatry 25*(4), 543–572.

Skuse, D. (1987) 'Extreme deprivation in early childhood.' In D. M. Bishop (ed.) *Language Development in Exceptional Circumstances.* Edinburgh: Churchill Livingstone.

Sloper, P. (2004) 'Facilitators and barriers for co-ordinating multi-agency services.' *Child: Care, Health and Development 30*(6), 571–580.

Smarsh-Hogan, T., Myers, B. and Elswick, R. (2006) 'Child abuse potential among mothers of substance-exposed and nonexposed infants and toddlers.' *Child Abuse and Neglect 30,* 145–156.

Smith, F. (2003) 'Safe-guarding the young.' *Paediatric Nursing and Midwifery 15*(10), 24–25.

Snowling, M. J. and Hayiou-Thomas, M.E. (2006) 'The dyslexia spectrum: continuities between reading, speech and language impairments.' *Topics in Language Disorder 26*(2), 110–126.

Spackman, M. P., Fujiki, M. and Brinton, B. (2006) 'Understanding emotions in context: the effects of language impairment on children's ability to infer emotional reactions.' *International Journal of Language and Communication Disorders 41*(2), 173–188.

Spangler, A. (1999) 'Frühkindliche Bindungserfahrung und Emotionsregulation.' (Experience of attachment and emotional regulation in early childhood) In W. Friedlmeier and M. Holodinski (eds) *Emotionale Entwicklung.* Heidelberg, Berlin: Spektrum, akad. Verlag.

Spencer, N. and Baldwin, N. (2005) 'Economic, social and cultural contexts of neglect.' In J. Taylor and B. Daniel (eds) *Child Neglect. Practice Issues for Health and Social Care.* London: Jessica Kingsley Publishers.

Spinhoven, P., Roelofs, K., Moene, F., Kuyk, J. *et al.* (2004) 'Trauma and dissociation in conversion disorder and chronic pelvic pain.' *International Journal of Psychiatry in Medicine 34*(4), 305–318.

Sroufe, L. (1996) *Emotional Development: The Organization of Emotional Life in the Early Years* New York: Cambridge University Press.

Stark, E. and Flitcraft, A. (1995) 'Woman battering, child abuse and social heredity: what is the relationship?' In N. Johnson (ed.) *Marital Violence.* London: Routledge and Kegan Paul.

Statham, J. (2004) 'Effective services to support children in special circumstances.' *Child: Care, Health and Development 30*, 567–570

Stern, D. N. (1994) 'The process of therapeutic change involving implicit knowledge: some implications of developmental observations for adult psychopathology.' *Infant Mental Health Journal 19*, 300–308.

Stevens, L. J. and Bliss, L. S. (1995) 'Conflict resolution abilities of children with specific language impairment and children with normal language.' *Journal of Speech and Hearing Research 38*, 599–611.

Stewart, D. E. and Cecutti, A. (1993) 'Physical abuse in pregnancy.' *Canadian Medical Association Journal 149*, 1257–1263.

Stobart, E. (2006) *Child Abuse Linked to Accusations of 'Possession' and 'Witchcraft'.* London: Department for Education and Skills.

Stop it Now! UK (2008) Publications, posters and leaflets on protecting children from sexual abuse can be ordered or downloaded from the website, www.stopitnow.org.uk/publications.htm (accessed 6/12/08).

Stratford, L. (1989) *Satan's Underground.* New York: Johanna Michaelson.

Stratford, L. (1993) *Stripped Naked.* Gretna, LA: Pelican Publishing.

Street, K., Harrington, J., Chiang, W., Cairns, P. and Ellis, M. (2004) 'How great is the risk of abuse in infants born to drug-using mothers?' *Child: Care Health and Development 30*(4), 325–330.

Sullivan, T. P., Lipschitz, D. S. and Grilo, C. M. (2006) 'Differential relationships of childhood abuse and neglect subtypes to PTSD symptom clusters among adolescent inpatients.' *Journal of Traumatic Stress 19*(2), 229–239.

Sussman, F. (1999) *More Than Words: Helping Parents Promote Communication and Social Skills in Children with Autism Spectrum Disorder.* Information Booklet: (The) Hanen Program®.

Svanberg, P. O. G. (1998) 'Attachment, resilience and prevention.' *Journal of Mental Health 7*(6), 543–578.

Swann, C., Bowe, K., McCormick, G. and Kosmin, M. (2003) *Teenage Pregnancy and Parenthood: A Review of Reviews.* www.nice.org.uk/niceMedia/documents/teenpreg_evidence_briefing.pdf (accessed 29/1/08).

Taket, A., Nurse, J., Smith, K., Watson, J., *et al.* (2003) 'Routinely asking women about domestic violence in health settings.' *British Medical Journal 327*, 673–676.

Taylor, J. and Corlett, J. (2007) 'Health practitioners and safeguarding children.' In K. Wilson and A. James (eds) *The Child Protection Handbook 3rd edn.* London: Sage.

Taylor, J. and Daniel, B. (2005) *Child Neglect, Practice Issues for Health and Social Care.* London: Jessica Kingsley Publishers.

Taylor, J. and Daniel, B. (2006) 'Standards for education and training for interagency working in child protection in the UK.' *Editorial, Nurse Education Today 26*, 179–182.

Taylor, J., Spencer, N. and Baldwin, N. (2000) 'Social, economic and political context of parenting.' *Archives of Disease in Childhood 82*, 113–120.

Taylor, R. and Selkirk, C. (2007) *TayStats leaflet:* Dundee: NHS Tayside.

Templeton, L., Zohhadi, S., Galvani, S. and Velleman, R. (2006) *'Looking Beyond Risk': Parental Substance Misuse Scoping Study.* Edinburgh: Substance Misuse Research programme, Scottish Executive.

Terr, L. (1979) 'Children of Chowchilla: a study of psychic trauma.' *Psychoanalytical Study of the Child 34*, 547–623.

Terr, L. (1991) 'Childhood traumas: an outline and review.' *American Journal of Psychiatry 148*, 1–20.

The Bridge Child Care Consultancy Service (1995) *Death Through Neglect.* London: BCCCS.

The Sonrise Program® (2001) *Information Pack.* Sheffield, MA: Autism Treatment Center of America™.

Thom, B. (2003) *Risk-taking Behaviour in Men: Substance Use and Gender.* London: NHS Health Development Agency.

Thompson, R. S., Rivara, F. P., Thompson, D. C., Barlow, W. E., *et al.* (2000) 'Identification and management of domestic violence a randomised trial.' *American Journal of Preventive Medicine 19*(4), 253–263.

Thompson, T. (2005) 'Churches blamed for exorcism growth.' www.guardian.co.uk/society/2005/jun/05/childrensservices.religion (accessed 20/7/08).

Tiegerman, E. and Primavera, L. H. (1984) 'Imitating the autistic child: facilitating communicative gaze behavior.' *Journal of Autism and Developmental Disorders 14*, 27–38.

Tjaden, P. and Tjaden, P. (2000) *Full Report of the Prevalence, Incidence and Consequences of Violence against Women* Washington, DC: National Institute of Justice: Centres for Disease Control and Prevention.

Tonmyr, L. (1998) *International Studies on the Incidence and Prevalence of Child Maltreatment. Selected Bibliography. Child Maltreatment Division.* Ottawa: Health Protection Board, Health Canada.

Toppleberg, C. and Shapiro, T. (2000) 'Language disorders: a 10-year research update review.' *Journal of the Academy of Child and Adolescent Psychiatry 39*(2), 143–152.

Tremblay, R. E., Japel, C., Perusse, D., McDuff, P., *et al.* (1999) 'The search for the "onset" of physical aggression: Rousseau and Bandura revisited.' *Criminal Behaviour and Mental Health 9*, 8–23.

Trevarthen, C., Aitken, K., Papoudi, D. and Robarts, J. (1999) *Children with Autism: Diagnosis and Interventions to Meet their Needs.* London: Jessica Kingsley Publishers.

Trickett, P. and McBride-Chang, C. (1995) 'The developmental impact of different forms of child abuse and neglect.' *Developmental Review 15*, 311–337.

Truman, P. (2004) 'Problems in identifying cases of child neglect.' *Nursing Standard 18*(29), 3–38.

Tsang, A. and Sweet, D. (1999) 'Detecting child abuse and neglect: are dentists doing enough?' *Journal of Canadian Dental Association 65*, 387–391.

Tudor Hart, J. (1971) 'The Inverse Care Law.' *Lancet 297*(7696), 405–412.

Tunnard, J. (2002) *Parental Drug Misuse – A Review of Impact and Intervention Studies.* Darlington. www.rip.org.uk (accessed 6/12/08).

Turton, J. and Haines, L. (2007) *The Child Protection Complaints Report.* London: Royal College of Paediatrics and Child Health.

Tuten, M., Jones, H. E., Tran, G. and Svikis, D. S. (2004) 'Partner violence impacts the psychosocial and psychiatric status of pregnant, drug-dependent women.' *Addictive Behaviors 29*, 1029–1034.

Tyler, K. and Cauce, A. M. (2002) 'Perpetrators of early physical and sexual abuse among homeless and runaway adolescents.' *Child Abuse and Neglect, 26*(12), 1261–1274.

UNICEF (2007) *Child Poverty in Perspective: An Overview of Child Well-Being in Rich Countries [Report Card 7].* Florence: United Nations Children Fund Innocenti Research Centre.

University of Glasgow and NHS Greater Glasgow (2005) *Child Protection and the Dental Team: An Addendum for Scotland.* Glasgow.

Vallance, D. D., Im, N. and Cohen, N. J. (1999) 'Discourse deficits associated with psychiatric disorders and with language impairments in children.' *Journal of Child Psychology and Psychiatry 40*(5), 693–704.

Vallely, P. (2007) 'Are Britain's fringe churches preaching a deadly message?' http://news.independent.co.uk/uk/this_britain/article299847.ece (accessed 3/5/08).

van der Kolk, B. A. (2005) 'Developmental trauma disorder: towards a rational diagnosis for children with complex trauma histories.' *Psychiatric Annals 35*, 401–408.

Van Fraser. J. (2005) 'How the masonic social services, police and justice systms are continually covering up ritual child abuse activities.' www.mindcontrolforums.net/rca_coverup.html (accessed 11/2/08).

van Weel, C., De Maeseneer, J. and Roberts, R. (2008) 'Integration of personal and community care.' *Lancet 372*, 871–872.

Velez, M. L., Jansson, L. M., Montoya, I. D., Schweitzer, W., Golden, A. and Svikis, D. (2004) 'Parenting knowledge among substance abusing women in treatment.' *Journal of Substance Abuse Treatment 27*, 215–222.

Velleman, R. and Templeton, L. (2007a) 'Substance misuse by children and young people: the role of the family and implications for intervention and prevention.' *Paediatrics and Child Health 17*(1), 25–30.

Velleman, R. and Templeton, L. (2007b) 'Understanding and modifying the impact of parents' substance misuse on children.' *Advances in Psychiatric Treatment 13*, 79–89.

Victorian Government Department of Justice (2006) *Management of the Whole Family when Intimate Partner Violence is Present: Guidelines for Primary Care Physicians.* Melbourne, Australia: Victorian Government Department of Justice.

Vincent, V., Fischer, W., Pahud, A.-L., Pascual, T. and Ladame, F. (1997) 'Multiple suicide attempts in adolescence, sexual abuse during childhood and borderline personality disorder.' *European Psychiatry 12*(2), 189s–189s.

Viner, R. M. and Barker, M. B. (2005) 'Young people's health: the need for action.' *British Medical Journal 330*, 901–903.

Virginia Future Forum (2007) *Competing in the 21st Century: Moving Virginia's Human Capital Meter.* www.future.virginia.gov/forum (accessed 6/12/08).

Volkmar, F. R., Lord, C., Bailey, A., Schultz, R. T. and Klin, A. (2004) 'Autism and pervasive developmental disorders.' *Journal of Child Psychology and Psychiatry 45*, 135–170.

von Feuerbach, A. R. (1832) *Caspar Hauser. An Account of an Individual Kept in a Dungeon, Separated from all Communication with the World, from Early Childhood to About the Age of Seventeen.* Boston: Allen and Ticknor.

Vulliamy, A. P. and Sullivan, R. (2000) 'Reporting child abuse: pediatricians' experiences with the child protection system.' *Child Abuse and Neglect 24*, 1461–1470.

Walby, S. and Allen, J. (2004) *Domestic Violence, Sexual Assault and Stalking: Findings from the British Crime Survey.* London: Home Office.

Wald, M. (1968) 'Child abuse in Wisconsin. The dentist's responsibility in reporting.' *Greater Milwaukee Dental Bulletin 34*, 113–116.

Walker, Z., Townsend, J., Oakley, L., Donovan, C., *et al.* (2002) 'Health promotion for adolescents in primary care: randomised controlled trial.' *British Medical Journal 325*, 524–529.

Walley, M., Lawn, J. E., Tinker, A., de Francisco, A., *et al.* (2008) 'Primary health care: making Alma-Ata a reality [editorial].' *Lancet 372*, 1001–1007.

Warren, S., Emde, R. and Sroufe, A. (2000) 'Internal representation: predicting anxiety from children's play narratives.' *Journal of American Child Adolescence Psychiatry 39*(1), 100–107.

Webb, E. (1998) 'Children and the inverse care law.' *British Medical Journal 316*(7144), 1588–1591.

Webster, R. (1998) 'Satanic abuse and McMartin: a global village rumour.' www.richardwebseter.net/speakofthedevil.html (accessed 11/11/07).

Welsh Child Protection Systematic Review Group (2008) *A Series of Systematic Reviews Defining the Evidence Base Behind the Diagnosis of Physical Child Abuse.* Cardiff: www.core-info.cardiff.ac.uk/ (accessed 6/12/08).

Wenegrat, B. (2001) *Theater of Disorder: Patients, Doctors and the Construction of Illness.* Oxford: Oxford University Press.

West, J. (1999) '(Not) talking about sex: youth, identity and sexuality.' *Sociological Review* 47(3), 525–548.

Whitelaw, S., Baxendale, A. and Bryce, C. (2001) 'Settings-based health promotion: a review.' *Health Promotion International* 16(4), 339–353.

Whitaker, D. J., Miller, K. S. and Clarke, L. F. (2000) 'Reconceptualising adolescent sexual behaviour: beyond did they or didn't they.' *Family Planning Perspectives* 32(3), 111–118.

Whittaker, A. (2008) *The Construction of Fatherhood Within the Context of Problem Drug Use* (PhD Thesis). Dundee: University of Dundee.

WHO, UNODC and UNAIDS (2004) *WHO/UNODC/UNAIDS Position Paper: Substitution Maintenance Therapy in the Management of Opioid Dependence and HIV/AIDS Prevention.* Geneva: World Health Organization, United Nations Office on Drugs and Crime, Joint United Nations Programme on HIV/AIDS.

Wilkins, C. (2006) 'A qualitative study exploring the support needs of first-time mothers on their journey towards intuitive parenting.' *Midwifery* 22, 169–180.

Williams, B. and Imam, I. (eds) (2007) *Systems Concepts in Evaluation: An Expert Anthology.* Point Reyes: EdgePress.

Williams, C. (2007) 'United Kingdom General Medical Council fails child protection.' *Pediatrics* 119, 800–802.

Willumsen, T. (2001) 'Dental fear in sexually abused women.' *European Journal of Oral Science* 109, 291–296.

Willumsen, T. (2004) 'The impact of childhood sexual abuse on dental fear.' *Community Dentistry and Oral Epidemiology* 32, 73–79.

Wilsnack, S., Vogeltanz, N., Klassen, A. and Harris, R. (1997) 'Childhood sexual abuse and women's substance abuse: national survey findings.' *Journal of Studies on Alcohol* 58(3), 264–271.

Wing, L. (1993) 'The definition and prevalence of autism: a review.' *European Child and Adolescent Psychiatry* 2, 61–74.

Wing, L. (1996) *The Autistic Spectrum.* London: Constable.

Wing, L. and Potter, D. (2002) 'The epidemiology of autistic spectrum disorders: is the prevalence rising?' *Mental Retardation and Developmental Disabilities Research Reviews* 8, 151–161.

Wolfe, D. A., Sas, L. and Wekerle, C. (1994) 'Factors associated with the development of post traumatic stress disorder among child victims of sexual abuse.' *Child Abuse and Neglect* 18, 37–50.

Women Equality Unit (2004) *The Cost of Domestic Violence: A Report by Sylvia Walby.* Leeds: University of Leeds.

Wood, P. (2006) Resources to support clinical governance in dentistry. Clinical Governance Support Team. www.cgsupport.nhs.uk (accessed 25/1/08).

World Health Organization (1978) Declaration of Alma Ata – International Conference on Primary Care USSR 6–12 September 1978. www.who.int/hpr/NPH/docs/declaration_almaata.pdf (accessed 23/9/08).

World Health Organization (2000) *Violence Against Women.* Factsheet No 239. Geneva: WHO.

World Health Organization (2002) *World Report on Violence and Health.* Geneva: WHO.

World Health Organization (2007a) 'A financial road map to scaling up essential child health interventions in 75 countries.' *Bulletin of the World Health Organization* 85(4), 305–316.

World Health Organization (2007b) *Chapter V. Mental Health and Behavioural Disorders International Classification of Diseases and Mental Health Problems 10th Revision.* Geneva: World Health Organization.

Yoshikawa, H. (1995) 'Long-term effects of early childhood programs on social outcomes and delinquency.' *The Future of Children* 5(3), 51–75.

Yule, W., Smith, P. and Perrin, S. (2005) 'Post-traumatic stress disorders.' In P. J. Graham (ed.) *Cognitive Behavior Therapy for Children and Families.* Cambridge: Cambridge University Press.

Zeedyk, M. S. (2008) *Promoting Social Interaction for Individuals with Communicative Impairments: Making Contact* London: Jessica Kingsley Publishers.

Zeedyk, M. S., Caldwell, P. and Davies, C. E. 'How rapidly does Intensive Interaction promote social engagement for adults with profound learning disabilities?' *European Journal of Special Needs Education* (in press).

Zielinski, D. S. and Bradshaw, C. P. (2006) 'Ecological influences on the sequelae of child maltreatment: a review of the literature.' *Child Maltreatment* 11, 49–62.

Zimmermann, P., Suess, G., Scheurer-Englisch, H. and Grossmann, K. (2000) 'Der Einfluss der Eltern-Kind Bindung auf die Entwicklung psychischer Gesundheit.' (The influence of parent-child attachment on the development of physical health) In F. Petermann, Niebank, K. and Scheithauer, H. (eds) *Risiken in der frühkindlichen Entwicklung.* Göttingen, Bern, Toronto: H

Subject Index

Author Index